Poverty and Health

Poverty and Health

A Sociological Analysis

Edited by John Kosa,
Aaron Antonovskv, and
Irving Kenneth Zola

A Commonwealth Fund Book

Harvard University Press

Cambridge, Massachusetts

1969

Foreword

Poverty is among the most familiar and enduring of human conditions. Yet, as John Kosa explains in the opening chapter of this book, each generation sees it differently and judges it according to a particular set of social values, which may be quite unlike those of an earlier era. The most recent "rediscovery" occurred in the early 1960's when Harrington and others pointed out that despite the unprecedented prosperity of the nation and the social legislation enacted since the Roosevelt era, mass poverty continued to exist and in fact seemed to be increasing in certain geographic areas. The social conscience of the nation was awakened, and a "war on poverty" was launched with considerable fanfare and some success.

In a way, *Poverty and Health: A Sociological Analysis* represents a rediscovery of the association between poverty and illness and interprets the association in terms of current sociological thought and the present state of medical knowledge. Not too long ago it was assumed that poverty and disease were inevitably linked, just as poverty itself was considered inevitable. Tuberculosis and the epidemic infectious diseases threatened all classes of society, but the poor were particularly afflicted.

With improved control of many epidemic diseases, attention refocused on the special connection between poverty and high rates of infant mortality, prematurity, and maternal maturity. But little attention was paid to the over-all association of poverty and health. In stark and unemotional terms this volume systematically analyzes the parameters of health and health services both for the poor and the affluent in our society. The evidence is overwhelming that just as the poor are deprived politically, educationally, and environmentally so are they deprived medically.

In recent years the nation has become aware of the importance of heart disease, cancer, and stroke as major killers, and it appears that coronary artery disease and other degenerative diseases of blood vessels are the diseases of an affluent society and have little to do with poverty.

This book should dispel the notion that health and poverty are unconnected. Undeniably, coronary artery disease presents a serious health problem for the affluent as well as the poor, but Monroe Lerner presents compelling evidence that the poor are considerably less healthy than the remainder of the population. Mortality rates for all ages and by age are higher for the poor, as is the incidence of serious illness. Similarly the level of dental health is related to social level, with the poor having the highest incidence of dental disease. Marc Fried states in the opening paragraph of Chapter IV that, "The evidence is unambiguous and powerful that the lowest social classes have the highest rates of severe psychiatric disorder in our society," and he provides the documentation for this categorical statement.

In every area that relates to health the poor are deprived. They are less well informed than other social groups about general health matters, they depend more upon lay advice, and they are relatively powerless in the medical care system. That part of the population who can afford the price can purchase directly, or indirectly via insurance, fee-for-service medicine and can exert some influence over the system, but the poor are dependent to a significant degree on "clinic medicine" which tends to be fragmented, dehumanized, and lacking in continuity. Not only does the poverty group receive a different quality of care for physical illness but even the stresses and anxieties associated with illness are treated differentially according to social class. Medical care is a middle-class commodity, and the poor are discriminated against medically just as they are educationally.

It would be naive to assume, however, that the inferiority of health services is the single cause of higher morbidity and mortality rates among the poor. The interrelationship between poverty and health is more complex than that and involves many factors ordinarily considered "nonmedical." Indeed, one special contribution of the sociologist to the medical field is the documentation of the interaction between health and the social environment.

Arthur Shostak, in Chapter IX, suggests that poverty can be alleviated (or even eliminated) gradually or with "dizzying speed." What the rate will be depends upon the willingness of the nation to cope with the problem financially and socially. If gradualism is the choice, the solution to the problem of health services for the poor is likely to be quite different than if rapid elimination of poverty becomes a national goal. At a time of increasing technological complexity, of rising medical costs, of relative shortages of health professionals, and at a time when the entire medical care system needs re-examination, the problems of medical care delivery may be further complicated by a perpetuation and extension of a two-class system of medical care. Therefore the speed with which the problems of poverty are solved may profoundly affect the medical care of the affluent as well as the poor.

Robert H. Ebert, M.D.
Dean, Harvard Medical School

January 1969

Preface

If we had chosen to prepare a reader on poverty and illness, life would have been much simpler for us, and this book would have been published earlier. A fair amount of published material has appeared since the social sciences discovered illness in the 1950's and since poverty was rediscovered almost a decade thereafter. We chose, instead, to try to prepare a book whose chapters would be linked by an overarching conception: the view of poverty and illness as the dynamic behavior of the human being which is culturally molded and located in social contexts. We have tried to place each author's contribution into an ordered structure, so that a sense of logic should flow from one chapter to the next, and the reader, on completion of the book, should feel an intellectual satisfaction that he has read a book.

Having made the initial decision to publish a yes-book in this era of non-books, we went a step further, although with much trepidation. We prepared a detailed outline of each chapter, as we would write it, and submitted this outline to the experts whom we asked to do the actual writing. We found, to our gratification, that this step did not give umbrage. The authors seemed to feel that the outlines enabled them to take off more easily, to divest themselves of the need to touch on every angle of the complex problem, and to write in the knowledge that they were writing for a book.

Two further prefatory points of substance should be made. First, it may seem to many that a book on illness and poverty should be an angry book. Can even the most insensitive respond with anything but passionate anger to this dual suffering in a nation with such an abundance of resources? We are sure we speak for our authors as well as ourselves when we say that, even though it does not show except here and there—and notably in Arthur B. Shostak's chapter—we are angry and we do care. But our professionalism is not supposed to add to the chorus of rage, much as we hope it will add to an effective pressure on the society. The problems are complex; if we have simply elucidated this complexity and enhanced our understanding, this will have been more of a service than ranting.

Finally, we wish to indicate our awareness of the geographic limitations of the book. One of us is an ex-Hungarian American; a second is an ex-American Israeli. We know that not only is America not the world, but that in many ways it is different from most of the world. We quite uncomfortably know that the sick and the poor in the contemporary United States constitute a very special historical case. Kwashiorkor gives way to dental caries and bilharzia to cervical cancer when one focuses on America. We initially weighed a world focus, historically and geographically, but decided to limit ourselves; otherwise the job would have been unmanageable. Nonetheless we do hope that an advance in understanding the problems of poverty and illness in America will also be germane to understanding these problems elsewhere. But there is no question in our minds that the American has much to learn for his own problems, particularly in the field of the organization of medical care, from experiences elsewhere.

This book was undertaken when the three of us were in the Boston area. John Kosa, as a member of the Family Health Care Program of Children's Hospital Medical Center, was in daily contact with the sick and the poor. Aaron Antonovsky had worked with the New York State Commission Against Discrimination and had directed research for the State Low Incomes program; during his stay here as Public Health Service senior research fellow, he was preparing a book on social class and illness. Irving Kenneth Zola brought along the experiences he gained during his affiliation with many major hospitals in Boston and his work on the cultural determinants of health behavior and decisions to seek medical care.

The initial idea had been Kosa's, but we became full partners as we worked through the detailed design of the book, mercilessly but pleasantly criticizing what each of us offered. Having finished the planning stage and deciding to whom we should turn for the papers, Kosa undertook the arduous organizational work, greatly helped by the encouragement of Dr. Charles A. Janeway and the generous cooperation of Dr. Joel J. Alpert. As papers came in, the three of us edited and commented. As the reader will note, Kosa undertook, alone or jointly, the writing of three chapters.

In the light of this division of labor, senior editorship accurately reflects the history of the book, while the two junior editors are listed alphabetically. Responsibility, of course, is shared by all of us.

John Kosa
Boston, Massachusetts

Aaron Antonovsky
Jerusalem, Israel

Irving Kenneth Zola
Waltham, Massachusetts

November 1968

Contents

Tables

Charts

Poverty and Health

I · The Nature of Poverty

by John Kosa

The biblical saying, "the poor always ye have with you" (John 12:8), hardly needs confirmation. Every epoch of history and every country of the world has had its share of the poor, although this name was given to groups of widely varying conditions. The slaves of the Roman Empire, the serfs of the Middle Ages, the peons of Latin America, the inmates of English poorhouses or (speaking of our country and time) the marginal farmers in Appalachia and the racial minorities in the urban ghettos were all called poor, even though they represented varying degrees of deprivation and different stages of forlornness. Small wonder that William Graham Sumner, a founder of American sociology and spokesman of the laissez-faire philosophy, claimed that there was no possible definition of "a poor man." He deplored the use of the phrase because it seemed dangerously elastic and capable of covering a host of "social fallacies." [1] Yet the usage of the word has survived.

If a common adjective has been applied to so many groups with varying ways of life, this must have happened because the word "poor" denotes an ancient concept for expressing social differences between man and man, a concept coined long before the social sciences came up with their notion of social stratification. This ancient concept has clearly distinguished one segment of the population from the rest and has gained general acceptance in our daily speech. Nowadays for many good reasons it cannot be replaced by such more precise terms as the lower class or the blue-collar class which, in spite of a considerable overlap, refer to a different classificatory system and are not interchangeable with "the poor." [2] For example, the blue-collar class includes industrial workers above the poverty level, but excludes the poor of the farming areas; similarly, the lower class excludes many of the elderly who spent their lives outside the lower class but have become destitute as an unfortunate consequence of aging.

The Unequal Distribution of Means and Privileges

As a more important difference, the word "poor" has an emotional appeal that the "lower class" lacks. "Poor" is usually taken as a synonym of "needy," and whoever is in need, can rightfully appeal to the help of the more fortunate ones. Poverty calls for help, evokes our commiseration, moves our instinct of nurturance, and claims our idealism. Quite in accordance with this emotional appeal, poverty is a relative term that reflects a judgment made on the basis of standards prevailing in the community. The standards change in time and place; what is judged poverty in one community might be regarded as wealth in another. Nevertheless, there is a reality behind the appeal to our nurturance, and the judgment is based on certain objective and even tangible criteria which are visible to the observer. Thus, the poor are those who, by the prevailing standards, are found to be deficient in means of subsistence and privileges of life.

In our economy the means of subsistence refers to money. Ours is a market economy in which money is the general medium for which the goods that people produce and the work that people render are institutionally exchanged. Money is accessible to all (although to varying extents) and buys everything that a person needs as well as many other things he does not need. In other communities of the past no market economy, or only an imperfect one, existed; money was not available to all, and each household unit produced what it could for the preservation of its life and resorted to barter but infrequently. Yet the material possessions, particularly the means of production such as land, work animals, and implements, were unequally distributed; the poor owned less, produced less, and subsisted on a precarious level.

The privileges of life can be described as intangible social and psychological possessions. They include a relationship to the social power, a participation in making decisions that affect the community, an ability to realize one's own decisions and plans, and a possession of knowledge; they include access to the pleasurable things of life and particularly to the services of others. In a primitive economy the services are rendered by servants whose main duty is to do heavy work and drudgery for the privileged ones; in our complex economy the most important services (medical care, education, police protection, and so on) are either institutionally marketed or dispensed by the government.

The privileges include access to health, wholesomeness, and all the conditions of a healthy life. It is by no means incidental that we tend to view health as a material possession and speak of "poor" health as if we were to speak of a lack of material possessions. Indeed, the privileged status implies the provision of health services, and from the time of Hippocrates up to our century these services have been directed mainly toward the privileged few.[3] Moreover, healthy life is a rational and planned way of living, not easily accessible to those within the range of poverty.

The means and privileges that are available in a community are interconnected, and the possession of one of them is likely to lead to the possession of another. In a primitive society without an efficient market economy, the poor have fewer means of production, gather in a poorer harvest, and are more vulnerable to the natural disasters of life such as famine and plague. In our society the doctor's son has a better chance than the tenant farmer's son to obtain a higher education, buy the pleasurable things, or take part in community decisions. It follows that within any group of people that is sufficiently large and has advanced beyond a rudimentary cultural development, the means and privileges are unequally distributed, and there is a class which possesses both and another class which is deficient in both. Thus, when speaking of poor versus wealthy we apply a rather simple and unidimensional division to the community and overlook the more complex forms of stratification which can be discerned with finer analytical tools. It is this disarming simplicity that recommends the concept of poverty and safeguards its currency in spite of the objections of many scholars and even more nonscholarly representatives of conservatism. It is a concept that can be applied to almost any society and understood by anybody; it helps to orient ourselves within any community because it makes one broad distinction between the wealthy and the poor.

The possession of means and privileges is visible and even conspicuous. The unequal distribution of worldly goods can be assessed and expressed without any special knowledge. A reasonably adequate judgment of the other person can often be formed without a personal acquaintance, and those who are familiar with their community can safely place their fellow citizens along the wealth-poverty line.[4] In fact, the designation of a person by his possession of worldly goods is an essential part of his full characterization, and writers of fiction seldom omit this trait when describing their fictional heroes. Compare F. Scott Fitzgerald with his fine differentiation among the wealthy and Erskine Caldwell with his compassionate rendering of the various shades of the poor; one gets the impression that while Caldwell urges us to help those in need, Fitzgerald does not seem to notice the existence of the poor. One could adduce many other examples of the fact that in spite of its visibility, poverty is not always perceived, and not only individuals but also entire communities might be seemingly imperceptive to it.

ATTITUDES TOWARD POVERTY

As a part of our social life we tend to judge our fellow beings by their wordly goods; we perceive some of them as poor and set them apart from the rest of us. This is a motivated judgment which bolsters the judge's social position by defining others as being inferior to him in worldly possessions. It is a social judgment based on common standards and the consensus of the community. Hence, within the community the individual judgments follow a common pattern and end up in a consensual evaluation; but the communities greatly differ among themselves in the perception of poverty and in responding to the emotional appeal of poverty.

Some communities regard poverty as part of a permanent social order established by nature, divinity, or a mythical hero. The social order is codified in unwritten customs or written laws which in a statutory way deprive one broad group of people of the means and privileges, relegate them to poverty, and enforce their deprivation. They establish slavery, serfdom, peonage, or any other of those disadvantaged statuses that exist in hierarchically structured feudal societies. Within the formally established social structure the status of the individual is often inherited, but in any case it is firmly assigned to him so that he can change it only in rare cases. The poor class owes permanent services to the privileged one and, in return, is supposed to receive some kind of protection which, however, does not protect him against perennial pauperism. As a matter of fact, poverty is not perceived as a separate phenomenon but is regarded as a relevant constituting element of a natural order.

Two examples may illustrate how institutionalized poverty is established within the total social structure. When in 1619 the first Negroes were introduced into the colony of Virginia, they were regarded as indentured servants. For the next three or four decades Negroes whose period of service had expired received land assigned to them in much the same way as white servants. Then the colony enacted a series of statutes which gradually excluded the Negroes from the privileges of the indentured servants, making the Negro a chattel and his servitude perpetual. By 1670 slavery as a legal institution was firmly established, and the statutes of Virginia became the models followed by the neighboring colonies.[5] Rather few of the statutes dealt with the means of subsistence; this was hardly necessary since the deprivation of privileges implied a commensurate deprivation of means also.

The other case of interest is Hungary where a semifeudal social structure prevailed up to 1945 and where the compulsory state health insurance was fashioned in accordance with the class privileges; in fact, the legislation establishing the health insurance scheme legally defined the main social classes of the country. The army officers, civil servants, and people in some of the free professions, constituting the ruling class, had separate health services of their own; two further health services were founded for the middle and the industrial working classes respectively; while the peasantry, constituting the lowest class, was deprived of the benefits of health insurance. The health insurance legislation corroborated and prolonged the long-lasting inequality among the classes and reflected the old principles; hence, the new privilege of insured health care was allotted in proportion to the previous privileges.[6]

As a contrast to feudalism, class societies regard poverty not as part of an immutable order but as a condition created essentially by men. They acknowledge the existence of several social classes, distinguished informally and without any legal barriers separating one from the other. The means and privileges, although unequally distributed, are legally available to all, but the legal freedom of acquisition does not imply that everybody is equally free to participate in the ensuing competition. Free competition hardly ever exists in human groups because it is restricted by several ubiquitous conditions, foremost by the unequal distribution of means and privileges. The possession of any of the means and privileges helps the acquisition of another one of them; that is, wealth helps and poverty restricts successful participation in competition. Moreover, numerous customs and prejudices (many of the latter reflect customs surviving from feudal times) further restrict the poor in any acquisition, and the case of the Negro in present-day America well illustrates the point.

Under such conditions poverty may, or may not, be perceived. But in any case the designation of being poor is informal and signals the recognition of a social distance separating the poor from the rest but no definitive exclusion from the means and privileges. Actually the elastic structure of a class society offers chances absent in feudalism: the poor might take part in competition and, if successful, might move upward on the social ladder. The elasticity of the structure and the rate of social mobility determine the success of the poor in upgrading themselves. An inelastic structure and slow mobility may perpetuate poverty within one segment of the population, as it has happened in the rural South of the United States and, notably, in its Negro community. On the other hand, an elastic structure and rapid mobility may cause a rotating poor class with many people moving upward while others are moving simultaneously downward or replenishing in any other way the poor class. The northern cities of the country, and notably their slums populated with the successive waves of old-stock and new-stock immigrants, Negroes and Puerto Ricans, present an example of this rotation.

The emotional appeal inherent in poverty may elicit a social response directed not toward the individual poor but toward poverty in general. The response takes one of two forms. It might be further deprivation or exploitation of the poor as the case of the early Negroes in Virginia illustrates, and it might take the form of help on some community-wide basis, but this happens only when the "poor" are equated with the "needy." Help to the poor is not a general response; it is present in some communities but conspicuously absent in others. Its presence or absence is dependent on a more general orientation of the community, namely, whether or not poverty is taken for granted. As a rule, feudalism takes poverty for granted as a stable and even immutable institution and, accordingly, does not deem any helping response necessary. A class society does not have a uniform response pattern because it may or may not take poverty for granted. It tends to respond in accordance with its moral sentiments and general conditions; if it views pauperism as a human condition subject to change, it is likely to extend help. To put it in plain words, it happens rather seldom that the sight of poverty leads to social help.

The perception and the response determine the attitudes that the communities take towards poverty. Their combinations yield four possible attitudes: (1) poverty is taken for granted and its existence is not perceived, (2) poverty is taken for granted, but its existence is perceived, (3) poverty is not taken for granted and its existence is perceived, and (4) poverty is not taken for granted, but its existence is not perceived. Let us examine the attitudes as they unfolded themselves during a historical development.

Poverty that is taken for granted and not perceived was a rather general attitude all through the ages—a simple attitude of agnosticism that required no response to the existing facts. Supported by the belief in an immutable social order, the existence of conspicuous poverty was silently accepted and tolerated, by the poor let alone the rich, without any manifest discontent or protest. The rich had few reasons, unless moved by their conscience, to voice protest; but one must note with some amazement the docile submission with which the masses of slaves and serfs tolerated their institutional deprivation for centuries and perhaps millenia without any serious effort to change it. Slavery in America produced some localized revolts but these were usually activated by slaves who were better off than the nonrevolting ones and were not infrequently led by white persons.[7] The remnants of this ancestral acquiescence might be still discovered among the poor of our day whom investigators are prone to describe as fatalistic, accepting deprivation as a natural part of life and showing relatively little inclination to diagnose and change the existing situation.[8]

Poverty that is taken for granted while its existence is perceived was another common attitude of the past. Poverty was to some extent reconciled with the given social order, and treated in a superficial way without changing the social order or the causes of destitution. One response of this kind was summed up in the saying of the Romans: *"panem et circenses."* It described a policy towards the numerous poor in the imperial city whose revolutionary discontent was placated by distributing bread among them and furnishing games for their entertainment.

Christianity formed a more sublimated response by positing charity towards the poor as one of the three theological virtues. It was a symbolic response given to a few selected charity cases which was not extended to the overwhelming majority of the poor excluded from the benefits of individual charity. The saints and heroes practiced charity, and their deeds were commemorated in many moving legends. The poor became the objects of charity, and their presence was needed for the daily practice of Christian virtues. Small wonder indeed that the Middle Ages did less than nothing to liberate the serfs and abolish the arrogant prerogatives of feudal lords; from time to time it displayed a bloody cruelty in putting down the peasant revolts.[9]

The Discovery of Poverty

The third community attitude, which does not take poverty for granted and perceives its existence, implies that poverty is a man-made condition, the result of human mismanagement of social affairs. It leads to a discovery of poverty in all its realistic details and to a desire to better the plight, not of a few charity cases, but of the whole class of the poor. The desire does not necessarily mean that the community advocates revolutionary changes in the social structure nor that it has the required means and the knowledge of social engineering to carry out the recommended reforms. The desire might be expressed in mere planning and scheming not followed by rational actions. Much of this planning may remain naive, impractical and even pettifogging, such as it was with many early communistic schemes, but the planning, whether good or poor, signals the readiness of the community to deal with pauperism as a social problem.[10]

The famous Poor Laws of England codified this attitude perhaps for the first time. They were intended not to abolish pauperism but to alleviate the plight of the poor uniformly across the country, and in a crude way they contributed much to that noble goal.[11] True enough, other countries did not seem to follow the English example, and England herself failed to adjust the Poor Laws to the changing social conditions. But the medieval notion that the existing social order was a part of a cosmic divine order, still held sway over people's minds and silenced the expression of any desire for social reforms. A general process of secularization was needed to change this mental disposition; when it came, it rejected the sacral notions surrounding the social order and contended that social structure was a human construct, free to be changed when change was desirable.

The modern discovery of poverty began with Adam Smith's notion that the *Wealth of Nations* was not a divine gift but rather the product of human labor which could be manipulated for the attainment of greater wealth. His book contained some sensible passages on the poor (such as, "Poverty sometimes urges nations to inhuman customs") and somewhat vaguely predicted that poverty would eventually disappear. His optimistic prophecy furnished food for thought to many who wanted to fulfill the vague prediction with concrete plans of their own making. Robert Owen proposed that poverty must be eliminated and recommended the Villages of Cooperation for this purpose. Saint-Simon outlined his hazy design of an industrial society without pauperism, and Marx developed an elaborate theory of socialism.[12] With the arrival of Marx, poverty became the central issue in European politics and social philosophy.

The fourth attitude mentioned above does not take poverty for granted but does not perceive its existence. Such a combination of the elements appears to be logically absurd, yet the attitude (either in a real or in an imaginary form) has exerted a tremendous impact upon present-day America. The writers who drew public attention to the problem in the early 1960's claimed that poverty was not known, and was ignored or hidden as if the nation wanted to close its eyes before a sight so disturbing to its conscience. Michael Harrington entitled the first chapter of his book: "The Invisible Land." [13] A reviewer of his book who was to shake up the social conscience of the readers of *The New Yorker,* summed up the point concisely: "For a long time now, almost everybody has assumed that, because of the New Deal's social legislation and—more important—the prosperity we have enjoyed since 1940, mass poverty no longer exists in this country." [14]

It might very well be that the claim of the writers referred to an imaginary attitude, but, under any circumstances, the claim appealed to the conscience of many and moved them to respond to the sight of poverty in an unprecedented way. It helped to launch the great national enterprise of the 1960's, the war on poverty, and if any attitude of not perceiving poverty had ever existed before, it certainly disappeared now. In an almost cathartic outburst of emotions the nation suddenly realized that large-scale, unattended poverty existed in the most affluent country of the world and set out with earnest dedication to resolve this "paradox." [15]

One may question whether it is really paradoxical that poverty should exist amidst wealth and whether it is normal that wealth should bring forth an equal distribution of means and privileges. But perhaps the paradox might be better understood if we examine the origin of America's wealth. This conspicuous feature of our country can be attributed to an interplay of economic and social conditions, and among the latter to the absence of feudalism as a social structure and to the effect of the Protestant ethic upon national development. The Protestant ethic, as embodied in the early beliefs of American Puritanism, emphasized "a devotion to the calling of making money," regarded money as the appropriate reward of man's work and recommended the application of men's best efforts to the pursuit of such a reward.[16] During the historical development of national growth, the originally non-Puritan segments of our society came to adopt this ethic as a part of their assimilation. Although the Puritan tenets of the Massachusetts Bay Colony changed much in time, their remnants can be still clearly recognized in the life style of the "middle class" or the "suburbanites," with its emphasis upon personal achievement, individual acquisition of means and privileges, high standard of living, and conformist behavior in the market economy.[17]

The Calvinist ethic left its imprint even upon the early discoverers of poverty in America. Benjamin Franklin, the Philadelphia freethinker and contemporary of Adam Smith, discovered the blessings of wealth for the New Englanders and taught them in witty sayings about wealth, thrift, and happiness. Robert M. Hartley, a contemporary of Robert Owen and chief mover of the New York Association for Improving the Condition of the Poor, invented ingenious ways of making poverty less disturbing to the middle-class conscience through the application of organized charity. And finally Henry George, the nearest American approximation of Karl Marx, presented in the idea of the single tax a simple recipe, free from any taint of socialism, for the elimination of poverty.[18] In fact, every generation of Americans has had to discover poverty for itself, and our experience of the 1960's has been just the latest in a long series, although more promising for the future than the previous ones.

A continual rediscovery of poverty was indeed necessary, because the traditions of the Protestant ethic set general standards for judging the poor, but the standards changed with changing times. The generation of Robert M. Hartley, for example, applied such standards as a means test combined with an inquiry into personal probity and respectability of character; accordingly, it divided the paupers into the "deserving poor" and "undeserving" ones; made charity available for the former and showed its charitable wrath to the latter. Yet, in all those actions for improving the conditions of the poor, Hartley's generation was dominated by a Puritan conscience with its particular principle of social justice and its middle-class determination to elevate the poor through the practice of philanthropy. It established organized philanthropy as a characteristic feature of American society and offered some kind of social nurturance to those who were deprived of their fair share of family nurturance. Nurturance, originating in deep-seated psychological motives, is essentially irrational; accordingly, philanthropy picked its recipients without any rational plan, selecting them incidentally from the local scene. This incidental and parochial character has greatly restricted the social effectiveness of our magnificent philanthropies, even of our highly bureaucratized state philanthropy, the welfare system—the most important social nurturance that we extend to the poor.

THE POVERTY-PRODUCING FACTORS

The social effectiveness of our philanthropy has been further limited by the fact that the Puritan conscience had firm standards of propriety but less firm definitions of poverty. This was perhaps not the fault of the Puritan conscience, but rather a consequence of the existing circumstances—the open class system and rapid social mobility in America. Such circumstances produced transitional poverty, mainly among the immigrant groups. Immigration, as it rose to its peak before World War I, brought an influx of the poor and destitute who in their new homes continued the life of poverty; they crowded into cheap tenements, worked in the least desirable jobs, and showed all the symptoms of social disorganization attendant on pauperism.[19] Yet in their case this state of deprivation lasted only for a while. In time they made their way out of poverty, sometimes in the first generation and at other times in the second. The descendants of poverty-stricken immigrants now make up an indistinguishable part of the suburbanite class.[20]

The rise of the immigrant groups into affluence represents an interesting chapter of the American rags-to-riches story and a spectacular example of our system of social mobility. But it was due to motives and conditions endogenous in the ethnic groups and absent from other segments of American society.

While the ascendance of the ethnic groups took place, others remained in their previous state of poverty or sank into poverty from a previous higher level.

It might very well be that social mobility in America is like Alice's Wonderland, where one has to run in order to stay in one place. In any case, it is reasonable to describe the poor of present-day America as a residual group which for some reason or another has not been able to take part in the general social mobility and acquire the means and privileges that ensure life above the poverty level; which has fallen short in personal achievements and other requirements of the Protestant ethic; and has been excluded from the country's general affluence.

The obvious failure of the poor cannot be described without inquiring into its causes. What keeps some people from ✕ acquiring the means and privileges that many others manage to acquire? We may dismiss moralizing answers which try to fix the blame for the failure and blame either the personal faults of the poor or the injustices of our social system. Poverty as a national phenomenon cannot be accounted for by one cause; rather it must be regarded as the product of a great many factors of diverse origin and impact. For the sake of convenience in discussion, we classify the factors into three main categories, geographical, social, and psychological.

It is an old observation that poverty is concentrated in certain areas of the country which can be clearly delineated on the map. For this purpose a division of the country into 119 subregions, made by Bogue and Beale, seems suitable since each subregion represents a natural economic and social unit.[21] Table I–1 lists the poorest one fifth of the subregions, i.e., those which had the highest proportion of families with an income of less than $500. The income data refer to 1949, but no similar regional survey of the country is available for a more recent date. Although the income of the nation has considerably increased since 1949, the indications are that the geographical location of poverty has not changed greatly, and the table is still useful in pointing out where poverty is located.

First it should be noted that the great urban slums of New York, Chicago or Detroit, on which nowadays the national attention is focused, do not appear in the table. Their exclusion is not due to the fact that the urban slums do not constitute natural subregions. They are excluded because the great urban slums show a relative (although conspicuous) poverty when compared to the suburbs but are much more fortunate in income and services than many nonurban areas. In fact, nonurbanized America is the seat of the real, long-lasting pauperism.

As the table shows, the nonmetropolitan areas have much higher proportions of poor than the metropolitan areas of the same subregion and, generally speaking, income is lower in rural than in urban areas. This difference is mainly due to the effect of geographical isolation which keeps out industrialization, restricts employment opportunities, and limits the marketability of farm products. As a second point, the poverty areas form two distinct clusters, one in the deep South, mainly in the plantation land, and the other in the Appalachian region. The former has retained many local remnants of a feudalism surviving from the time of slavery and strictly observed through local statutes and customs; the latter, through its marginal farming and mining, has developed a distinct local culture perpetuating poverty.[22]

As it appears, the geographical factors of poverty refer, not to the infertility of the land or its distance from the seaboard, but to a combination of localized social and economic conditions which man has created or failed to create and which restrict high-return work opportunities. The combination of local conditions tends to produce further aggravating factors such as the unequal distribution of government services in education, transportation, and particularly in welfare. The state and county governments with the proportionally greatest number of poor provide the least of those services that may alleviate poverty. For example, in January 1967 the average family on ADC received $198.25 in Massachusetts but only $38.30 in Mississippi, although the Mississippi family on welfare was somewhat larger than its counterpart in Massachusetts. The poverty-producing factors work in associations, generating vicious circles. If one of them is permitted to operate unchecked for some time, it tends to introduce another factor into the same area. The end result is likely to be an endemic poverty which the local residents can hardly eradicate without outside assistance. The person unfortunate enough to be born or come to live in a poverty area is likely to be condemned to poverty—unless he moves elsewhere.

Table I–1. Geographical factors in poverty: subregions of the United States with the highest proportion of low-income families.

Subregion of the Country	Percent of families having income of less than $500 (1949)		
	Total	Metro-politan	Nonmetro-politan
Alabama-Mississippi-Black Prairie	27.4	11.2	33.3
South Carolina-Georgia Upper Coastal Plain	29.7	—	29.7
Mississippi-Alabama Piney Woods & Brown Loam	25.2	13.9	27.2
Tennessee-Mississippi River Hills	18.0	8.1	27.0
Georgia-Alabama Central Coastal Plain	25.3	—	25.3
Alabama-Upper Coastal Plain	25.0	—	25.0
South Carolina-Georgia Fall Sand Hills	12.6	9.7	23.4
Middle Tennessee Valley and Sand Mountain	22.5	—	22.5
Eastern and Western Highland Rim (Kentucky-Tennessee)	22.1	—	22.1

Table I–1. (*Continued*)

Subregion of the Country	Percent of families having income of less than $500 (1949)		
	Total	Metro-politan	Nonmetro-politan
Mississippi Delta	20.5	8.4	21.9
Tennessee-Mississippi Fall Line Slopes and Pine Hills	21.8	—	21.8
Southern Piedmont (South Carolina-Georgia-Alabama)	15.0	7.4	20.0
South Carolina-Georgia Atlantic Flatwoods	15.3	11.5	19.5
Southern Blue Ridge Mountains	17.3	8.9	19.4
Ozark Plateau	17.1	6.9	19.3
Middle Arkansas Valley and Ozark Slopes	14.9	9.5	18.4
Crowley's Ridge and Arkansas Prairies	18.3	—	18.3
Virginia-North Carolina Coastal Plain	17.9	—	17.9
Georgia Florida Lower Coastal Plain	17.7	—	17.7
North Carolina Upper Coastal Plain	15.5	8.4	17.2
Pee Dee and Lumbar River (North & South Carolina)	17.0	—	17.0
South Central Indiana and West Central Kentucky Hills	16.6	—	16.6

Source: Donald J. Bogue and Calvin L. Beale, *Economic Areas of the United States* (New York: Free Press of Glencoe, 1961), pp. VII–XL.

The social factors involved in poverty (such as race, sex, age, education, family structure, work status) determine the individual's place within the acquisitive society. Each of them is linked to acquisition through the generally accepted standards and each of them has a specific role in helping or hindering any person to acquire the means and privileges. To explain their role, Table I–2 summarizes the effect of some social factors upon the prevalence of poverty in the United States.[23]

Race is a major category of deprivation which in its total constellation blocks the acquisition of means and privileges. The nonwhite family is about three times as likely as the white to be in any of the poverty groups, and the difference persists even when matching categories of white and nonwhite families are compared. Although sex in itself does not represent a category of deprivation, the female is greatly restricted in her acquisitive freedom by the fact that the important money-making activities are preempted by the males; hence, the family with a female head is again three times as likely as the family with a male head to fall into the group of the poor.

Family structure and work status are factors of a different order. Each of them is a composite of many subfactors some of which are, to a greater or lesser extent, subject to the volition of people and can be freely changed. For example, the simple dichotomy of working versus nonworking makes a basic contribution to poverty, but this contribution is greatly affected by the reason that puts any person out of work as well as by such contingencies of the work career as occupation, education, and age. The poverty of the unemployed varies by the ups and downs of business cycles, but the poverty of the chronically ill remains much the same even in times of greatest boom. A developing disability will in all likelihood cause poverty for a laborer but not necessarily for a businessman or professional.

As for family structure, the nuclear family, with a planned number of children, is the ideal acquisitive unit since it implies the optimal state of having a male breadwinner and an optimal ratio of breadwinner and dependents. Any deviation from this ideal model is likely to increase the risk of poverty. The "unrelated individual," being totally deprived of the eco-

Table I–2. Social factors in poverty: percent of families and unrelated individuals with 1963 income below specified levels.

Social characteristics	All families			All unrelated individuals		
	Total number thousands	Per cent with incomes below		Total number thousands	Per cent with incomes below	
		economy level [a]	low-cost level [b]		economy level [a]	low-cost level [b]
Race of head:						
white	42,663	12.0	19.3	9,719	41.8	48.0
nonwhite	4,773	42.5	55.6	1,463	57.6	61.8
Type of family:						
male head	42,554	12.3	20.0	4,275	33.7	39.4
female head	4,882	40.1	49.3	6,907	50.3	56.3
Work status of head:						
worked in 1963	40,753	11.3	18.2	6,729	26.4	30.8
did not work in 1963	6,683	38.3	51.9	4,453	70.4	78.5
ill or disabled	1,745	46.5	59.9	974	79.8	86.4
keeping house	1,603	49.7	57.8	2,076	71.5	79.8
could not find work	202	49.3	60.5	128	83.3	87.5
Number of earners:						
none	3,695	53.4	70.2	4,204	73.8	82.0
1	20,832	15.7	24.7	6,978	26.0	30.4
2	17,306	8.7	14.4	—	—	—
3 or more	5,603	7.4	12.3	—	—	—
Number of related children under age 18:						
none	19,119	12.7	20.1	—	—	—
1	8,682	12.1	17.7	—	—	—
2	8,579	11.3	17.5	—	—	—
3	5,554	17.4	26.8	—	—	—
4	2,863	22.8	34.8	—	—	—
5	1,429	35.8	53.0	—	—	—
6 or more	1,210	49.3	63.5	—	—	—
Total	47,463	15.1	23.0	11,182	43.9	49.8

Source: Mollie Orshansky, "Counting the Poor," Social Security Bulletin, 28 (January 1965), 12.

[a] Incomes ranging from $1,580 for a single person under age 65 to $5,090 for a family of seven or more persons.

[b] Income ranging from $1,885 to $6,395.

nomic advantages of the nuclear family, represents the greatest deviation as well as the greatest risk of poverty, while the absence of an earner or the presence of too many children, producing a partial deprivation of economic advantages, affects the risk in proportion to the deviation from the ideal. As a final point it should be noted that the factors of poverty tend to cluster in families much the same way as in geographical areas. For example, the nuclear family is usually described as characteristic of the middle class, while broken families with their poverty-producing environment appear to be common in groups disadvantaged by race and low education.[24]

PSYCHOLOGICAL FACTORS IN POVERTY

In order to understand the psychological factors of poverty we must consider the family environment from another point of view. In our market economy every person is supposed to learn the standard acquisitive skills, and the basic part of this learning experience takes place within the family during the socialization process of childhood. The middle-class family (the usual model of the good in our American way of thinking) puts a heavy emphasis upon imparting those skills and teaches them with fair success. To be sure, the social, financial, and emotional stability that characterizes the middle-class family is a help, because the intactness of the family as well as the active participation of both father and mother in the socialization process greatly contribute to its success.

In contrast, poverty as an environment does not favor, or outright prohibit, the acquisition of those personality characteristics which would be useful in breaking away from poverty; it perpetuates and reinforces the personality of the pauper. The poor family seems to have a pattern of socialization in which the skills of acquisitiveness do not have a steady place and cannot be easily transmitted to the children. As one study concluded, the "task of the lower-lower class person is to evolve a way of life that will reduce his insecurity and enhance his power in ways that do not depend on achievement in the universalistic sector and on command of a rich and sophisticated variety of perspectives." Another study, dealing mainly with female-centered families, pointed to such "focal concerns" in their socialization process as a preference for using one's wits rather than doing steady dull work, a dislike of formal intellectual and scholastic activities, and an admiration of card sharks, gamblers, and con-artists as popular heroes.[25]

One essential element in the middle-class socialization process is a tendency to build up a disposition for putting off the immediate gratification of wants for the sake of those ulterior gratifications that can be obtained at a later time.[26] This delayed gratification pattern operates under conditions when rational planning for the future is possible, when actions and their contingent rewards can be assessed, and the ulterior reward is deemed to be attractive enough to prevail over the impulse of immediate gratification. Such planning, when applied to career, financial management, marriage, and family, helps to assure the acquisitive success of the middle class. For example, the pursuit of higher education implies that the young man and his family postpone immediate gratifications for the ulterior reward of a higher income and a more prestigious job that can be gained upon completing education.

The poor family is seldom in a position to impart this pattern because its environment lacks the necessary favorable conditions. As was noted, the lower-class child "lives in a world of anxiety about the immediate provisions for his basic needs of food, clothing, and shelter" and learns to seek immediate gratification in all his actions.[27] Accordingly, he is likely to drop out of school and rationalize his behavior by referring to a discrimination on the part of his teachers. While discrimination and mistreatment must not be entirely discounted, his behavior is just as much motivated by the fact that in his unstable environment he is unable to assess his actions and their contingent rewards; consequently he regards the ulterior gratifications that higher education can give as too uncertain to renounce for their sake his immediate gratifications.[28]

An unwillingness to defer gratifications seems to be a common characteristic not only of the budgeting and spending habits but also of the sex behavior of the poor class. It was found that males with college education show the lowest and males with grade-school education the highest incidence rates of premarital intercourse, while the incidence rates of masturbation are just reversed among the educational groups.[29] Dating and engagement were found to be more prevalent among youths of higher socio-economic level than among those of lower level. In fact, dating and engagement were described as typically middle-class rituals designed to prolong the preparatory stage to marriage. They were contrasted to the corresponding behavior of young people of the lower class who tend to "drift" into marriage, often under indications of premarital pregnancy, at a comparatively early age. A corresponding deferment of marriage can be observed: college-educated people tend to marry at a later age and are more likely to stay single than people with less education.[30]

According to a popular belief, sexual irregularities are common in the poor class, and a best seller of our poverty-conscious decade seems to teach that the wages of sex are poverty.[31] While marriage brings a happy ending in novels, in the life of the poor it is often followed by marital instability, broken families, and sexual behavior which is contrary to middle-class standards. Those upsetting events, crises, and stresses which may threaten daily life in any class, appear to be accentuated in the poor family which, at any rate, has its undue share of "troubles"—brushes with the representatives of authority, including law, school, and welfare administration, as well as a high rate of delinquency, serious mental illness, and other difficulties which sociologists like to call social problems.[32]

One might rightly ask to what degree the social problems of the poor should be attributed to their deprivation of privileges and to what degree to their imperfect observance of the inhibitory system. The agencies of social control adjudge and treat deviants with due regard to their social status and community power; law enforcement and medical care do adjust their rules of operation to the practical requirements of community life. Accordingly, they treat the same act as an offense by a poor person but not as an offense by a respectable citizen and may label the same symptomatology as a psychosis in the former case but not in the latter. Drunkards in the city jail and patients in the state hospital are likely to be poor, and in all likelihood they have been adjudged by standards which do not wholly apply to their more fortunate fellow citizens. Hence, a comparison across class lines of rates of delinquency, mental illness, and many other social problems invariably turns out to be unfavorable for the poor.

At the same time, however, one cannot entirely overlook the differences anchored in the personality structure. The inhibitory system that keeps people out of trouble and makes them conform to communal standards is closely linked to the socialization process, and it operates differently in different social classes. Some of the taboos observed by the middle class are not known in the poor class, and other taboos are less firmly internalized and less rigorously observed. In any case the observance of the taboos is reinforced with far greater efficiency in the middle class, where observance brings higher rewards and infringement causes heavier punishments. A jail sentence for public drunkenness may bring inestimable social loss, perhaps ruinous effects upon career and success, in the middle class, but may hardly affect the prestige and earning power of a poor man.

In their total effect the factors of poverty add up to what can be best described as a stigma, imprinted upon every poor person as a visible sign of his state, that accompanies him all the time and every place, and unfavorably influences his personality, behavior, presentation of himself, and chances to achieve a change for the better.[33] Since the factors determine a specific behavior for the poor, it can be expected that this behavior manifests itself in the field of health also. The role of poverty in health status and care will be examined in the following chapter, but as a point of beginning it is safe to assume that the poverty-producing factors are bionegative in their nature and determine poor health conditions for the poor.

So far we have been speaking of the poor as a homogeneous class of people, seemingly overlooking the fact that they are not equal in their poverty nor are they people of the same kind. The poverty-producing factors bring forth a variety of poor. For example, physical disability and age-connected unemployment are often of progressive nature; the loss in the earning power that they cause at their onset may fall anywhere between "small" and "great" and increase with the passing of time; and their total impact is further modified by the person's financial status at the time of onset.[34] The combination of several factors (such as disability, race, and occupation) introduces even greater variations. Therefore, a definition of several types of poverty might be useful.

THE TYPES OF POVERTY

The old moralistic typology of the deserving and nondeserving poor, although it has survived among some sociologists for a remarkably long time, is obviously inadequate and meaningless.[35] A phenomenological typology is more relevant for descriptive purposes because the degrees of deprivation mark meaningful differences among the poor. Thus, a distinction between "economy level" and "low-cost level" of poverty (see Table I–2) delineates two empirical categories which greatly differ in size and social characteristics; or the distinction made by Galbraith between insular poverty and case poverty clearly points out the environmental and personal causes of poverty.[36]

Other authors have developed more elaborate sets of typology, based usually on a combination of the causes as well as visibility of poverty. The listing presented below summarizes their ideas.[37]

Michael Harrington (a messianistic philosopher instrumental in mobilizing our consciousness of poverty) and Hubert H. Humphrey (often described as an ebullient spokesman of liberal ideas) used a practical reconciliation of causes and visibility and concentrated on types of the poor that the public can easily recognize. S. M. Miller applied a sociological typology based on the combination of economic security and familial stability. His types run from the stable poor (characterized by regular employment and stable family life) through the strained (economic security but familial instability) and the coper (economic insecurity but familial stability) to the unstable or "hard-core" poor (economic insecurity and familial instability).

Types of Poverty as Seen by Three Authors

Harrington (1962)	Humphrey (1964)	Miller (1964)
The unemployed	Urban poverty	The stable poor
Marginal farmers and farm workers	Rural poverty	The strained
	Depressed areas	The copers
Negroes	Negroes	The unstable
Deviants (beats, alcoholics, urban hillbillies)	Welfare recipients	
	The undereducated	
	The unemployed	
The aged		
The mental health problems		
Slumdwellers		

Within the theoretical framework of this book we propose a relatively simple typology. We shall distinguish on the basis of different deprivation processes between chronic and acute poverty. The first, exemplified by the Negro in the rural South and the northern slums as well, implies a long-established—lifelong or perhaps multigenerational—deprivation process; the second, exemplified by the elderly, implies deprivation following a period spent above the poverty level. In the first case the acquisitive abilities have been chronically restricted and poverty is regarded as the usual and known state of life, often as the normal or natural life, viewed without much realistic hope for changing it. The chronically poor person has no personal knowledge of how to live above the poverty level and, if given some unexpected aid from a charity organization, he cannot live up to the expectations; perhaps, as has been suggested, he has to be taught the rudiments of middle-class life and spending habits.

In the case of acute poverty there has been a loss of acquisitive power. The loss is not necessarily complete; in many cases it amounts to "reduced means" and the retention of some of the privileges which may present quite a contrast to the deprivation of the chronically poor. The memory of olden days is much alive and stimulates an active desire and effort to restore the former state, and any help given in these efforts is likely to be acknowledged and utilized.

Chronic poverty is self-perpetuating and preserves all the negative traits of pauperism mentioned above. Its characteristic response to the existing state of affairs is either acquiescence or periodic and essentially futile rebellion. Acute poverty is largely free of the negative traits so shocking to the middle class, and its usual response to the existing state of affairs is either resentment at being déclassé or a refusal to identify oneself as poor. The bashful person who does not apply for welfare benefits is a case in point.

The typology might be helpful in assessing the changes that take place among the country's poor and in answering the question whether the number of the poor is generally increasing or whether we are witnessing just a shift from one type of poverty to the other. Two important social forces, cybernetics and the aging of the population, function in a way as to lead continually new masses into poverty. Cybernetics, as a sophisticated form of increasing mechanization, eliminates many unskilled jobs in services and industrial production. It regularly dislocates a great number of laborers whose chances to find new jobs on a shrinking market are in proportion to their educational and industrial skills; the undereducated among them are likely to face chronic unemployment.

The general increase in the number of the aged, a common phenomenon in the industrial civilizations of the western world, poses a similar problem. The chances of being able to provide for old age and keeping oneself above the poverty level, are proportionate to the educational and acquisitive skills of people; the chance is not given to the chronically poor and hardly given to the many marginal people remaining near to the poverty line.

At the same time, other social forces work in the opposite direction and help to reduce the number of poor. Social mobility is still conspicuous in our society and its usual road, the learning of acquisitive skills through higher education, is quite open to young people whose parents did not have the same opportunity. General economic progress, rising incomes, extended welfare programs and related governmental services, the civil rights movement and other measures to ensure equality for minority groups help to reduce poverty. But again, the benefits that anyone may derive from such social forces are proportionate to his status and skill, and the poorest can benefit the least. One cannot entirely dismiss the total impression that the social forces, as they naturally operate in our society, may help to reduce acute poverty but tend to increase, or at any rate perpetuate, chronic poverty.

This was the background about 1960 when a number of conditions never before present in American history were manifest. The country reached an unprecedented affluence, but chronic pauperism seemed to grow. The Puritan conscience, or its traditions surviving in public opinion, felt troubled by this paradox, and its shame was heightened by the conviction that our industralized society possessed the financial means and social-engineering skills to eliminate poverty. If any further stimulus was needed to make the conscience work, this was given by the first great successes of the civil rights movement. The stimuli coming from different directions reinforced one another and created a psychological readiness to do something of lasting impact about the seemingly eternal poverty.

THE WAR ON POVERTY

The intellectuals of the country expressed the general mood; they argued for the necessity of a new approach to the old problem, and produced many new ideas and concrete propositions as their personal contribution to a national enterprise. Economists of both liberal and conservative persuasion set out detailed plans about possible governmental services and writers and social practitioners added practical as well as ideological suggestions.[38] Among the philosophers of activism Saul Alinsky proved to be the most practical with his emphasis on organizing the poor to exercise direct political power against the bureaucratic efforts of local governments. Michael Harrington's theory about the decadence of the poor from their position as the major revolutionary force of the last century appealed to the romantic imagination, while the ideas of the civil rights movement (such as Martin Luther King's program of nonviolence and Stokely Carmichael's principle of black power) gave additional weight to activating the Negro masses.[39]

The intellectual ferment played a major part in mobilizing public opinion and gathered enough support to initiate governmental action. The transit from intellectual planning to governmental action did not take a long time but lasted long enough to go through the usual motions of American reform movements—the reconciliation of the independent and often contradictory ideas into a practical compromise in which the leadership of the various kinds of social and political practitioners could prevail. Under such leadership the new action program became essentially nonideological and pragmatic; in fact, the prevalence of activists over the more meditatively oriented planners has been a characteristic feature, and perhaps shortcoming, of the whole poverty program. Yet, at the same time it turned out to be a vigorously antitraditional program in treating the poor.

Pragmatic as it was, the action program recognized that the treatment of acute poverty is a relatively simple task because it deals with people who, on the whole, anxiously endeavour to shake off their poverty; such supportive measures as health insurance for the elderly or job training and placement services for dislocated laborers are greatly effective in keeping these people above the poverty line. Chronic poverty, however, needs more than supportive actions; it needs massive intervention programs which are activated by the power structure residing outside poverty and are designed to alter radically yet systematically the general conditions existing among the poor.

Now public opinion and government were ready to initiate supportive measures as well as interventions. The total program amounted to a large-scale social manipulation aimed at changing a basic psychological need as well as the underlying objective situation. The involvement of the federal government in the direct handling of poverty followed a long line of development which saw the extension of the federal authority over many new areas, in the present case, over the social manipulation of broad masses of our society. The federal government made funds available for nationwide coordinated programs; it aroused the attention of the nation and obtained safeguards against the political vagaries of local governments; and furthermore, it made possible the participation of formerly apathetic individuals and formerly nonexistent organizations.

The charity organizations of the past and the welfare structure of rather recent vintage were limited in their ability to handle the specific tasks of the new program. Private and church charity as well as welfare administration were too parochial in their interests and too static in their goals. They aimed at maintaining an existing situation, helping the deserving poor, fighting the chiselers, but stopping short of any radical action that may affect the poor as a group. Thus, when it came to implementing the plans, the program could resort to new and often ad hoc organizations willing to assume new responsibilities, working under great pressure, and disadvantaged by a lack of experience and a necessity for extemporizing. But by their structure the new organizations were independent from the local centers of power, were free of bureaucracy and eager to experiment with new methods of solving the poverty problem.[40]

With the help of this organizational setting, the intervention program took a very American direction. While it remained non-ideological and notably aloof from any socialistic scheme (so distasteful to the American mind), it worked toward an indirect redistribution of the means and privileges by furnishing the poor with the standard acquisitive skills. It undertook to teach those skills, not so much to the adult generation, persevering in its way as it is wont to do, but rather to the young people. Thus, it designed compensatory educational programs which would enable the children of the poor to reach out for higher income and take their places in the acquisitive life. It launched community action programs that would establish a participatory democracy, make the poor active partners in civic actions and, in their psychological implications, end their powerlessness, apathy, forlornness, and enable them to cope with the tension and anxieties of an acquisitive society.[41] It initiated health programs that would transmit to the poor the rational and planned ways of healthy living, including family planning, as the important conditions of a middle-class life.

The war on poverty (as this very peaceful activity came to be called for reasons of publicity) is far from having accomplished its task or its formally announced goals; yet, as it is bound to happen amidst so much public attention, it has been evaluated and criticized many times.[42] We do not wish to add one more piece to the critical evaluations of an unfinished business but certain questions must be raised that refer to the theoretical considerations of this book: Is this national intervention program able to counterbalance the poverty-producing geographical, social, and psychological factors? Is it capable of correcting the effect of those social forces that perpetuate chronic poverty?

It is evident that poverty, as well as wealth or affluence, are man-made conditions that human work and planning can change for the better. But any intervention affects each of the poverty-producing factors in a different way, coping efficiently with some of them but remaining inefficient against others. Geographical factors such as isolation and local remnants of feudalism are easily amenable to manipulation; they are now removed with relative ease through roadbuilding programs in Appalachia and voter registration in the South. On the other hand, some of the social factors are resistant to any action program; old age and the female sex will always constitute deprived categories in acquisitive competition, and no change can be expected in such hard facts of life. The psychological factors present a different problem: they are closely tied to the socialization process which works through the cycle of generations and cannot be changed in less time than that of a generation.

The psychological lag that is concomitant to any intervention program helps to explain the persistence of the poor in their ways of life. The hard-to-reach or hard-core family has been observed in social work and medical practice for quite a long time because of its conspicuous reluctance to change its way of life under professional guidance.[43] Such a resistance to reasonable change can be understood: to many poor people any change may appear as a threat to that personal security that they perceive within the existing familiar order. Small wonder that the poverty program has repeatedly encountered such resistance; still, it has better chances to overcome the same reluctance than the previous fragmented and individualistic actions.

The long-range limitations of the poverty program are defined by its problems. An adjective restricts the meaning of its noun: compensatory education is less than education proper and participatory democracy is less than democracy; qualified education and qualified democracy are actually substitutes for more basic entities. Compensatory education is designed to be a substitute for the middle-class socialization process, and participatory democracy is a similar substitute for the civic activity and political interest generally shown by the middle class. It remains to be seen how effective a substitute will be: whether the subtle effect of the total family environment upon the child can be replaced with some kind of formal education given at a much later stage of life; whether the required participation in community action or the instituted compliance with health programs will work out among the poor the same way as the spontaneous activities of similar nature do in the middle class.

Yet it should not be forgotten that participatory democracy is a tremendous step forward when compared to the patterns of previous welfare administration and charity management. It is a part of the often praised, and just as often criticized, feature of the poverty program—of not distributing money among the poor in charity fashion but working toward more essential goals. The achievements of the program consist of moving toward those goals. The poor of the country have been placed on the road of social mobility and prompted to participate in the acquisitive life; the children of the poor have been influenced, and even prepared, to aspire for the means and privileges represented by the affluence of the middle class. These social efforts have been well supported by the related achievements of the civil rights movement in assuring equality to the minorities and of the federal legislation extending minimal health care to every citizen.

Such achievements reach beyond the purely emotional goals of lessening misery, humiliation, and deprivation. They work toward that idealistic aim, a more equalitarian society, which gives fair chances to everybody for starting out in life. To be sure, no perfectly equalitarian society can be conceived, and the equal chances at start turn into unequal achievements later in life. It is perhaps a vain hope that in the more affluent society of tomorrow poverty, measured by the relative standards prevailing at that time, will be viewed as absent; in all likelihood poverty will always be with us. But the present intervention program, or call it war on poverty if you like, is at work at a major restructuring of American society, at the reduction of the conspicuous differences in means and privileges and the establishment of an ideal structure which, without establishing a ceiling to anybody's affluence, establishes a bottom below which no family can fall in its standard of living.

II · The Social Aspects of Health and Illness

by John Kosa and Leon S. Robertson

The practicing physician, a proverbially busy person, tends to regard health, illness, disability, and death in their concrete relevance. For him the problem is how to diagnose the specific complaint presented by the patient and how to apply the treatment that is appropriate under the given circumstances. His attention centers around such practical details as the heart murmur of a middle-aged man, the examination of a healthy child, or the emotional difficulties of a suburban housewife. Amid such preoccupations definitions of health and illness appear to him as matters all too abstract and removed from the current problems.

When, however, we have to move beyond the clinical appearances of health and illness, to a level where they cease to be unique events and become parts of a complex social situation or a national policy, their conceptual clarification becomes necessary. If a national health policy has to be considered or the relationship of health and poverty to be assessed, the unique clinical observations need to be synthesized into a general conceptual framework where health and illness become social as well as medical phenomena. Accordingly, this chapter aims to present, first, a critical review of the existing models and definitions, and then, a theoretical framework for the interpretation of health and poverty.

THE MEDICAL VIEW

One definition, found in medical writings throughout the ages, is broadly utopian. Galen, writing *On Health Care* in the second century, described health as a "condition in which we neither suffer pain nor are hindered in the functions of daily life," that is, when we are able "to take part in government, bathe, drink, and eat, and do other things we want." [1] In our times, the World Health Organization placed the following definition in the preamble of its constitution: "Health is a state of complete physical, mental and social well-being and not merely the absence of disease or infirmity." [2] The striking similarity of the two statements indicates an old tradition in medicine. Yet, this tradition always had its disputants. One critic, reading the definition of the World Health Organization, exclaimed, "This sounds more like a coma than health." [3] To be sure, it is a policy definition incorporated in a constitution which spells out the aims of an action-oriented organization. It is far too general to be useful in understanding the etiological, therapeutic, and behavioral aspects of health phenomena.

Physicians engaged in clinical work have always been greatly interested in the specific theories of illness which promised to explain their bedside observations and promote better methods of treatment. The fanciful theories of the prescientific age hardly need to be described here; it is sufficient to concentrate on the main ideas that have developed in modern medicine since the time of Louis Pasteur. [4] The germ theory of disease helped to vanquish many dreaded infectious diseases; the traditional epidemiological theory, which viewed illness as a battle of three interacting entities, the host, the agent, and the environment, helped to defeat the epidemics; the cellular concept of disease, emphasizing the changes within the cell as the basic components of disease, was associated with the rapid progress of biological sciences in our century; and the mechanistic concept, which viewed the body as a machine and viewed disease as a defective part of the machine, reflected a similar progress in surgical procedures. All four theories were overwhelmingly specific, concerned with unravelling the mysteries of given pathological conditions and applying this knowledge to a clinical conquest of the pathology. In an era in which infectious diseases posed the major threat to mankind, the specific approach was indeed useful. But once society has moved beyond this state, a fully comprehensive theory, applicable to all groups of infirmities, is essential.

Two comprehensive, although simplistic, views have gained wide acceptance among medical authorities and lay people as well. One of them regards as illness any state that has been diagnosed as such by a competent professional. It certainly reminds us of Occam's razor, but its simplicity is deceptive. Many illnesses and infirmities are never brought before professionals for diagnoses; in many other cases the professionals are by no means unanimous in their diagnoses.[5] Let us consider two hypothetical patients: one with high blood pressure and electrocardiographic evidence of left ventricular strain who has not missed a day's work and insists that he feels great; and another whose father dropped dead at an early age and who ever since has led a life of restricted activities in spite of the negative findings of innumerable laboratory procedures. Both patients are likely to receive contradictory diagnoses from different professionals who may disagree about which one of the patients is ill.[6]

The other widely accepted view defined illness in the patient's terms: whoever feels ill should be regarded as sick. The importance of such a subjectively based concept should not be underestimated because it calls attention to that personal feeling that leads the patient to the doctor and initiates medical action. However, the use of such a subjective criterion raises a problem of its own, that of distinguishing between a bionegative feeling and an objective state of disease. The problem was well posed by the question whether the experience of grief, which ordinarily follows the loss of a loved person, a valued possession, or an ideal, should be regarded as a disease.[7]

Psychologically oriented authorities have consistently rejected the specific explanations of diseases, and have preferred to view disease in its relationship to the whole person, regarding it as a situation that naturally arises in life; as a phase of life that alternates with phases of health, as a part of a continual adjustment to the momentary exigencies of life; as a dynamic process taking place in an ever changing environment; or a natural course of changes resulting from an accumulation of stress.[8] These views tend to emphasize that disease is more than a symptom and prefers to speak of sick people rather than of diseases.

Influenced by the advances of psychiatry, medical thinking has come to consider that a great many social and psychological variables are involved in sickness. These variables could be well reconciled with the clinical concept of sickness, so much so that an entire school of investigators has pointed to certain combinations of organic and nonorganic factors as the real determinants of illness. Their views appear to be prevalent in present-day medicine, but the variables named by them are too numerous to be adequately reviewed in this context. Therefore we select only those which refer to stress and hormone production and discuss them at some length. This discussion, we believe, will illustrate both the strengths and weaknesses of the multifactor theory of disease etiology.

THE DETERMINANTS OF ILLNESS

The traditional epidemiological model of illness focuses on those factors which result in a noxious agent coming in contact with a tissue and producing a change which is defined as morbid. Social variables such as occupation, family characteristics, and ethnic background have been shown to be important in this model with respect to a number of diseases. Graham has illustrated the value of such a model in research on scrotal and lung cancer, and has cited numerous other examples of relationships between social variables and various chronic diseases. However, the specific noxious agents involved in most of these diseases have not been specified. This may be a partial result of over-emphasizing exogenous agents. Quoting Graham, "most diseases are the result of a pathologic environmental agent brought into contact with a host individual genetically susceptible to this agent." [9]

Only the broadest definition of "a pathologic environmental agent" allows the inclusion in the model of stress, the factor which increasingly is hypothesized as playing a major role in most chronic illness and perhaps in the onset of some acute infectious diseases as well. Some of the findings in recent research on stress and illness and basic research on stress suggest that an exogenous physical agent is often necessary but not sufficient for illness to occur. Indeed there are some diseases in which no such agent is present. In view of this, an alternative to the epidemiological model is offered by King.[10] The model focuses on the possible interaction processes of genetic predispositions, exogenous and endogenous physical agents, and stress and coping mechanisms which may result in the onset or avoidance of disease. The specific interaction processes which result in illness have not been specified, and it is hoped that the model will suggest hypotheses which will lead toward that end.

Stress has been implicated in a remarkable variety of pathological conditions. However, all writers do not agree about what constitutes stress. Selye concentrates on physical agents (heat, cold, infection) as stressors and uses stress to denote the condition which results from these agents. Stress itself does not refer to a specific state such as nervous tension but is an abstraction "manifested by a specific syndrome which consists of all the nonspecifically induced changes within a biologic system." Included in the changes are fluctuations in endogenous elements such as the "anti-inflammatory hormones" (adrenocorticotropic hormone, cortisone, cortisol), the "pro-inflammatory hormones" (somatotrophic hormone, aldosterone, desoxycorticosterone), the adrenalines and thyroid hormone.[11]

Maladaptation occurs when the secretion of these hormones is out of balance with the requirements of the organism in adjusting to the stressor. This maladaptation, along with dietary, hereditary, and other factors, is posited as important in the development of the following diseases: high blood pressure, heart and blood vessel diseases, kidney diseases, eclampsia, rheumatic and rheumatoid arthritis, inflammatory diseases of the skin and eyes, infections, allergic and hypersensitivity diseases, nervous and mental diseases, sexual derangements, digestive diseases, metabolic diseases, cancer, and diseases of resistance.

Advocates of the psychogenic theory of illness accept the proposition that excessive or insufficient hormone productions is the factor promoting the onset of various illnesses, but they emphasize psychological rather than physical stress as the major source of changes in hormone secretion. Simmons argues that disease results from a "weakness of the adult personality structure," which is a function of "defective relationship patterns in childhood." [12] Stress, although not carefully defined, is said to be the result of extreme and/or prolonged emotional reaction to a situation which is unusually meaningful for the person. A precise link between the personality structure and stress is not offered except for the statement that "emotional stress plays the role of catalyst." The disease-producing hormone changes are thought to be consequences of the intensity and duration of emotional stress rather than a maladaptation of response to stressors.

The weakest aspect of the psychogenic theory is the position of a weak personality structure as the central factor. Personality traits often are correlated with a higher incidence of certain ill-nesses. Eysenck cites a number of studies which show higher than usual extroversion on the part of persons with heart disease and cancer.[13] Extroversion is also high in heavy smokers, indicating the possibility that a more complex relationship than the simple smoking-cancer or smoking-heart disease relationships may be plausible. King, in a review of the literature on rheumatoid arthritis, points to studies which characterize arthritics as shy, feeling inadequate and inferior, self-sacrificing, overconscientious, unable to express anger overtly, obsessive, and compulsive.[14] However, the critical mind demands that the process whereby personality traits, stress and hormone overabundance or inadequacy combine to produce or exacerbate illness be specified. To say that persons become ill because of weakness, approaches tautology.

The behavioral scientist must leave research on the hormone-illness relationship to medical and biological scientists. Nevertheless, the hypothesis that sustained overproduction or underproduction of hormones cause disease or lower resistance to infectious agents gives the behavioral scientist a task on which he can work. The most appropriate task would seem to be to specify the process by which personality traits, stress, and other possible factors result in sustained levels of hormone production.

Social situations must also be considered as possible factors in disease. Indeed many of the factors which Simmons terms psychogenic might more appropriately be called sociogenic. Interpersonal relations, divorce, and financial reverses are not exclusively psychological. The prevalence of such events preceding the onset of illness is striking. One study compared the two-week period before and the two-week period after the appearance of streptococcal infections and found that the incidence of crises (such as death of grandparents, change of residence, father's loss of job, unusual pressures on the infected person) were four times as frequent before the illness as after it.[15] Chronic family disorganization and the sharing of bedrooms by children also appear to be related to increased susceptibility. There is evidence that a concentration of social stresses exists before the onset of various illnesses.[16] Sanatorium employees who contracted tuberculosis were compared to a matched sample of healthy employees with respect to social stresses in a ten-year period, and the stresses of the ill group were found to be skewed significantly in the two years before illness. Similar studies of cardiac patients, persons with skin disease, inguinal hernia patients, and both married and unmarried pregnant females show the same results.

THE DEVELOPMENT OF STRESS-RELATED ILLNESSES

Basic research on stress also points to the importance of social factors in the mode of reaction to stress. Funkenstein and his associates show that college male subjects in an experiment designed to induce stress manifest cardiovascular responses much like those which occur when either epinephrine or norepinephrine (adrenal hormones) are injected in subjects not under stress. The subjects' verbalized emotional responses are related to physiological reactions. An angry response is more often accompanied by a norepinephrine-like response, while self-blame or anxiety are more frequent when the response is epinephrine-like. These reactions, as the psychogenic theory would predict, are also related to the subjects' recall of childhood relations with parents. When the father is characterized as a stern and distant authority and the mother is warm and affectionate, blame of others is more frequent. Self-blame occurs more often when father is a mild and affectionate authority and mother is the primary source of affection. When mother is both authority and source of affection, the response to stress more often is anxiety.

The psychogenic theory is not supported, however, when the reactions to two subsequent encounters with the stress are observed. The Funkenstein group classifies the reactions to the three stress situations in the following ways: (1) mastery, i.e., no severe anxiety in the first two encounters and performance anxiety or no emotion in the third encounter; (2) delayed mastery, i.e., severe anxiety in the first or second encounter and no emotion or performance anxiety in the third encounter; (3) unchanged reaction, i.e., the same reaction excluding severe anxiety in all three encounters; and (4) deteriorated reaction, i.e., severe anxiety in the third encounter regardless of the first two responses. There are no relationships between this classification and the above mentioned initial reactions or the recall of relationships with parents. Mastery of stress in this context is found to be related to scales designed to measure the degree to which the subjects' concept of himself differs from his view of his peer groups' feelings about him. While the mastery group's view of self is congruent with their estimate of peers' impressions of them, the delayed mastery group indicates feelings of being overevaluated by peers, and the deteriorated group show feelings of being underevaluated by peers.[17]

A number of studies demonstrate the physiological correlates of group characteristics and interpersonal relations. One of them reports differences in free fatty acid in plasma of subjects in groups with varying cohesion, conformity, and leadership.[18] Others find that the heart rates of patient and therapist in psychotherapeutic interviews are alike depending on the content of their interaction.[19] Another research project demonstrates a relationship between positive, neutral, and negative sociometric pair choice and degree of covariation in galvanic skin response during five discussion sessions.[20] Each of the physiological indicators in these studies is related to hormone output. These findings suggest that it is not a personality characteristic per se which determines the individual's mode of handling stress but perhaps the degree to which the personality is congruent with the social environment.

The emphasis in the theory of hormone nimiety or deficiency as a cause of illness is on the sustained nature of the hormone condition. Presumably, a pathological state develops only when hormone production is beyond certain limits for an extended period of time. One theory of mental illness, for example, suggests that hallucinogenic derivatives of epinephrine may be factors in producing the symptoms so labeled.[21] Funkenstein reports that patients diagnosed as paranoid manifest an excess of norepinephrine while those diagnosed as depressive show an overproduction of epinephrine. These physiologic reactions are sustained for the patients but are not so for the student subjects in the experiment discussed earlier. Whether or not the reactions would have become prolonged for those who did not master the stress in subsequent encounters is, of course, unknown.

Feedback is one of the possible processes which might result in a sustained level of stress with the noted physiological consequence. If some combinations of personality trait and social environment causes stress which, in turn, reinforces the personality trait and/or social environment toward producing more stress, then the basis for a prolonged state of stress exists. Recent research on affiliation suggests the possibility of such a process.

Schachter's experiments show that the only and first-born children in a condition presumed to provoke fear (as in this experiment threat of electric shock in a forbidding environment) express a desire to wait with others (affiliation), while later-born subjects prefer to wait alone.[22] No significant birth order differences occur among subjects in the nonfear condition. Interpretation of the results is based on another finding that the only and first-born children have higher dependency needs than later-born children.[23] Assuming that this is true, what happens if persons with such needs are socially isolated or, conversely, if nonaffiliative persons are in situations where social contact is inescapable? A partial answer to this question is provided by Dohrenwend.[24] When subjects are isolated in a sensory deprivation experiment, the only and first-born children display higher symptoms of stress while later-born children show lower stress symptoms than they displayed before the experiment. However, in a slum area with crowded living conditions, the later-born respondents report a significantly higher number of stress symptoms than do the only and first-born respondents.

These findings suggest that two types of persons will develop stress-related illness: (1) affiliative persons who are in isolation from which they cannot escape and (2) nonaffiliative persons in situations where social interaction is unavoidable. Further, it is suggested that a feedback process is operating in these two cases. Stress increases the need of the affiliative person for social interaction. If the interaction is not available, the person is again stressed and the process continues until interaction becomes available or the sustained stress with its accompanying hormone state produces illness. The following analogous chain is hypothesized for the nonaffiliative person: stress—need for isolation—isolation not available—stress—need for isolation—and so on.

Similar feedback processes involving other personality traits, stresses, and social situations are probably equally plausible. At present, however, the theory cannot answer certain important questions that its critics may justly raise. It cannot specify the types of illnesses which develop from such a process because this specification may need, as a basis, the presently unavailable knowledge of genetic predispositions with respect to susceptibility to endogenous or exogenous agents. In addition, it may be necessary to know whether or not the hormonal predisposition is connected with specific emotions under stress and whether or not particular types of hormones are affected by given emotions. In spite of such shortcomings in knowledge, it is likely that the riddle of disease etiology will be solved by exploring feedback or other processes involving social and personality variables rather than by relying on such vague concepts as a "weak personality structure."

A Sociological View of Illness

The behavioral sciences, not being directly involved in clinical work and not necessarily oriented toward an organic view of illness, have been mainly interested in a model for human behavior in health and illness—a model that fits the statistical requirements of empirical research. Statistics dissects any broad concept into measurable components which can be established on the basis of empirical observations and applied to a quantitative interpretation of the whole concept. Thus the National Health Survey, when studying the relationship of family income and health, selected for measurement three types of health characteristics: disability, hospitalization, and injury; it subdivided each characteristic and classified, for example, disability into four subcategories: restricted activities, bed rest, inability to work, and inability to attend school.[25] Such a treatment of the topic (just as the contemporary medical views of disease) suggests that health is a multidimensional variable. It is a concept so broad or abstract that in its totality it is not available for immediate observation; its clarification must consider a great many facets.

Psychology illuminates rather well the many-faceted nature of health, and its contribution to the topic leads us back to the definitions of Galen and the World Health Organization. Psychological studies have found that avowed happiness had three general correlates: youth, health, and good education. While a low socio-economic status is associated with unhappiness, materialistic luxury and good treatment, as implied by the wealth and education of one's parents, are not related to the avowed happiness of students. On the other hand, health has a stable relationship to happiness, even in populations that are, on the average, probably quite healthy.[26]

Sociology might be the useful discipline to deal with the

many facets of health because it places illness and health in a social context in which not only the sick person but his whole environment, and particularly those significant persons who try to heal him, find their places. It regards the problems of health as parts of a dynamic interaction process, views illness in its relativity, and assumes that the extent and meaning of any illness can be understood only in relation to other healthy and sick people.

The great pioneer of medical sociology, Henry E. Sigerist, presented the concept of the "special position of the sick." As he reasoned, "To be ill means to suffer," and every culture defines its stand toward suffering. While many cultures of the past tended to view illness as a punishment of the wicked, modern civilization grants, as a general rule, a privileged position to the sick and manifests a systematic concern with the healing and welfare of sick people.[27]

✕ Talcott Parsons elaborated this reasoning and placed it in the framework of a theory of social systems. In his conception, a person's illness needs to be legitimized by the authority of the medical profession, his intimates or other people having influence over him. When the illness is legitimized, the person assumes a special sick role which replaces, or modifies, his usual occupational or familial roles. The sick role permits him to observe specific norms such as freedom from the usual obligatory duties; at the same time it imposes specific norms on people near to him such as family members or attending physicians.[28]

This theory has gained wide popularity in sociology; however, empirical studies have found a limited usefulness for it. Role playing implies a relatively stable and lasting position that a person takes in the stream of social interrelationship. Occupational and family roles last for many years, and people usually wish to maintain their accepted roles; for example, many workers are unwilling to relinquish their occupational roles at the mandatory age of retirement. But illness is seldom lasting and even less seldom stable in its effects; as a rule, it is not associated with endeavors for its unrestricted prolongation. Because of such differences one may ask whether there is any state to which the name of sick role can properly be applied; at any rate, its use needs to be restricted by sheer logic to the chronic illnesses in a more-or-less stationary state.[29]

More recent theories have attempted to fill this gap and offer a broader explanation of health-related phenomena. King emphasized the perceptual component of illness and described "one crucial variable" in any health-related action: the way in which man "sees or perceives the situation of disease and all of the social ramifications that accompany it."[30] Mechanic built on such a basis the concept of illness behavior, concerned with "the ways in which given symptoms may be differentially perceived, evaluated, and acted (or not acted) upon by different kinds of persons."[31]

Following a different chain of thought, Suchman presented a theory of stages of illness and medical care which discerns five stages "demarcating critical transition and decision-making points in medical care and behavior." The five stages are symptom experience, assumption of the sick role, medical care contact, dependent-patient role, and recovery or rehabilitation.[32] Finally, Kasl and Cobb distinguished health behavior, illness behavior, and sick-role behavior, reasoning that "the likelihood that an individual will engage in a particular kind of health, illness, or sick role behavior is a function of two variables: the perceived amount of threat and the attractiveness or value of the behavior."[33]

The last four theories agree on certain points. They relegate the stationary sick role to a restricted place, emphasize the dynamic nature of health-related episodes and regard the alternations of good and ill health as a continuous process evolving within a social context. In the present discussion we are attempting to build upon their concepts, reconcile those concepts with the views commonly held by the medical profession, and formulate a sufficiently broad and flexible theory to explain the health-related phenomena. In this attempt it is necessary to re-examine the usual dichotomy of health versus illness. This dichotomy was formulated in old times, when epidemics and other serious illnesses were common, when the generally inefficient medical care could hardly offer any real help beyond a placebo effect, and when any illness was likely to last for a long time. Since then the advent of scientific medicine and the improvement of health care have basically changed all those conditions. They have vanquished many of the life-threatening diseases, made reasonable health care available to practically all people, and greatly reduced the duration of many common ailments. As a result, man in his life cycle now enjoys a long period of good health (roughly from the age of 15 to 45 and perhaps beyond) during which he survives for many years without presenting any serious illness to his physician. The health problems that he presents are, in all likelihood, not the serious organic damages of the past epochs, but illnesses with psychosomatic components, emotional and social complaints or problems of a preventive nature.[34]

One is reminded of the stimulating idea of Thomas S. Szasz that the word *illness* should not be applied to *mental illness*.[35] It would not be quite proper to apply this idea to physical health. However, it is evident that the most common health-related actions and experiences of our times cannot be clearly labeled as *illness* or *health*. This dichotomy does not accommodate the preventive measures which are so common among healthy people and include such activities as daily physical exercise, a reducing diet, or a check-up with physicians. It does not accommodate the small incidents of life (abrasions, lacerations, common colds) which temporarily may upset the family but have no significant duration and consequences. It does not fit many common forms of disability which are compensated, rehabilitated, or corrected either naturally or with professional help by wearing eyeglasses, dentures, protheses or tooth fillings. Finally, it excludes a whole set of complaints that stretches from the psychosomatic component of every illness to the nonincapacitating and not-treated but serious psychoneuroses.

THE CONCEPT OF MORBID EPISODE

As an appropriate concept that includes the measures, conditions, and disabilities mentioned above as well as the traditional symptoms and illnesses, we present the term *morbid episode*. *Episode* refers to man's persistent view that such an act or condition must be an interruption of the normal or desired course of events because the normal or desired state is characterized by freedom from such episodes. One may argue that physiological normality does not exclude repeated occurrences of symptoms, illnesses, and disabilities, but (as will be presently discussed) the health behavior of people seems to be governed by the belief in a desired state of health rather than by the teaching of biological sciences.

All these episodes (including the preventive measures) have reference to morbidity. The extent of the morbidity present in any episode cannot escape attention; it is assessed crudely by the patient or other layman helping him and more exactly by professional health personnel. This assessment initiates a social-psychological process of handling the morbid episode. The process is an integral part of the usual pattern of social interactions in which the patient and other significant persons are involved. Its regular course can be broken down into four elementary parts: (1) the assessment of a disturbance in, or of a threat to, the usual functioning of physiological-psychological health; (2) the arousal of anxiety by the perception of such an incidence; (3) the application of one's general medical knowledge to the given disturbance; and (4) the performance of manipulative actions for removing the anxiety and the disturbance. Let us discuss each element separately.

The disturbance or threat is assessed by the patient or somebody near to him such as a family member. What a "layman" perceives is a comparative difference between the present (acute) functioning of health and its previous or usual functioning. The felt difference is communicated in the relative terms of symptoms which furnish rather imperfect clues to the total disturbance and (with a few exceptions such as fever) cannot be quantified by the layman. Given the broad range and limited quantification of disturbances, the layman tends to use subjective criteria in judging whether an observed phenomenon should be assessed as a symptom, and those criteria vary according to the circumstances.

Any disturbance must reach a certain degree of seriousness or duration in order to be assessed as a symptom; below that degree a person may experience a cough, pain, a discomfort without perceiving them as symptoms (subliminal symptoms). This perceptual threshold changes with the circumstances: it is lower in summer when people do not expect illnesses and higher in winter when respiratory ailments and other illnesses are frequent; it is lower on work days and higher over the weekend when the usual pattern of recreational activities acts as a psychological block to the usual assessment of disturbances; it is lower for children and higher for adults.[36] Furthermore, one may expect that the perceptual threshold changes with social class and income level, and low-income and high-income groups differ in their assessment of a given disturbance as symptom.

Any threat to one's security and physical and psychological well-being evokes anxiety which, in case of health disturbances, is aggravated by the ultimate anxiety of death. Thus, any morbid episode appeals to the deepest fear of man, the fear of death, and sets more powerful psychological forces into motion than the word *episode* would indicate. On a psychological level disturbance and threat are inseparable. The experience of fever and pain or the expectation of fever or pain evokes as its psychological response a specific anxiety which tends to be proportionate to the seriousness of the symptom or threat. The symptom is assessed by the measure of anxiety it arouses, and the anxiety introduces the many subjective variations in setting the perceptual thresholds.[37]

Any threat to a beloved person, such as a family member, evokes an essentially similar anxiety and causes the emotional involvement of several people in the morbid episode. Every disturbance of health originates a specific anxiety in the patient as well as in people near to him. Thus, an episode seldom remains the affair of only one individual, the patient; usually it involves other people also, initiates a chain of interactions between the patient and the others, and the extent of the interactions tends to be proportionate to the seriousness of the episode. At the same time, a threat releases general or floating anxiety, usually present in the psychological mechanism of every person, and focuses it on the threatened person. This anxiety is pre-existent to, and independent from, the morbid episode; it is a function of psychological and social factors. In contemporary American families the child is the most likely focus of anxiety; the relative living in the household, the least likely focus; while self and spouse are in between. Accordingly, when mothers were asked to report all symptoms experienced by family members within a month, children were most frequently mentioned as having had symptoms, relatives least frequently, with mothers and fathers falling in between. The more serious symptoms (those requiring two or more days of restricted activities), when separately examined, did not show a similar frequency distribution.[38]

RESPONSES TO ANXIETY

Evidently, any sickness is likely to direct the floating anxiety toward the sick person and allot to him the "special position" described by Sigerist. Threatening events, unrelated to health, may also release the floating anxiety, focus it upon one person, and affect the morbid episode. Such an extraneous event as the loss of the father's job may either focus anxiety on the child's illness and cause unreasonable concern about it, or may act just the other way, detract from the anxiety focusing upon the sick child and result in a neglect of his illness. Thus the degree of the floating anxiety does not necessarily correspond to the seriousness of the health disturbance. The total anxiety, present at the time of a morbid episode, is not a simple outcome of the perceived disturbance but a fusion of two independent anxieties; hence, it is in its extent and manifestation always individualistic and subjective.

The natural response to a feeling of anxiety is the endeavor to remove or relieve whatever its cause might be. In daily life, however, the cause of anxiety can seldom be ascertained unambiguously. The feeling of anxiety and the response to it are linked through a vague and uncertain causal relationship that is common in the realm of psychology. To any given anxiety people respond in many ways, and the relieving effect of any of the alternative responses depends on many individual circumstances. One frequent response is the instinctual one which often follows the dictates of the avoidance-escape mechanism. In case of health disturbances this kind of response means an attempt to forget about the matter and put it out of one's mind—a common enough response that can be observed in delaying health care, breaking appointments, and refusing to participate in reasonable health plans.[39] Another frequent form of the instinctual response seeks the help of superhuman powers and uses magic or superstition in an attempt to remove the cause of anxiety.

Very often the instinctual response has a useful function in relieving anxiety; so it is in bereavement where forgetting is a common reaction. Health disturbances, however, present a special case. Here the instinctual approach may immediately alleviate the existing anxiety but lead in the long run to dangerous consequences—neglect of treating an acute and curable disease. The danger is great. Fortunately enough, there exist control systems which subject the instinctual response to the censorship of higher order psychological functions (learning, reasoning, judgment) and work to bring forth a reasonable response that is judged to be beneficial to health. Such control systems are, on one level, personal knowledge and, on another level, the social organizations of the family and professional medicine.

Since morbid episodes occur regularly, their course can be observed and their treatment explored; thus, people acquire a general body of knowledge about health, illness, and therapy. This knowledge corresponds to the cultural level existing in the community, and it might be described as magic belief in one community, folk medicine in another, and medical science in a third.[40] On each level knowledge is likely to include some kind of classification of morbid episodes, evaluation of the nature and seriousness of the common illnesses, and predictions relating to the eventual outcome and possible handling of the symptoms. On every cultural level this body of knowledge is available in two forms—a popular one accessible to the average person and an esoteric form accessible to the professional healers. The popular form of knowledge depends on the professional one for its source and authority; in many instances it attempts to imitate the professional know-how existing in the community. Although popular, it is not an equally general knowledge; those persons who have the special duties of nurturance (mothers, older women) are its usual repositories.[41]

This knowledge, acquired to a great extent from past experiences, is applied to assess morbid episodes. It functions as a rational censorship of anxiety and prompts people to consider the whole situation in the light of their available knowledge. It influences them to make judicious decisions about taking actions for the removal of the cause of anxiety and the possible elimination of the health disturbance. The soundness of the decision depends on the medical knowledge available, but knowledge is never equally distributed among the social classes. Thus one may expect that low income and other underprivileged groups handle health-related anxiety and decision-making differently from the privileged groups.

When this knowledge is applied to the state of good health, it tends to act in accordance with the floating anxiety and initiate preventive actions. For centuries, popular knowledge has recognized that disturbances in health can be prevented and has recommended such preventive measures to healthy people as "an apple a day keeps the doctor away." Furthermore it has prescribed a great number of harsh and even painful preventive treatments (purgation, bloodletting, circumcision), a practice which can be hardly understood without considering the interplay of floating anxiety.

When the same knowledge is applied to a disturbance in health, it helps to assess the total situation, particularly, the level of seriousness and the necessity of taking actions. In many cases no action is taken, in others only a psychologically supportive response is given to the patient because it is believed that the episode will run its usual course and resolve itself without the necessity of any outside interference. In other cases again, the disturbance is treated at home by the patient or by a member of his family, while the more serious cases are brought to the attention of professional healers.

The actions that people take are of manifold nature and effectiveness, but all of them have two characteristics in common:

they take part within the framework of the usual interaction pattern, and aim at the satisfaction of a basic psychological need (such as relief from anxiety) by changing the underlying objective situation (the disturbance in health). Such complex goal-directed actions are best denoted as manipulations, and the name can be properly applied to the health-related actions, many of which do not have a rational relationship to therapy in its general sense.

THE MANIPULATIVE ACTIONS

The social interaction pattern is involved, first of all, in the person of the manipulator. The manipulative action is carried out either by a lay person or a professional healer. The former is affected by anxiety and is emotionally involved in the total episode but has no special knowledge of health; the latter does not share the anxiety and emotional involvement but has a special knowledge commensurate to the cultural level of the community. The duality of the manipulators implies that simple actions (such as home treatment) are carried out by lay persons and complex actions by professionals; however, the duality does not necessarily coincide with the therapeutic or nontherapeutic nature of the action. Medically not approved practitioners (in our society as well as in other societies) manipulate the anxiety without proper therapy for the disturbance, while lay people often take therapeutically sound actions.[42]

The authority of performing manipulative actions is, on the whole, ambiguously defined. Both personal involvement in the anxiety and special knowledge of health entitle people to take such actions, and the perceived seriousness of the episode designates the point where the authority of the lay person is supposed to yield to the authority of the professional healer. This general ambiguity leads to many dilemmas, particularly when it comes to selecting one out of several alternative manipulative actions;

at the same time, it prompts the professional healers to impart a popularized form of their special knowledge upon the lay public.[43]

Manipulative actions aim at simultaneously removing both the health disturbance and anxiety. The achievement of this ideal goal is not always possible because disturbance and anxiety are to a certain extent independent in their origin as well as behavior, and the alleviation of one does not automatically alleviate the other. While the alleviation of a disturbance is likely to reduce the specific anxiety (although it may leave unaffected the floating anxiety), the alleviation of the anxiety, as a rule, does not reduce the underlying physiological disturbance. Other times anxiety may linger on after the apparent cessation of the disturbance, for example, in the form of a fear of its reoccurrence.

It is, therefore, practical to classify the manipulative actions according to their intended effectiveness in dealing with the health disturbance only. On such a basis we may distinguish between therapeutic and gratificatory actions. The therapeutic action aims at the removal or arrest of the disturbance, giving, at the same time, proper consideration to the anxiety surrounding it, in accordance with the standards set by the competent healing profession. It is likely to be the outcome of a reasoned judgment which establishes priorities among the possible aims and actions and proceeds consistently toward the desired end.

Gratificatory manipulation is essentially nonrational and has a main aim other than the professionally defined cure of the disturbance. It may aim at a relief of the anxiety without the underlying disturbance, or at the gratification of wishes and needs not directly related to the morbid episode. Certain specific instances of it are particularly common, such as the escape-avoidance of painful or threatening therapy or the unwillingness to give up a pleasurable activity for the sake of health. The patient's desire for prolonging the sickness is frequent in mental and psychosomatic illnesses; for example, patients use hysteria for the gratificatory aim of dominating their family and, accordingly, to resist professional therapy.[44] Faith healers and cultists are likely to gratify various needs not related to the disturbance; the gratificatory nature of their manipulations helps to explain the popularity they enjoy with the public.

The manipulation of one symptom may include several actions; hence, therapeutic and gratificatory actions can be taken simultaneously. In the health care of the American middle class, manipulatory gratification has an adjunct role, secondary to the therapeutic one, and shows up, for example, in the usual pampering that patients give themselves or receive from others. In an adjunct role the medical profession also uses gratificatory manipulations (by "sweetening the pills," recommending bed rest or a "change of air") either as the signs of nurturance given by the healing professions or as psychologically effective means in the total therapeutic management.

To summarize the preceding discussion, Chart II–1 shows the schematic representation of the morbid episode as the patient's experience. From the patient's point of view, the four elements (perception, anxiety, knowledge, and manipulation) are interrelated; each of them affects all the others and, at the same time, is affected by them. Thus existing medical knowledge, while functioning as a rational censorship of anxiety, modifies the perception and manipulation; and, in turn, this knowledge is modified by the experience gained in each morbid episode.

It must be realized, however, that the patient, although the center of the episode, is seldom able to handle it by himself. He needs the assistance of persons in his immediate environment, particularly, in his family. He finds further help in the more distant environment—in his community where professional health care is organized for giving support and nurturance in case of need. The resolution of the morbid episode requires interactions on the levels of his primary and secondary groups,

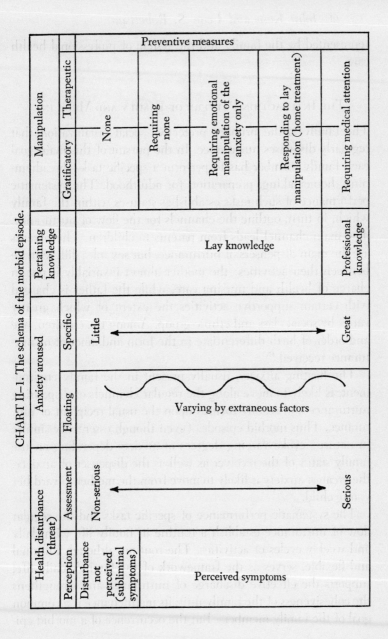

CHART II-1. The schema of the morbid episode.

Health disturbance (threat)		Anxiety aroused			Pertaining knowledge	Manipulation	
Perception	Assessment	Floating	Specific			Gratificatory	Therapeutic
Disturbance not perceived (subliminal symptoms)	Non-serious		Little		Lay knowledge		None
							Requiring none
Perceived symptoms		Varying by extraneous factors				Requiring emotional manipulation of the anxiety only	
						Responding to lay manipulation (home treatment)	
	Serious		Great		Professional knowledge	Requiring medical attention	

Preventive measures

represented by the family and the system of professional health care.

THE INTERACTION PATTERN OF FAMILY AND MEDICINE

The family is the primary protective social organization that regularly dispenses nurturance. In the pursuit of this main goal each family member has to perform a specific task—breadwinning, homemaking, preparation for adulthood. The systematic performance of such tasks establishes statuses within the family which, in turn, outline the channels for the flow of nurturance. The main channel leads from parents to children. The parents are the main dispensers of nurturance, but sex roles differentiate between their activities: the mother almost invariably is put in charge of health and nursing care, while the father is charged with certain supportive activities the extent of which greatly varies by social class and ethnic group. Among the children, age and order of birth differentiate in the form and amount of nurturance received.[45]

The floating anxiety, usually present in the family environment, is likely to move along the regular channels of dispensing nurturance and readily focuses upon the usual recipient of nurturance. Thus morbid episodes (even though essentially similar in nature) evoke varying degrees of anxiety depending on the family status of the receiver as well as the dispenser of anxiety; the greatest anxiety is likely to move from the mother toward her young child.

The systematic performance of specific tasks and the regular flow of nurturance establish a routine in family life with daily and weekly cycles of activities. The routine, although informal and flexible, serves as the framework of the family's daily life, supports the effective discharge of nurturance and strengthens the cohesiveness of the family unit; its maintenance is a common goal of the family members. But the occurrence of a morbid episode disrupts the established routine. It demands a rearrangement in the usual flow of nurturance so that special care can be focused upon the afflicted member, and sometimes it demands a rearrangement of the usual tasks so that the family members can be free for the performance of manipulative tasks.

The family has to find ways to minimize the disruption and maintain the routine. This is achieved by varying those criteria which are used in judging the seriousness of symptoms and selecting manipulative actions. The systematic changes of those criteria mark weekly and seasonal cycles as well as variations by family status among morbid episodes.[46] In this way the family censors the experience of the patient and adjusts it to the necessary routine. While this is usually done with reasonable care, in its total effect it amounts to the family operating as an inhibitory system against the wishes and desires of the sick person. In particular, the family tends to enforce the primacy of the routinelike tasks over the immediate gratification of pleasurable needs, restricts the gratificatory manipulation of morbid episodes in favor of therapeutic ones and, more generally, aims to decrease the number and duration of morbid episodes.

Professional health care in our society is part of an extremely complex system.[47] It is comprised of a network of practitioners with special skills and knowledge and of institutions with trained manpower and special equipment. Some of the practitioners and institutions are independent, others are formally coordinated, forming numerous subnetworks. While the whole system essentially follows the directives of the medical profession, it is by no means hierarchical in its structure. The principle of "fee for service" and the entrepreneurial spirit that permeates the whole organization permit any patient to select freely a practitioner or institution of his own choice or select none of them.[48] The organization is structured for the purpose of giving service to the patients and satisfying the health needs of the community. It gives institutional nurturance as well as therapy not available outside the organization. The patient who enters this network (or often is caught in it) expects to receive the benefits of nurturance and therapy as given to him in diagnosis and treatment.

The diagnostic procedure aims not simply for the exploration of possible organic disturbances but also for a convenient labeling of the patient, and such a labeling helps the communication among the members of the national organization of health care. An English authority reminds us that "there is no disease of which a fuller or additional description does not remain to be written; there is no symptom as yet adequately explored." [49] In accordance with the available level of medical knowledge the diagnosis classifies the symptom into one of the professionally approved categories for which standard management procedures are available. The system of professional health care, in the effective discharge of its duties, has to follow a specific routine and categorize the personal complaint of the patient so it can be handled uniformly by any unit of the organization.

The diagnosis is the beginning of a routinization.[50] It imposes upon the patient an inhibitive system that controls his primary responses to anxiety and leads him toward a professionally approved, therapeutic management of his complaint. The facilities of professional health care are structured accordingly. It provides for the efficient handling of the patients' medical needs two separate subnetworks which coexist in each community: the private practice of physicians and the public clinics maintained by institutions. The two networks are interlocked in various ways: many physicians work in both simultaneously and many patients use both alternately; yet they are distinguished by important structural differences. Private practice operates on a fee-for-service basis and is utilized primarily by patients in higher income brackets who are willing to pay for such desirable qualities of medical care as the continuity of services, the personal relationship between doctor and patient, and the immediate availability of service. Public clinics operate on a service basis with no fees, or with graduated fees and are used primarily by patients in lower income brackets who receive there competent but impersonal and discontinuous care.[51]

STRAINS AND STRESSES IN THE HEALTH CARE SYSTEM

The private practice of medicine is sensitive to the patient's personal anxiety and is willing to consider his wishes regarding therapy; it functions in a way as to complement and accommodate the patient's manipulative actions. The public clinic system, lacking the needed time, facilities, and privacy, cannot develop a similar personal relationship with the patient and cannot pay due regard to his manipulative actions. Frequently, it leaves a gap between the professional and the lay system of manipulating health disturbances; in particular, it is likely to leave unattended the problems of anxiety.

In spite of such differences, private practice and public clinics exert the same kind of control over the morbid episodes of the public. One line of control is implied in their service pattern which, in face of the haphazard needs of the public, sets up a systematic routine-like cooperation of many agents in the management of diseases, the schedules and circumstances of physician-patient contacts, and the preventive measures applied to the general population. The routine eliminates wasteful individual variations, increases the efficiency of organized work, and insures a fairly uniform treatment of a large mass of patients. The popular joke about hospital patients being awakened to receive their sleeping pills caricatures the general shortcomings inherent in every routine; but, as more positive achievements, the same routine enables us to administer various screening tests to large populations or to obtain comparable tests and analyses from almost any agent of the health care system.

As another line of control, professional health care influences the public toward adjusting the lay system of manipulating health disturbances to the professional standards of therapy. This is mainly done through the formal and informal teaching that members of the health professions carry out in public as well as in private contacts with patients, and this teaching furnishes another inhibitory system to the instinctual responses to health disturbances. The routine and the inhibitory system of professional health care carry the danger of ignoring the anxiety element of morbid episodes; any increase in routine and efficiency tends to increase this danger and cannot fail to evoke criticism from patients.

Cure is the ultimate aim of every manipulative action, but one should remember the old wit's saying, "When trying to cure illnesses, medicine sets its aim too high." Cure is indeed a complex, and often unattainable, goal because it refers to a reasonable combination of the following outcomes: (1) the cessation of the health disturbance, if possible; (2) if not possible, a reasonable control over the disturbance; (3) the cessation of the anxiety accompanying the disturbance or, if not possible; (4) a reasonable control over the anxiety, and (5) the cessation of, or control over, the physical and social disabilities that serious illnesses are likely to leave behind.

The current standards of medicine try to adjust the professional practices to this complex aim. They recommend treating the patient rather than the symptom and utilizing the whole process of social interaction for the achievement of the medically ascertainable cure. In any case they use relatively objective criteria in judging whether a cure has been accomplished.

The layman applies more subjective standards to his judgment of what constitutes a cure. For him the morbid episode for all practical purposes ends at a psychological threshold where he does not discern any anxiety-arousing health disturbance or where his felt anxiety is at a level comparable to the level that existed before the perception of the disturbance.[1] In case of minor symptoms this state is often achieved "naturally," and the patient claims that the cold or other ailment "has gone." More serious illnesses require a more careful assessment of whether or not a cure has been achieved. Since gratificatory manipulations often alleviate the symptom and bring results which by lay standards come near to cure, the patient feels healed and may end the therapy without completing the cure. Other times, however, the patient is willing to make a more balanced judgment of whether or not he has been cured, and in this judgment he is led by his medical knowledge and feelings of anxiety. Thus his perception of being cured is a psychological counterpart of his initial perception of a health disturbance, an assessment of the comparative difference between the previous (sick) and the present (cured) functioning of his health.

To summarize the reasoning above, Chart II–2 gives a schematic representation of the place of morbid episodes in the social interaction pattern. It indicates that the morbid episode, individualistic and unique in its physiological as well as psychological origin, in the course of its treatment and cure has to be fitted into the social interaction pattern of the patient with his primary group (as represented by the family) and his secondary group (as represented by the system of professional health care). Both groups have their routines for dealing effectively with morbid episodes, and, in order to obtain their help, the patient has to comply with the demands originating in the inhibitory system and other stable features of the social organizations.

XThe compliance imposes strains and stresses upon the patient which manifest themselves in expressed dissatisfaction and criticism directed against the attending family members, physicians, and the whole health care system. Such strains may be common and perhaps unavoidable whenever personal needs have to be fitted into an organizational routine, yet, one may logically assume that they are more common and more pressing in the low-

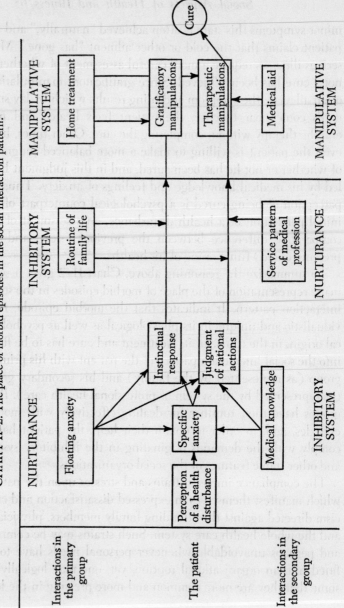

CHART II-2. The place of morbid episodes in the social interaction pattern.

	NURTURANCE	INHIBITORY SYSTEM	MANIPULATIVE SYSTEM	
				Cure
Interactions in the primary group	Floating anxiety	Routine of family life	Home treatment	
			Gratificatory manipulations	
	Instinctual response		Therapeutic manipulations	
	Judgment of rational actions			
The patient	Specific anxiety		Medical aid	
	Perception of a health disturbance	Medical knowledge		
Interactions in the secondary group		Service pattern of medical profession		
	NURTURANCE	INHIBITORY SYSTEM	MANIPULATIVE SYSTEM	

income groups which rely on public-clinic facilities. In all likelihood the existing health care system, while offering competent care, treats the strains and anxieties surrounding the morbid episodes differentially according to social class. It creates thereby a specific problem that will be discussed in the following chapters.

Within the framework outlined above the problem of health and poverty will be discussed. The described interaction of the patient, his family, and the medical care organization assures the health care that our medically advanced age can offer. But the sight of poverty suggests that the interaction of the three parties works optimally when the patient possesses the necessary means and privileges and that poverty in itself tends to detract from the smoothness and efficiency of the interaction.'

It would be easy indeed to verify this assumption and compare the poor and the non-poor if there was a uniform index of health that could measure in a simple way all the differences that can be observed in the course of morbid episodes. But no such index exists because the pathological, the psychological, and the social components of any morbid episode are to a great extent independent and cannot be reduced to a common denominator.

The following chapters investigate the social aspects of morbid episodes in the sequence that they present to, and are treated by, the health care organization. Chapters III and IV describe the observable social differences in physical and in mental health, Chapter V deals with preventive behavior, Chapter VI with the perception of health disturbance and the first actions taken. Chapters VII and VIII discuss the main aspects of the manipulative system, while Chapters IX and X attempt to assess the present efforts and future possibilities for overcoming poverty and providing a better health care. Chapter XI sums up the problem, while the Appendix takes up the issues of methodology, aiming, not at promoting pedantry, but at warning against the many pitfalls of treating emotionally loaded issues. Emotions, of course, surround all our actions. They surround our hope that this presentation will help to explain and bring nearer to a reasonable solution what is a pressing problem of our epoch.

III · Social Differences in Physical Health

by Monroe Lerner

This chapter systematically surveys the existing empirical data that compare the physical health of the poor with that of the rest of the population. Its aim is to generalize on the basis of existing data; its discussion focuses on the United States, and within this country its primary emphasis is on the national health situation. However, local data are used to clarify relationships in those instances where appropriate national data are not yet available. Although the primary emphasis is on the poor as an over-all category, some consideration of the Negro as a specific subcategory of the poor has been included. Other subcategories of the poor, such as the Puerto Rican or Mexican populations or other generally poor ethnic minorities, the aged, the migratory laborers, or the rural poor in Appalachia and the Deep South, are not discussed separately.

How can we best measure with any substantial degree of validity or accuracy, the level of a population's physical health? This is a complex conceptual problem and especially so because health is a multidimensional characteristic for which no standard definition appears to be completely satisfactory.[1] But another factor adding to the difficulty is that the achievement of health is often considered as a major index of the moral worth of a community's social and political organization. As a result of the intense desire to achieve superiority in this dimension of moral worth, partisan considerations may well enter at each step of the measurement process.* Nevertheless, in the absence of any better procedure, levels of physical health will be considered for present purposes as adequately measured by mortality rates and by that proportion of this nation's morbidity, impairments, and disability which manifests itself directly as, or is due directly to, "physical" as opposed to "mental" illness.

Mortality rarely, if ever, has other than a physical condition as its immediate cause, at least in the philosophical sense in which the concept of "cause" is customarily used in mortality statistics. As a result, mortality rates are quite legitimately used as at least partial indicators of a population's level of physical health, and to do so here involves no particular stress. However, the distinction between physical and mental causation or involvement is much less clear with regard to morbidity, impairments, and disability; the decision to confine the present discussion to the physical aspects of these conditions is purely arbitrary and is justified only by the usefulness of the distinction for analytical purposes. Finally, no attempt will be made in the present discussion to combine mortality with morbidity, impairments, and disability into any sort of over-all ratio; each of these dimensions of physical health will be considered separately and on its own merits.

Another problem concerns the definition of the poor. Concepts of poverty are obviously relative, varying with time and place, and numerous standards have been used to define poverty

---

* Prominent political leaders frequently deplore our inability to achieve this dimension of moral superiority. The late Senator Robert Kennedy, for example, once called America's health care programs "a national failure . . . We are providing poor quality care at high costs." He termed the cost of health care "staggering . . . more than six percent of our gross national product." Despite this huge outlay, he said, "in 1950, we ranked fifth in the world in our infant morality rate. Today we rank fifteenth—below all of the industrialized nations of Europe. Twelve other nations have higher life expectancy rates than we do" (New York Times, November 20, 1967).

and to measure the "poor" population. But poverty may perhaps best be thought of as *relative deprivation,* using some standard for comparison, while subjective elements are crucial in the definition of its own situation by a nation, group, family, or individual. As a result, the problem of measurement becomes enormously complicated. In any case, and almost regardless of what definition of poverty is used, mortality statistics have never been collected for the country as a whole in a way which might distinguish between the poor and the rest of the population. It has been necessary, as a result, to use the data from special studies based on limited areas or populations, to infer the mortality experience of the poor. However, for morbidity, impairments, and disability, some national data have been collected in recent years on the basis of family income, and these data have been used extensively in the present discussion.

MORBIDITY AND THE POVERTY GROUP

On an *a priori* basis, there appear to be adequate reasons for expecting substantial differentials between the health level of the poor and that of the rest of the population. It follows from the fact that good health is a universal value, usually desired by all, except perhaps a small number of deviant individuals. However, the supply of health services, which are usually assumed by definition and regardless of their form to be the most direct means for the attainment of health, is finite, and therefore available only in limited degree to the entire population. Since this is the case, the means for the attainment of health may be thought of, in the terminology of economics, as a scarce good. In any society, whatever the prevailing system of social stratification, the scarce goods of life are likely to be distributed unequally. As a result, the upper strata of the society, however defined, will in all likelihood have the power and means to obtain a larger share of the total than their sheer numbers would warrant, while the lower strata are likely to be able to obtain far less than their "fair" proportion.

This situation results in better health for the more affluent only to the extent that health services actually do provide better health for their recipients. The extent to which this has been the case in the past is unknown. Even at present, there are far too many lacunae in medical knowledge to assume that anything approaching complete control of an individual's health is possible. There are still too many unknowns in the etiology and/or therapy of some illnesses and causes of death. In some instances, even if all etiological factors of all illness conditions were known and therapy were available for all of these, complete control might still be impossible, since massive changes in the customary behavior patterns of the population might have to take place. The current impasse in the smoking-lung cancer problem is only one, albeit very dramatic, instance of this. Although good health is surely a universal value, evidently our attachment to this value is not strong enough to orient all of our behavior, at the expense of alternative satisfactions, toward the attainment of perfect health.

Actually, there appears to be very little question that poverty and ill health have been closely related, certainly in our immediate past. This has been especially true for the major communicable diseases—the leading causes of death until very recently in human history and possibly through the first quarter of this century in the United States. Pond has recently reviewed some of this literature:

> Historically, the healthiest nations have been those with the highest incomes and the lowest illiteracy rates. At the beginning of this century life expectancy at birth was greater in the United States, Great Britain, and the Scandinavian countries than it is today in many parts of the world . . .

Throughout history communicable diseases have struck most severely among the poor. Even today, it is the serious communicable diseases that present the greatest threats to the health of people in underdeveloped lands. Many diseases that are virtually unknown or non-existent in the United States and other economically favored nations are the main causes of death and disability among large population groups elsewhere on the globe.[2]

Typhoid fever and tuberculosis are obvious cases in point, but the same is true also for the communicable diseases of childhood, gastrointestinal diseases, leprosy and plague, smallpox, typhus and other louse-borne diseases, and syphilis.[3]

During the periods when the communicable diseases were the major causes of death, they must also have been the major causes of morbidity and impairments, and therefore also of disability. If this is indeed the case (and there seems to be little reason to doubt it), then the poor, most affected by these diseases, must have been less healthy than the well-to-do along the entire measurable spectrum of ill health, i.e., along each of its measurable dimensions. The main health problems of the entire population of each community must have been public health problems of the traditional kind—poor sanitation, water supplies, and so on. It seems reasonable to suppose that the well-to-do populations must have been able, at least in some degree, to counteract their poor sanitary environments, for example, by better nutrition, better access to medical care, less crowded housing, and better working conditions.

What was described above is clearly still true in large parts of the world, especially where public health facilities remain inadequate, where water supplies are contaminated, or food impure. But it is probably also still true even where traditional public health services are relatively adequate, for example, in the slums of large cities in this country. Here the symbiotic relationship between poverty and ill health continues to exist. Mortality rates, particularly during infancy, childhood, and even the younger adult years, appear to be higher here than for the rest of the population, especially from the communicable diseases. Morbidity, impairments, and disability must also be more prevalent here than in the surrounding communities. The same is likely to be true for other pockets of poverty in this country— the Deep South, Appalachia, Indian reservations. By and large, whatever the public health situation of these populations may be, they surely do not have access equal to that of the rest of the population for adequate personal health services, nor do they have adequate nutrition and housing. Cultural factors and knowledge of how to use these services are all relevant in this context. The lower level of use of primary health services is perhaps most clearly evident in the area of dental care, possibly the most neglected aspect of health.

During the second quarter of this century the major communicable diseases declined as leading causes of death in this country, to be replaced by the "degenerative" diseases—heart disease, cancer, and stroke—and accidents. Medical advances, especially development of the antibiotics, and the improving social conditions of the general population have surely played a major role in this transformation. In contrast to the communicable diseases, which take their major toll of life during the younger years, heart disease, cancer, and stroke are largely associated with the aging process and take their major tolls at the later years. What is most important, however, is that by and large the burden of these conditions, as expressed in excess mortality, apparently does not now fall much more heavily, if at all, on the poor than on the rich, although this was surely the case some years ago, before antibiotics. There are some specific exceptions to this relationship, especially among various components of the broader disease categories, e.g., cervical cancer, cancer of the digestive system, infectious diseases of the heart, but it appears to be generally true of the broad disease categories.

As a partial explanation of these statements, which seemingly fly in the face of common sense, some of the newer and more important forms of ill health may to some degree be an actual concomitant of the degree of affluence which is today characteristic of the upper middle and upper strata in the United States. These strata, perhaps in recalling past deprivations, whether real or imagined, or for other reasons, may overcompensate in their drive to achieve high status. High status, in turn, so often involves sedentary (executive and white collar) occupations, mechanized transportation (two cars and now perhaps even three in every garage), and richer foods. The unintended consequences of the affluence achieved by these strata may well include obesity, excessive strains and tensions, excessive cigarette smoking and, resulting from these, perhaps ultimately premature death from coronary artery and arteriosclerotic heart disease, from cancer, or stroke. Males aged 45–64, especially white ones, appear to be particularly vulnerable to coronary artery disease and respiratory cancer. Women among the middle and upper strata, on the other hand, appear to be less affected by these affluence-related forms of ill health than men, possibly because of innate resistance, for example to coronary artery disease and lung cancer; because social pressures upon them are greater to avoid obesity and take better care of their health generally; because they may lead generally less stressful lives, or perhaps because of some combination of all of these factors.

During infancy and the younger years, however, while differentials in mortality among the various socio-economic strata of the nonpoverty population have probably narrowed, those between the poverty and nonpoverty populations have remained substantial, despite the decline in absolute mortality rates for both groups. For example, Robert M. Woodbury, studying infant mortality during the period 1911–1916 in seven cities in this country, found that infants born to families with an annual income of $1,250 or over had an almost three times better chance to survive their first birthday than infants in families with annual income of less than $450; the infant mortality rates were 59 and 167 per 1,000 respectively.[4] While these rates are not nearly as high today for either group, the comparative ratio between the two groups continues to be substantial, although not as great as formerly. The sharpest contrasts today in infant mortality and in mortality during childhood and the younger years are probably between the nonwhite population, in both the Deep South and the large-city poverty areas, and the white nonpoverty population, especially its more affluent strata.

The differentials in morbidity, impairments, and disability between poverty and nonpoverty populations, apparently quite clear and well defined during the communicable disease era, are probably considerably less clear today if both relatively severe and relatively minor conditions are considered separately. Thus they continue to exist for the relatively severe conditions, particularly chronic conditions, causing some form of activity restriction over a long period of time. These conditions are most prevalent during the later years of mid-life and old age. Very likely the poverty population experiences more severe illness to begin with, or is much more vulnerable to it when it does appear. But even if this were not the case, if they experienced only the same amount of illness and degree of vulnerability as everyone else, their illnesses are much more likely to remain untreated and ultimately to result, at least for some conditions, in higher mortality among them. It seems reasonable to expect that the traditional poverty-nonpoverty differentials for severe illness still exist today, although possibly the comparative ratios may not be as high as in former years.

For minor illness, however, especially for conditions which by their nature are self-limiting and do not result in mortality, the situation may be considerably different. Considering the entire

United States population as a whole and with no distinction between rich and poor, there appears to be relatively more minor illnesses today than in former years, at least as reported in household interviews. This was one of the principal findings that emerged from an earlier study of acute disabling illness by Lerner and Anderson.[5] For serious acute illnesses, on the other hand, that study found that there had been a substantial decline in prevalence since earlier in the century, especially for the communicable illnesses serious enough to be reportable to the U. S. Public Health Service. As part of the general decline in the major communicable diseases, the proportion of many of these illnesses terminating in death (their case-fatality rates) had declined sharply.

The Lerner and Anderson study also compared early data (July 1958—June 1959) on the prevalence of acute disabling conditions derived from the household interviews by the U. S. National Health Survey with combined data from five separate periodic-visit household enumerations of illness between 1938 and 1943. According to this comparison, the prevalence of acute disabling conditions in this country had risen substantially— better than a 200 percent increase—from the earlier to later surveys, during the period of approximately a generation. As a counteracting tendency the average duration of each illness had declined sharply, by almost 50 percent. Thus many more disabling conditions of relatively short duration were being reported in household enumerations of illness. Was this a "real" increase, or merely an artifact of better data-gathering techniques and improved survey procedures? The suspicion that it may have been real was in some degree strengthened by data on illness among industrial employees, which showed that their annual rate of illness cases disabling for one day or longer was substantially higher in 1952 (when the series was terminated) than during the 1930's.[6]

It is difficult to accept and explain the notion that there may have been a real increase in the volume of minor illness in this country over the last generation. The following hypotheses are offered tentatively. If in fact the increase uncovered in that study was real, it may have resulted from a whole complex of changing social conditions and structural features of our society. For example, more liberal policies regarding "sick leave" than in former years, the growth of insurance against medical costs and loss of income due to illness, the relatively full employment since World War II—all of these may have reduced the economic and social penalties for short absences from employment or other restrictions on usual activities. The average person is better educated, more sophisticated about the uses of medical care, and probably far more aware today than in former years of the need to acknowledge and seek treatment for even minor cases of illness which might have been ignored in the past. Finally, the increased use of physicians' services and the increase in hospital admissions, along with shorter stays, may both indicate a larger volume of illness, at least as defined in terms of people's awareness of illness and perceptions of their need for services. All these factors, and others not specified here, may add up to a real increase in the volume of illness, but especially of those relatively minor conditions which are self-limiting.

The assumption that the increase is real was further strengthened by the data from the above study on "condition group" (diagnostic condition) of illness. Thus the largest increases from the earlier to the later surveys were for the upper respiratory conditions (common cold, acute sinusitis, pharyngitis, tonsillitis, laryngitis, and tracheitis). These conditions increased in prevalence by over 500 percent and accounted for almost 40 percent of all illness conditions in the National Health Survey data. Large increases were also registered for lower respiratory conditions (influenza and grippe, bronchitis, pneumonia, pleurisy), and for accidental injuries. In the more recent of the two surveys data, about 60 percent consisted of fractures, dislocations, sprains, strains, contusions, and superficial injuries. The infectious-parasitic condition group also increased, but again the increases were confined to the relatively minor conditions in this group. Smallpox, pertussis, typhoid fever, diphtheria, scarlet fever, malaria, undulant fever, and some others—the more serious of the conditions in this group—actually declined sharply. The average duration of illness declined for each of the major condition groups enumerated in these surveys.

These increases in relatively minor illnesses are real, for the reasons enumerated earlier. But also, the major changes specified here have taken place primarily in the relatively affluent middle classes, or at least in the nonpoverty population. The middle classes are least likely to encounter social and economic penalties for any relatively short excursion into the sick role. In general, the middle classes tend to work in more protected jobs than the poverty population, are more likely to be better educated, more sophisticated about the uses of medical care, and more aware of the need to seek treatment for even minor cases of illness than the poverty population. As a result, this group is likely to report more relatively minor illness than the poverty population, although the latter is likely to report more relatively severe illness. Since the statistics on illness do not usually distinguish adequately enough for this purpose between minor and severe illness, the resulting picture is likely to be confusing to the observer.

DIFFERENTIALS IN MORTALITY

Mortality in this country, as elsewhere throughout the western world, has declined substantially during the twentieth century. This is true regardless of whether crude or age-adjusted mortality rates are used to measure the decline, and it appears to be true for both the total population of the country and for each of its major segments. However, a levelling off began to take place prior to 1954 in the downward trend of the crude rate for the total population, and since that time this rate has more or less rested on a plateau. Thus the crude mortality rate for the total population of this country dropped from 17.2 per 1,000 population in 1900 to 9.2 in 1954, but the rate rose to 9.5 in 1960 and in 1966.* While the severe influenza epidemic of 1918–1919 caused the mortality rate to rise sharply, the rise was only temporary. The mortality rate fell at a particularly rapid rate after 1939, largely in response to the introduction of new medications (sulfas, antibiotics) and other life-extending medical advances.

The crude mortality rate of a population is clearly inadequate in most instances for comparing the mortality experiences of one population with that of another or of the same population at different points in time. This is primarily so because mortality is a function of age, and age-compositions vary substantially among populations. Therefore, it is customary to compare populations in terms of age-adjusted mortality rates, and this is usually done by using the 1940 population of the United States as the standard to which adjustment is made. The change in the age-composition of the United States population between 1900 and the present was generally in the direction of an increase in the high-risk groups at the expense of the low; thus the age-adjusted death rates prior to 1940 were much higher than the crude rates, while since that time age-adjusted rates have been much lower. The decline in age-adjusted death rates from 1900 to the

* The rate for 1900 was based on data from the "death-registration states" only (ten states and the District of Columbia in that year). However, for comparison purposes this rate is customarily taken to represent that of the entire country. The rate for 1966 is provisional, based on a 10 percent sample of death certificates received each month. See U.S. National Center for Health Statistics, "Births, Deaths, Marriages, and Divorces, Annual Summary for the United States, 1966," *Monthly Vital Statistics Reports: Provisional Statistics,* vol. 15, no. 13 (July 26, 1967).

present was therefore much sharper than the comparable decline in crude rates; however, there has been little or no decline in age-adjusted rates since 1960.*

Unfortunately for the present purpose, no mortality statistics have ever been collected specifically for the poverty population of the entire United States. Obtaining data for this population separately would require that death certificates contain the information necessary to classify the deceased in terms of at least some objective indices of socio-economic status, i.e., income, educational attainment, occupation during the major portion of their working life, size of family. An innovation of such major dimensions in the vital-statistics' record-keeping system on a nationwide basis is unlikely to occur, at least in the near future.† As a result of this inadequacy in our vital statistics, we do not know whether the poverty population in this country has shared equally with the rest of the population in the overall mortality decline since earlier in this century. Comparisons of the mortality experience of the poverty population with the mortality experience of the rest of the community must necessarily rely on the results of studies of limited populations. In the present instance, much of the discussion is based on a study of the mortality experience of poverty and nonpoverty populations in Chicago.[7] However, this is supplemented by a study of mortality contrasts in high and low-income states and a study of mortality in three geographic divisions.

* The discussion in this paragraph owes much to an earlier treatment of this subject. See Monroe Lerner and Odin W. Anderson, *Health Progress in the United States, 1900–1960* (Chicago: University of Chicago Press, 1963).

† Moriyama has pointed to the possibilities inherent in the matched records' technique, such as that used by the University of Chicago in the study of Social and Economic Differentials in Mortality in 1960, and in record linkage. See Iwao M. Moriyama, "Vital and Health Statistics of the Future," Milbank Memorial Fund Quarterly, 44 (July 1966), part 1, 318–321.

Table III–1. Selected measures of over-all mortality (all ages combined) and infant mortality by place of residence (poverty and nonpoverty areas) and race, Chicago, 1964.

Selected measures of over-all mortality and infant mortality	All races			White population			Nonwhite population		
	All places of residence	Poverty areas	Non-poverty areas	All places of residence	Poverty areas	Non-poverty areas	All places of residence	Poverty areas	Non-poverty areas
	1	2	3	4	5	6	7	8	9
Over-all mortality (all ages combined) rates per 1,000 population									
All causes of death	11.9	12.1	11.8	12.6	14.0	12.2	10.0	10.7	7.4
By cause									
Heart disease	4.6	4.4	4.7	5.1	5.7	4.9	3.1	3.3	2.4
Cancer, all sites	1.7	1.5	1.8	1.8	1.7	1.9	1.3	1.3	1.0
Cancer, by site (rate per 100,000 population)									
Colon	19.4	15.9	21.2	21.2	20.4	22.4	12.7	12.0	12.6
Breast	16.0	11.1	18.7	17.8	11.2	20.3	9.7	10.5	3.8
Cervix	4.4	6.6	3.2	3.6	5.3	3.0	7.3	7.2	6.0
Infant mortality rates per 1,000 live births									
All causes of death									
Entire year of infancy	30.0	38.5	22.2	22.2	25.1	21.3	43.0	45.5	29.6
Neonatal period	21.1	25.6	17.0	16.6	17.3	16.4	28.7	29.9	22.0
Post-neonatal period	8.9	12.9	5.2	5.6	7.8	4.9	14.3	15.6	7.6

Table III-1. (*Continued*)

Selected measures of over-all and infant mortality	All races			White population			Nonwhite population		
	1 All places of residence	2 Poverty areas	3 Non-poverty areas	4 All places of residence	5 Poverty areas	6 Non-poverty areas	7 All places of residence	8 Poverty areas	9 Non-poverty areas
Entire year, by cause									
Influenza and pneumonia	5.0	7.9	2.2	2.6	4.4	1.9	8.9	9.8	4.4
Congenital malformations	1.1	1.3	1.0	0.9	0.6	1.1	1.5	1.6	1.1
Gastroenteritis, colitis	—[a]	1.3	—[a]	—[a]	0.6	—[a]	—[a]	1.6	—[a]

Source: Chicago Board of Health, Planning Staff of the Health Planning Project, *A Report on Health and Medical Care in Poverty Areas of Chicago and Proposals for Improvement* (Chicago: Board of Health, 1965), p. 24–25.

[a] Less than 0.05 per 1,000.

Differentials in the Chicago Poverty Study

One study used an earlier division of Chicago into poverty and nonpoverty areas by the Chicago Committee on Urban Opportunity as the basis for analyses. It defined poverty as the concentration of populations with the following characteristics within specific areas of the city: low income, low education, poor housing, large proportions of the population on public assistance, and high unemployment and juvenile delinquency rates. On the basis of this definition, Chicago's 75 community areas were divided into 24 poverty and 51 nonpoverty areas. The residents of the poverty areas were, on the average, considerably younger than the nonpoverty population, and about one half were non-white.

Since the younger population resided in Chicago's poverty areas, it would be expected that, if poverty made no difference and if the age-specific or "real" mortality experience of these two groups were identical, the crude mortality rate in the poverty areas should be much lower than the comparable rate in the nonpoverty areas. This proved not to be the case. The overall crude mortality rate in the poverty areas (12.1 per 1,000 population) was actually slightly higher (by less than 3 percent) than the comparable rate of 11.8 in the nonpoverty areas (see columns 2 and 3 of Table III–1). If it had been possible to compute age-adjusted mortality rates for this study and compare the "real" mortality experience of these two groups, a substantial differential would have been found, with rates much higher among the poverty population. The conclusion is, on the basis of these data, that poverty does make a difference in the risk of mortality.

This contrast in over-all mortality rates between the poverty and nonpoverty areas is confirmed and made more evident in the age-adjusted mortality data for 1960 available from the *Chicago Local Community Fact Book* and adapted for present purposes.[8]

The data are expressed in terms of the standardized mortality ratio, a measure of the extent to which the age-adjusted mortality rate for community areas exceeds or is less than the comparable rate for the city as a whole. According to these data, the age-adjusted mortality rate in the poverty areas exceeded the comparable rate for the entire city of Chicago by about 23 percent, while the same mortality rate in the nonpoverty areas was less than the comparable rate for the entire city by about 12 percent. To put it in other terms, the age-adjusted mortality rate in the poverty areas exceeded that in the nonpoverty areas by about 40 percent.

The effect of differences in age-composition are evident also when comparing the white and the nonwhite population of the city. The crude mortality rate for the white population (12.6) exceeds that for the nonwhite (10.0) by about one fourth. Again the implication is clear that age-adjusted mortality rates would have shown an entirely different picture. Finally, when race is held constant (and this holds some proportion of the age differences constant also), the effect on mortality of residence in the poverty areas is seen. The crude mortality rate for the white population was 14.0 in the poverty areas as against 12.2 in the nonpoverty areas, an excess of 15 percent in the poverty areas, while for the nonwhite population the comparable rates were 10.7 and 7.4, respectively, an excess of almost 50 percent in the poverty areas. Again, these differences would clearly have been of much greater magnitude if age-adjusted rates had been used.

Table 1 also shows data on mortality rates from heart disease and cancer, the two major causes of death which had rates of at least 0.05 per 1,000 population. Both of these causes are strongly associated with the aging process. Because of the older average age of the nonpoverty population compared to the residents of the poverty areas, and of the white population compared to the nonwhite, the mortality rates from heart disease and from cancer (all sites) were found to be higher for the nonpoverty population and for the white population than for their opposite numbers. The mortality rate from diseases of the heart in the nonpoverty areas, 4.7 per 1,000, exceeded the comparable rate in the poverty areas, 4.4, although only by a relatively slight margin (about 6 percent). The comparable figures for the mortality rates from cancer of all sites were 1.8 and 1.5 per 1,000, respectively. The very narrowness of these differentials, despite the wide differences in age-composition of the two populations, suggests that the influence of poverty on the population residing in the poverty areas raises the mortality rates from these causes of death far above where they would otherwise be. Thus the nonwhite population residing in poverty areas had substantially higher mortality rates than that residing in nonpoverty areas. The same relationships held for the white population, at least for heart disease; but for mortality from cancer of all sites, the white population residing in nonpoverty areas had somewhat higher rates.

Particular interest attaches to the mortality from cancer of three specific sites: the colon, breast, and cervix because, in the opinion of authorities, a large proportion of deaths from cancer of these sites is preventable through the proper application of modern medical knowledge. However, mortality rates from cancer of these sites was relatively high among all four population groups considered here. Only for cancer of the cervix was the mortality rate for the poverty population (6.6 per 100,000) clearly and substantially higher than the comparable rate for the nonpoverty population (3.2 per 100,000), and the rate for the nonwhite population (7.3) clearly and substantially higher than that for the white population (3.6). For cancer of the colon and the breast, the higher average age of the white population and of the nonpoverty population than of the nonwhite and poverty populations could have resulted in higher mortality rates among the former and therefore makes the evaluation difficult. An excess risk comparable to that for cancer of the cervix, however, was clearly not demonstrated.

Restricting the mortality rates shown in Table III–1 only to data for the two major causes of death, heart disease and cancer, obscures the importance of the communicable diseases as major health problems in the poverty areas of Chicago. Andelman has recently pointed out the magnitude of tuberculosis as a problem in that city:

National rates and statistics in the field of tuberculosis are frequently most misleading . . . It is recognized that health statistics must of necessity be collected and reported on governmental subdivisions because the state, county and city health departments are the reporting agencies. However, in every one of these reporting units we must analyze the data carefully to understand the significance of each local situation.

The national new TB case rate is about 29 per 100,000 persons per year. For the purpose of illustration let us say that in a specific state that same rate may be 37. On that basis it may appear that tuberculosis is not too serious in that state. Then, let us look at the figures for a large city in that state. We find that the new case rate in that city is 75 per 100,000 persons per year. We will see that other cities have even higher new case rates, so rationalize that this 75 is only two-and-a-half times the national average and only twice that for the state . . .

Now we look at the new case rate of 75 in the city under consideration and learn that in some parts of the city there are no new cases or only one or two a year, while in some community areas there is a new TB case rate anywhere from 150 to 200 per 100,000 per year. This analysis points up the real tuberculosis situation in the city. It shows that there are well-defined pockets of tuberculosis in the city. This condition prevails in nearly every big city in the nation.[9]

MORTALITY IN HIGH- AND LOW-INCOME STATES AND GEOGRAPHIC DIVISIONS

It may be useful, for purposes of the present discussion, to supplement the data available from the Chicago study with those available from a study of the convergences and contrasts in mortality between high- and low-income states in this country. The latter study compared the mortality patterns of the ten states (including the District of Columbia and excluding Hawaii and Alaska) ranking highest in average per capita personal incomes with the ten lowest states during 1930, 1940, 1950, and 1957.[10] The composition of these groups of states varied somewhat over the years, but in general the high-income group consisted largely of the most industrialized and urbanized states, especially those in the Northeast and including some in the Middle and Far West. In contrast, the low-income states were generally but not exclusively in the South, rural in character and with large non-white populations. The range between these groups of states in average per capita income narrowed between 1930 and 1957, as did the differentials in some of the health facilities available to their respective populations.

The generally superior health facilities available to the population residing in the high-income states were reflected in lower mortality rates only to a relatively small extent even in 1930, but this differential has actually declined since then. Thus in 1930 the age-adjusted mortality rates of the low-income states exceeded the comparable rates in the high-income states by 13 percent, but by 1940 this margin had dropped to 7 percent, to 5 percent in 1950, and to less than one percent in 1957. However, the trends and differentials in mortality rates between these two groups of states varied sharply in accordance with the age of their populations. Thus in 1930 mortality rates had been substantially higher in the low-income states at ages under 45, and especially during childhood and infancy; by 1957, although these differentials were much reduced, they were nevertheless still substantial. At ages 45–64, mortality rates had been somewhat higher in the low-income states in 1930; by 1957 there was almost no difference. Finally, at ages 65 and over, relatively little difference in mortality rates between the two groups of states had existed in 1930; however, by 1957 the low-income states were favored with a substantially lower mortality rate.

The changing relationship of mortality in the low- and high-income states has resulted largely from the general decline of the major communicable diseases (influenza and pneumonia, tuberculosis, gastritis, and other major infectious diseases of the gastro-intestinal system, the major communicable diseases of childhood, and certain diseases of early infancy) as leading causes of death. These diseases were primarily responsible during the early years of this century for the higher mortality rates prevailing in the low-income states; in later years they were replaced as leading causes of death by heart disease, cancer, and stroke. The latter conditions, strongly associated with the aging process, were generally far more prevalent in the high-income states. Because of these trends, the rates for the leading causes of death converged in the two groups of states.

A parallel convergence in mortality from some of the leading specific causes of death accompanied this convergence in the over-all mortality rate. Thus the mortality rate from diseases of the heart in 1930 was only 71 percent as high in the low-income states as the comparable figure among the well-to-do states; by 1957, however, this percentage had risen to 86. The comparable mortality from cancer rose from 59 to 77 percent; mortality from *diabetes mellitus* rose from 57 to 80 percent; and for suicide the percentage went from 59 to 91.

Another study compared mortality rates in three geographic divisions of the United States—the heavily urbanized Middle Atlantic states (New York, New Jersey, and Pennsylvania); the relatively prosperous and rural West North Central states (Minnesota, Iowa, Missouri, North and South Dakota, Nebraska, and Kansas); and the relatively poor and rural East South Central states (Kentucky, Tennessee, Alabama, and Mississippi).[11] Between 1940 and 1959 age-adjusted over-all mortality rates converged among these three groups of states; nevertheless, in 1959 the relatively well-to-do midwestern rural states still had the lowest mortality rates, while the heavily industrialized and urbanized northeastern states had the highest mortality rates. Mortality rates in the East South Central states were close to those of the Middle Atlantic.

In general, the relatively well-to-do rural midwestern states had not only the lowest over-all mortality rates, but their experience was uniformly favorable at all ages and from the leading causes of death. Thus in 1950 (the latest year for which these data were available at the time of the study), they had the lowest mortality rates not only from the major communicable diseases (e.g., influenza and pneumonia, tuberculosis, major communicable diseases of childhood, certain diseases of early infancy) generally most prevalent at the younger ages, but also from the so-called degenerative diseases associated with the aging process (heart disease, cancer, stroke). These states consisted largely of well-to-do rural populations, with relatively small proportion of poverty populations.

The relatively poor, rural southern states, on the other hand, had the highest mortality rates at ages under 45, and especially during infancy and childhood. Their mortality rates were highest at all ages from the major communicable diseases and from accidents. However, their mortality rates among the population aged 65 and over and their over-all age-adjusted mortality rates from heart disease, cancer, and stroke were not as high as the comparable rates in the Middle Atlantic states. Their mortality patterns for the entire geographic division were characteristic of rural poverty populations. Although these patterns tend to be similar in most respects to those of urban poverty populations, the latter constitute only part of the total population in the Middle Atlantic states, so that the over-all mortaliy patterns within the two divisions accordingly differed somewhat.

Finally, the heavily urbanized and industrialized Middle Atlantic states had the highest mortality rates at the middle and upper ages, especially from heart disease, cancer, and stroke. Their mortality from accidents was lowest among the three groups of states. And because large poverty populations resided in these states, even as far back as 1950, their mortality from influenza, pneumonia, and tuberculosis was substantially higher than in the West North Central states, i.e., the relatively well-to-do midwestern states.

The Problem of Infant Mortality

Perhaps the most sensitive single index of health conditions within a community is the infant mortality rate (deaths of children under one year of age per 1,000 live births). This rate has traditionally been widely used to classify communities or populations in terms of their over-all levels of health, particularly where morbidity data have not been available. Further, the infant mortality rate has generally been used as an indicator of the level of social and economic well-being within a country. This has been so, according to Stockwell, because "in the past, the decline in infant mortality was so marked as soon as a nation began to undergo economic development that the infant mortality rate began to be looked upon as the most sensitive index of level of living and sanitary conditions that we possessed. As such, it was often used as a means of comparing the relative levels of social and economic well-being characterizing different countries.

Since infant mortality was such an extremely sensitive index of economic differences among countries, one would logically expect it to have been equally sensitive to economic differences that existed among different segments of the population within a single country, and so it was." [12]

However, some question about its usefulness for either of these purposes has arisen in recent years, because the formerly sharp relationship between socio-economic status and infant mortality rates apparently began to blur. Thus Willie, who studied this relationship in Syracuse, New York, for 1950 concluded:

> Under the conditions of this study, little association was demonstrated between infant mortality rates and the socio-economic status level of ecological areas in Syracuse, N. Y. Family income was significantly associated with both distributions of neonatal and post-neonatal mortality rates while the socio-economic status index consisting of occupation, education, and housing variables was significantly associated with post-neonatal mortality rates only. These associations were negative. In all instances, however, family income or socio-economic status factors accounted for less than 15 percent of the variance in the ecological distribution of neonatal or post-neonatal mortality rates. The fact that sectors of high and low rates were found in all socio-economic areas and that variations in rates by socio-economic areas were not statistically significant cast further doubt upon the hypothesis that socio-economic status factors are primarily associated with the ecological distribution of neonatal or post-neonatal mortality in Syracuse today as in years gone by.

It was further suggested that if this relationship no longer held for Syracuse, it might also no longer exist elsewhere, and that perhaps our theories should be revised:

Scientific theories must be revised and updated with changes in the social order. When the inverse relationship between socio-economic status and infant mortality was first discovered, unsanitary conditions prevailed in many cities. Today these conditions have changed and it is timely to determine if there has also been a change in the association between infant mortality and socio-economic status. In scientific knowledge as in other dimensions of the social order cultural lags may exist.[13]

Stockwell's study of infant mortality in Providence, Rhode Island, during 1949–1951 also suggested the need for a revision of some of our long-held concepts:

It is apparent that, at least in one city, infant mortality is no longer the extremely sensitive index of differences in socio-economic status that it was in the past. The erratic pattern that was observed when total infant mortality was related to socio-economic status was found to be a reflection of the fact that the majority of the deaths under one year of age today occur during the first few hours or days of life, and are due to causes that are associated with biological rather than socio-economic factors. On the other hand, for those few deaths that take place between the ages of one month and one year, where the major causes of death are farther removed from the physiological processes of gestation and birth, infant mortality continues to be inversely related to differences in socio-economic status.

. . . We might now be at a point where it is time to reconsider the assumption pertaining to the infant mortality rate being the most sensitive index we possess of the level of social and economic well-being characterizing a given population group. Although this may still be true on an international level, the evidence . . . indicates that it is apparently no longer true in modern urban-industrial society—certainly not true to the extent that it was in the past.[14]

Both studies were based on the experience of relatively small and homogeneous northern cities where nonwhites constituted only a small proportion of the total population. Thus according to the U.S. Census, nonwhites made up 3.5 percent of the total population of the city of Providence and only 2.3 percent of the city of Syracuse. The disparities in social and economic levels among the populations of the various ecological areas in these cities may not have been very great, certainly not of the magnitude of those in New York or Chicago, and obviously not large enough to be associated with significant differentials in infant mortality. In short, these two cities may not have had the enormous pockets of utter poverty that we now see in our large metropolitan areas. But even in 1950, and despite the studies of Willie and Stockwell, substantial differentials in infant mortality were very much in evidence between the white and nonwhite populations among the states and within the very large cities and metropolitan areas, and they continue to be very much in evidence today. It is, in fact, quite possible that at least the differentials within the large cities may have widened since that time, partly because of the continuing influx of migrants from southern rural and mountain areas. In any case, the differentials certainly do exist today, and infant mortality rates should continue to be used as an index both of general health levels and of levels of living.

DIFFERENTIALS IN INFANT MORTALITY

In Chicago in 1964, according to the data of the Chicago poverty study shown in the lower tier of Table III–1, the differential in infant mortality between the populations residing in the poverty and nonpoverty areas was substantial. For example, the infant mortality rate for the population residing within the poverty areas, 38.5 per 1,000, was about 75 percent higher than the comparable rate of 22.2 within the nonpoverty areas. Moreover, the differential by racial group was also substantial. Thus considering the population of the city as a whole, the infant mortality rate of the nonwhite population was almost double that of the white, 43.0 and 22.2, respectively. The same relationship—higher infant mortality rates among the nonwhite population than among the white—was evident in both poverty and nonpoverty areas. For example, the nonwhite infant mortality rate of 29.6 in all nonpoverty areas exceeded the comparable rate of 21.3 for white persons residing in these areas by about 40 percent. For residents of the poverty areas, the comparable rates were 45.5 and 25.1, an excess in nonwhite infant mortality over white of about 80 percent. Thus, to judge by these figures, the impact of race alone, at least for infant mortality, was greater on the residents of the poverty areas. The disabilities which are usually associated in our society with membership in a minority group—discrimination, inability to obtain access to adequate medical care, and so on—fell most heavily on the nonwhites residing in the poverty areas.

Racial group membership alone did not account for the differentials in the infant mortality rate within Chicago because, even with each racial group considered separately, there was still a substantial differential between those in the poverty areas and those in the nonpoverty areas. Thus the infant mortality rate of the nonwhite population residing in all poverty areas combined was over 50 percent higher than the comparable rate of the nonwhite population residing in the nonpoverty areas; for the white population, however, the comparable excess was only about 18 percent. These figures indicate that the association of high infant mortality with residence in poverty areas, although by no means negligible for the white population, was far greater for the nonwhite population. In short, the nonwhite population residing in poverty areas experienced the disability associated with both major social disadvantages—minority group membership and residence in the poverty areas—and as a result had by far the highest infant mortality rate of the four population groups considered here.

Even though infant mortality rate is a sensitive indicator of health levels, the post-neonatal mortality rate (deaths of infants who have survived their first month of life per 1,000 live births) is perhaps even more sensitive. This measure eliminates from consideration the large number of deaths of new-born babies, some proportion of which results from biological factors whose control is either extremely difficult or impossible in the present state of medical science. Such deaths occur apparently in almost equal degree among babies born to mothers of all social classes; that is, they appear to be largely independent of social and economic status.

The post-neonatal mortality rate for the entire population of Chicago in 1964 was 8.9 per 1,000 live births. Post-neonatal deaths thus accounted for about 30 percent of all infant deaths. As expected, the rate for residents of the poverty areas, 12.9 per 1,000, was more than double the comparable rate of 5.2 for residents of the nonpoverty areas. Similarly, considering the experience of residents of poverty and nonpoverty areas combined, the rate for the nonwhite population, 14.3 per 1,000 live births, was two and a half times the comparable rate for the white population, 5.6. The highest rate among the four population groups was again that for the nonwhite population residing in the poverty areas, 15.6; this rate was double that of the white population residing in poverty areas (7.8) and just over double that of the nonwhite population residing in the nonpoverty areas (7.6); it was over three times as great as that of the white population residing in nonpoverty areas (4.9).

Among the major causes of infant death, the combined disease category of influenza and pneumonia played a leading role in all segments of the population. This category accounted for 5.0 infant deaths per 1,000 live births in the city as a whole. However, as a clear indication of the extent to which mortality from influenza and pneumonia reflected social and economic conditions, the comparable mortality rates from this cause in the poverty and nonpoverty areas were 7.9 and 2.2, respectively, while for the nonwhite and white populations in the city as a whole they were 8.9 and 2.6. These are substantial differences. Even more substantial is the fact that the infant mortality rate from this cause was more than five times as high for the nonwhite population in the poverty areas as for the white population in the nonpoverty areas. Influenza and pneumonia accounted for over 20 percent of all infant deaths among the nonwhite population in the poverty areas, against less than 10 percent of all infant deaths among the white population in the nonpoverty areas.

Congenital malformations as a cause of infant death also reflected differences in social and economic conditions in the city, but not nearly to the same extent. The rate in the poverty areas was 1.3 infant deaths from this cause per 1,000 live births, compared to 1.0 in the nonpoverty areas. Similarly, the infant mortality rate from this condition was 1.5 for the nonwhite population, compared to 0.9 for the white population. Somewhat surprisingly, the infant mortality rate from this condition was among the white population higher in the nonpoverty than in the poverty areas. Finally, gastroenteritis and colitis as a cause of infant deaths is shown in the table only for the poverty areas because the rate in the nonpoverty areas was less than 0.05 per 1,000. In the poverty areas the nonwhite rate, as expected, was considerably higher than the comparable rate for the white population.

The relationships between poverty and infant mortality found in the Chicago poverty study correspond generally to those between racial group membership and infant mortality found in a study of the health experience of the ten largest cities in this country during 1962.[15] While the nonwhite and poverty populations in this country do not coincide, they overlap a good deal, and the analysis in the following pages is offered as suggestive rather than definitive.

As the data in Table III–2 show, the nonwhite population of the ten largest cities experienced an infant mortality rate of 39 per 1,000 live births compared to 23 per 1,000 for the white population, an excess of 67 percent. (As reported earlier, the comparable figures in Chicago during 1964 were 38.5 per 1,000 for the poverty population and 22.2 for the nonpoverty, an excess of 73 percent, and 43.0 for the nonwhite population compared to 22.2 for the white, an excess of 94 percent.) The comparable ratio of nonwhite to white infant mortality rates was larger among the deaths due to factors presumed to be of postnatal origin (an excess of 104 percent) than among those due to prenatal or natal origin (an excess of 49 percent). The general direction of this relationship was similar to that found in Chicago.

Table III–2. Infant mortality by cause, 1962, in ten largest cities (according to 1960 U.S. Census).[a]

Cause category [b]	Category number [b]	Deaths under 1 year per 10,000 live births		
		White	Non-white	Percent excess of nonwhite
All causes	—	230.8	386.0	67.2
Prenatal and natal	—	154.6	230.4	49.0
Immaturity and certain other prenatal and natal causes	769,774,776	44.0	87.8	99.5
Postnatal asphyxia and atelectasis	762	48.9	81.4	66.5
Congenital malformations	750–759	36.0	31.8	−11.7

Table III–2. (*Continued*)

Cause category [b]	Category number [b]	Deaths under 1 year per 10,000 live births		
		White	Non-white	Percent excess of nonwhite
Birth injuries	760–761	18.8	25.7	36.7
Hemolytic disease of newborn (erythro-blastosis)	770–771	6.9	3.7	–46.4
Postnatal	—	76.2	155.6	104.2
Ill-defined, peculiar to early infancy	772–773	18.0	30.6	70.0
Influenza and pneu-monia (except newborn)	480–493	18.5	41.3	123.2
Certain infections	053,340, 470–475 500–527, 763–768	17.0	41.8	145.9
Disease of digestive system	530–587	7.8	11.7	50.0
Accidents	E800–E962	3.8	10.1	165.8
Other postnatal causes, including residual	—	8.2	10.8	31.7
Symptoms and ill-defined conditions	780–795	3.0	9.5	216.7

Source: Eleanor P. Hunt and Earl E. Huyck, "Mortality of White and Nonwhite Infants in Major U.S. Cities," *Health, Education, and Welfare Indicators* (January 1966), p. 15.

[a] Baltimore, Chicago, Cleveland, Detroit, Houston, Los Angeles, New York, Philadelphia, St. Louis, and Washington, D.C.

[b] According to the Seventh Revision of the International Statistical Classification of Diseases, Injuries, and Causes of Death, World Health Organization, 1955. Categories are listed in rank order according to United States rates, 1962, for corresponding categories.

Among the mortality factors of postnatal origin, the ratios were particularly high for accidents (166 percent), certain infections (146 percent), and influenza and pneumonia, except of the newborn (123 percent). Among the factors of prenatal and natal origin, the ratio was particularly high for immaturity and certain other prenatal and natal causes (almost 100 percent), and postnatal asphyxia and atelectasis (67 percent). The high ratios for the categories lacking in diagnostic content—symptoms and ill-defined conditions, and immaturity and certain other prenatal and natal causes—indicate, in the opinion of the authors of the study, a lower degree of completeness of reporting of causes of death for nonwhite infants. This incomplete reporting may also have been a partial factor in the lower rates for nonwhite than white infants of the somewhat more specific diagnostic categories "hemolytic disease of the newborn" and "congenital malformations."

DIFFERENTIALS IN MORBIDITY, DISABILITY, AND IMPAIRMENTS

In contrast to death, by its very nature a clearly defined event, morbidity and impairments, as well as the disabilities associated with these conditions, are often relatively nebulous categories, and therefore difficult to measure. They may be thought of as states of being which lie beyond a point on a continuum. Frequently of long duration, many separately identifiable states of impairment may coexist within the same individual at the same point in time; in some instances it may be very difficult, if not impossible, to classify these separately identifiable states along a hierarchy of importance. Because of the resulting difficulties of measurement and because death records, having important legal consequences, have to be carefully kept in any well-ordered society, the development of statistics on morbidity, disability, and impairments has generally lagged far behind the development of mortality statistics. This situation in the United States, due largely to the efforts of the U.S. National Center for Health

Statistics (NCHS), has improved greatly within recent years. For the first time we are now beginning to have some systematic data on these conditions.

Nevertheless, from the point of view of comparing the health levels of poverty and nonpoverty populations, the adequacy of morbidity data still leaves much to be desired. For example, in contrast to the relative availability of mortality statistics, we still have no series of data on morbidity, disability, or impairments by state or by any geographic area smaller than national. The few available data along these lines are fragmentary, scattered among different sources and in many instances collected on different bases. As a result, we cannot as yet directly analyze differentials in these conditions by state or within a state, and certainly not between poverty areas within a city.

Some data on morbidity and disability by family income are available from the National Health Survey of NCHS.[16] They are based on household surveys of the civilian noninstitutional population, and their degree of generalizability should be considered as limited. Furthermore they gloss over important differences which are germane to the present comparison, since they do not pinpoint the poverty population accurately. To do this, for example, family income needs to be related to such characteristics as size of family, place of residence (rural, urban, or suburban, and geographic areas), race, availability of health facilities and costs of services. These modifications were not made in the present data; nevertheless, they are by far the best data available.

Table III–3 presents one of the best-known tabulations of data demonstrating a reasonably clear inverse relationship between disability in its major forms and family income in the civilian noninstitutional population of the United States. As the top row of the table shows, days of restricted activity per person per year dropped from 22.4 among persons in families with incomes less than $2,000 to 14.1 at incomes of $10,000 or over. However, between those with family incomes under $2,000 and those over \$2,000—very roughly, a poverty cutoff—the break was fairly abrupt (22.4 and 17.7 days, respectively), while at the higher incomes an apparent leveling off occurred (14.3 days at \$7,000–\$9,000 and 14.1 at \$10,000 or over).

Similar relationships were evident for days of bed-disability: a decrease with rising income, a relatively abrupt break at the poverty cutoff, and a leveling off among the two higher income groups. For days lost from work, however, although the decrease with rising income and the leveling off were there, the break at the poverty cutoff was more gradual than for the other major forms of disability.

Table III–3. Days of disability per person per year by major form of disability and family income, United States, July 1963—June 1964.

		Family Income				
Major form of disability	All incomes (includes unknown incomes)	Under \$2,000	\$2,000– \$3,999	\$4,000– \$6,999	\$7,000– \$9,999	\$10,000 or over
Restricted Activity [a]	16.2	22.4	17.7	15.2	14.3	14.1
Bed disability [a]	6.0	8.1	6.6	5.9	5.5	5.6
Lost From Work [b]	5.5	8.2	7.1	6.0	4.4	4.2

Source: U.S. National Center for Health Statistics, "Disability Days, United States, July 1963–June 1964," Vital Statistics: Data from the National Health Survey, ser. 10, no. 24 (Washington, D.C.: U.S. Government Printing Office, November 1965), pp. 8, 29–33. Data are based on household interviews of the civilian noninstitutional population.

[a] All figures except those in "All incomes" have been adjusted to the age and sex distribution of the total civilian noninstitutional population of the United States.

[b] Per currently employed person per year. Persons aged 17 years and over. All figures except those in "All incomes" have been adjusted to the age and sex distribution of the currently employed population of the United States.

The above relationships are evident for the total population, i.e., all ages combined (actually, except for "all incomes," age-and-sex-adjusted rates were shown in the tabulation.) When, however, the data are examined by age, these relationships are not equally consistent. For example, the inverse relationship-decrease of disability days with rise in family income—seems to be most consistent among the three major forms of disability during the adult years, beginning with the 15–24 age group and ending at 65–74 (see Table III–4). For persons at ages under 5, 5–14, and 75 and over, at least for restricted-activity and bed-disability, the inverse relationship is either inconsistent or completely reversed. For days lost from work the relationship is consistent prior to the retirement age, but inconsistent for the 65-and-over population. Finally, the relationship is most inconsistent for days lost from school per school-age child per year.

Another well-known set of tabulations demonstrating a similar inverse relationship is presented in Table III–5, which shows the percentage of persons with one or more chronic conditions in the civilian noninstitutional population of the United States. The group of chronically ill is subdivided into persons with and persons without limitation of activity, and the former may be considered the more severely ill. The proportion of one or more chronic conditions among persons of all ages drops significantly with rising family income from 57.6 percent among those with family incomes under $2,000 to 42.9 percent at $7,000 or more (see the top tier of Table III–5). The same relationship is much more pronounced for relatively severe chronic illness (characterized by limitation of activity), with the comparable percentages dropping from 28.6 at less than $2,000 to 7.9 at $7,000 or more. However, the proportion of persons with one or more chronic conditions but without limitation of activity (the less severely ill), instead of dropping, actually rises with increasing family income from 29.0 percent to 35.0 percent. These patterns were consistent for all age groups (as the lower tier of the table shows) but the relative magnitudes of the differences were sig-

Table III–4. Days of disability per person per year by major form of
disability, family income, and age group, United States,
July 1963—June 1964.

Major form of disability and age-group (in years)	All incomes (includes unknown incomes)	Family income				
		Under $2,000	$2,000– $3,999	$4,000– $6,999	$7,000– $9,999	$10,000 or over
Restricted activity						
Under 5	10.6	9.6	10.0	10.8	10.8	11.7
5–14	10.6	8.8	8.6	10.8	11.4	12.1
15–24	10.5	11.3	12.0	10.4	10.2	9.0
25–44	13.5	19.4	15.9	13.7	12.3	11.6
45–64	22.2	43.6	26.6	19.7	16.8	16.1
65–74	34.0	43.4	36.8	27.4	23.3	19.5
75 and over	46.1	47.6	48.4	39.1	44.1	54.2
Bed disability						
Under 5	5.0	5.7	5.9	4.9	4.3	5.5
5–14	4.5	4.2	3.7	4.6	4.8	4.7
15–24	4.6	4.8	4.8	4.6	4.4	3.9
25–44	5.0	7.2	6.2	5.1	4.4	4.1
45–64	7.0	14.4	8.0	6.1	5.0	5.1
65–74	11.1	11.4	12.8	10.1	7.1	10.7
75 and over	19.0	16.8	18.7	21.5	26.5	24.9
Lost from work [a]						
17–24	3.9	2.5	5.2	3.9	3.5	3.0
25–44	4.7	6.8	6.5	5.3	3.5	3.5
45–64	7.0	11.1	7.9	7.3	5.8	5.6
65 and over	7.3	6.2	8.9	9.5	5.1	4.4
Lost from school [b]						
6–16	5.0	5.2	5.0	4.7	5.3	5.3

Source: U.S. National Center for Health Statistics, "Disability Days,
United States, July 1963–June 1964," *Vital Statistics: Data from the
National Health Survey,* ser. 10, no. 24 (Washington, D.C.: U.S.
Government Printing Office, November 1965), pp. 29–33. Data are
based on household interviews of the civilian noninstitutional population
of the United States.

[a] Per currently employed person per year.

[b] Per school-age child per year.

nificantly greater in older ages and almost nonexistent among children.

As for the more severe forms of chronic illness, the proportion of persons with one or more chronic conditions causing activity limitation was inversely related to family income for such major illnesses as heart conditions, arthritis and rheumatism, mental and nervous conditions, high blood pressure, visual impairments, and orthopedic impairments (except paralysis and absence of limbs). Each of these conditions was far more prevalent among the older than among the younger, although the inverse relationship to family income was evident among all age groups except children under 15 where the prevalence of these conditions was too small for any relationship to be evident.

For acute conditions receiving medical care or resulting in activity limitation a constant inverse relationship to family income was clearly not evident. In fact, inference from the data could be made more readily to a direct than to an inverse relationship. For example, the age-adjusted incidence of medically attended or activity-restricting acute conditions per 100 persons per year dropped from 215.9 at incomes under $2,000 to 204.5 at $2,000–$3,999, but thereafter the rate rose to 216.2 at $4,000–$6,999 and 232.5 at $7,000 and over.[17] By specific condition group, a rising rather than a falling gradient with family income was evident for infective and parasitic diseases as well as upper respiratory conditions, but no gradient for influenza and other respiratory conditions. Only acute conditions of the digestive system showed a clear inverse relationship to family income.

By age group, considering all medically attended or activity-restricting acute condition groups combined, an inverse relationship to family income was much more pronounced in old age (65 and over) than in mid-life (ages 45–64). During early adulthood (ages 15–44), family income was apparently unrelated to the incidence of acute conditions, but during childhood

Table III-5. Percent distribution of the population by severity of chronic illness by family income and age group, United States, July 1962—June 1963.

Age group and severity of illness	All incomes (includes unknown incomes)	Family income			
		Under $2,000	$2,000–$3,999	$4,000–$6,999	$7,000 or over
	Percent distribution				
All age groups					
All persons	100.0	100.0	100.0	100.0	100.0
Persons with one or more chronic conditions	44.5	57.6	46.5	40.6	42.9
With limitation of activity	12.4	28.6	16.0	8.9	7.9
Without limitation of activity	32.1	29.0	30.5	31.7	35.0
Persons with no chronic conditions	55.5	42.4	53.5	59.4	57.1
Under 15 years of age					
All persons	100.0	100.0	100.0	100.0	100.0
Persons with one or more chronic conditions	19.5	19.2	19.4	18.8	20.8
With limitation of activity	2.0	2.9	2.1	1.8	1.9
Without limitation of activity	17.5	16.3	17.3	17.0	18.9
Persons with no chronic conditions	80.5	80.8	80.6	81.2	79.2

Table III-5. (Continued)

Age group and severity of illness	Family income				
	All incomes (includes unknown incomes)	Under $2,000	$2,000–$3,999	$4,000–$6,999	$7,000 or over
15–44 years					
All persons	100.0	100.0	100.0	100.0	100.0
Persons with one or more chronic conditions	45.9	48.4	45.3	46.1	46.6
With limitation of activity	8.0	13.4	10.6	7.4	6.1
Without limitation of activity	37.9	35.0	34.7	38.7	40.5
Persons with no chronic conditions	54.0	51.7	54.7	53.8	53.4
45–64 years					
All persons	100.0	100.0	100.0	100.0	100.0
Persons with one or more chronic conditions	64.3	76.8	68.3	62.3	61.1
With limitation of activity	20.7	41.2	26.2	17.5	13.8
Without limitation of activity	43.6	35.6	42.1	44.8	47.3
Persons with no chronic conditions	35.7	23.2	31.7	37.7	38.9
65 years and over					
All persons	100.0	100.0	100.0	100.0	100.0
Persons with one or more chronic conditions	81.2	86.4	81.5	77.2	76.3
With limitation of activity	48.9	58.1	47.8	43.3	39.7
Without limitation of activity	32.3	28.3	33.7	33.9	36.6
Persons with no chronic conditions	18.8	13.6	18.6	22.8	23.8

Source: U.S. National Center for Health Statistics, "Medical Care, Health Status, and Family Income, United States," *Vital Statistics: Data from the National Health Survey*, ser. 10, no. 9 (Washington, D.C.: U.S. Government Printing Office, May 1964), pp. 53–64. Data based on household interviews of the civilian noninstitutional population.

this incidence rose sharply with income. Thus children in well-to-do families experienced many more acute conditions than the children in low-income families.

DENTAL MORBIDITY AND THE UNMET NEED FOR DENTAL CARE

The level of dental health is regarded as an important aspect of the general level of health and well-being of the population. Nevertheless, in many nations of the world, and especially in those with poor health facilities, inadequate nourishment and endemic debilitating communicable diseases, infections of the teeth and oral tissues represent a considerable burden on the population and substantially depress the general level of health. In the United States, where dentistry has attained a high level of development, the critically serious sequelae of dental disease are seen only infrequently and the major dental diseases (caries and periodontal disease) are rarely direct causes of death.

Nevertheless, the sheer accumulation of untreated dental conditions in the United States is staggering: they are among the most common of all diseases afflicting the American people. One authority estimated that in 1960 the average American had four unfilled cavities in his mouth, while current evidence suggests that this figure continues to increase, rather than decrease, with the passage of time.* Dental morbidity is not self-limiting; dental caries and periodontal disease are not likely to cure themselves without proper care, although uncared-for teeth may either be extracted or fall out.

Regular dental care undoubtedly contributes to better health,

* If only those with one or more primary or permanent teeth are taken as the base for this computation, the figure is 4.5. The figure of 4 was derived by using the entire population as the base for the computation. See Wesley O. Young, "Dental Health," in Commission on the Survey of Dentistry in the United States, *Survey of Dentistry, Final Report,* Byron S. Hollinshead, Director (Washington, D.C.: American Council on Education, 1961).

but in the country's population a considerable disparity exists between the need for and the receipt of dental care. Americans apparently give a low priority to dental care, and the shortage and maldistribution of practicing dentists as well as the inability of many patients to pay for the needed care also exert an unfavorable influence. The burden of these factors, of course, falls most heavily on the poor.

However, the addition of fluoride to a community's water supply materially lessens the amount of dental decay among children, and this simple preventive measure—convenient, inexpensive, and safe—benefits the poor and the affluent alike. It is performed by the community, requiring no effort on the part of the individual. As a result, that segment of the poverty population which drinks fluoridated water may have a lower level of dental caries than those non-poor who are not served by fluoridated water supply. But when the effects of fluoridation are held constant, the impact of socio-economic status on dental health is considerable.

A recent study of nearly 4,000 5-year-old children of Contra Costa County, California, showed that the prevalence of dental caries was inversely related to socio-economic status.[18] Children in the lowest socio-economic group had 60 percent more carious teeth (decayed, teeth indicated for extraction, and filled teeth) than those in the highest group, while a much lower proportion of the former were free of caries altogether. Similar results were found in a survey by Szwejda of school children in Buffalo, New York.[19] The same author studied the caries experience of white and nonwhite children, at ages 6 through 11 and of differing socio-economic backgrounds, in fluoridated and nonfluoridated communities in North Carolina.[20] In the nonfluoridated community, the white children of upper socio-economic status had a much lower dental caries rate than children of either race in the low socio-economic group. In the fluoridated area, there were only negligible differences in the permanent teeth of all groups;

among the primary teeth, however, the caries rate for the upper socio-economic groups was better than for the others.

The amount and type of dental care that a person receives varies significantly by family income. According to data of the National Health Survey for the twelve-month period ending June 1959, the rate of dental visits per person per year was for persons with family incomes of $7,000 or more over three times the rate of persons with less than $2,000 income (2.3 visits as against 0.7 visits).[21] For children under age 15 the comparable ratio was about five times as high for the $7,000-and-over income group as for the under-$2,000 group; for persons aged 15–64, about three times as high; and for persons 65 and over, almost twice as high. While in the highest income families 42 percent of those interviewed had not visited a dentist during the year, the comparable proportion was 78 percent in the lowest income group; in the highest income families 32 percent of children under 15 had never visited a dentist, but the comparable figure was 74 percent in the lowest income group; among persons aged 15–44 only 7 percent in the highest income group had not seen a dentist in five years or more, but the comparable figure was 29 percent in the lowest income group.

What kinds of services do people receive when they see a dentist? According to NHS data for July 1957—June 1958, preventive care services such as fillings, cleaning or examinations, and straightenings accounted for a much larger proportion of the visits by persons in upper-income families than those with lower incomes, while for therapeutic work—extractions and denture work—the reverse was true. Generally the percentage for each of these items increased as family income rose. For example, for persons of all ages the proportion of visits for fillings rose from 27.4 percent at under $2,000 to 45.7 percent at $7,000 and over; for cleaning or examinations, the comparable percentages were 12.2 and 21.8; and for straightenings they were 1.2 and 5.3 percent. For extractions, however, the comparable proportions dropped from 37.1 to 9.9 percent, and for denture work, from 14.2 to 7.9 percent. There was some variation in each of these patterns by age, but on the whole they were remarkably consistent.

Clearly the poverty population is considerably less healthy than the rest of the population of this country. It still experiences substantially higher rates of over-all mortality (all ages and by age, and especially from the communicable diseases), infant mortality, and severe illness.* Its level of dental morbidity is higher and its need for dental care much greater. However, a countervailing tendency may operate here and the more affluent strata of the nonpoverty population may be subject to new environmental hazards which may increase its mortality, especially from coronary artery diseases and lung cancer. The same strata of the nonpoverty population may experience a larger volume of relatively minor illness conditions, subjective or real, than the less affluent nonpoverty strata. Considering total mortality (from all causes) and total morbidity (from all conditions and with all degrees of severity), one can expect a U-shaped curve: over-all mortality and morbidity may be highest, or most prevalent, among the poor and the well-to-do, and lowest, or least prevalent, among the middle strata of our population.

It seems likely that, as the programs to alleviate poverty in this country succeed, the health level of the poverty population will closely approximate that of the lower strata of the nonpoverty population. As the poor move into the mainstream of the dominant middle-class pattern of American life, they are likely to experience substantial reductions in over-all mortality from the communicable diseases, especially at the younger ages, in infant mortality, and in severe illness; in other words, they

* An important factor here may be "drift" across social class lines due to severe illness. The severely ill may drop in social class position. This would particularly affect the statistics if annual income is used as the indicator of social class.

are likely to move to the bottom of the U-shaped curve. This, however, requires massive changes in their life styles which the health levels of the poor will reflect with a substantial lag of time only. Hence, we can expect a considerable time to elapse before this improvement in the mortality and morbidity of the poor will become observable.

IV · Social Differences in Mental Health

by Marc Fried

The evidence is unambiguous and powerful that the lowest social classes have the highest rates of severe psychiatric disorder in our society. Regardless of the measures employed for estimating severe psychiatric disorder and social class, regardless of the region or the date of study, and regardless of the method of study, the great majority of results all point clearly and strongly to the fact that the lowest social class has by far the greatest incidence of psychoses. It is striking that, despite the strength and consistency of this finding and the infrequency of such results in the social sciences, it remains in the limbo of facts that continue to be understated, challenged, and rarely examined for clarification.[1]

Although the evidence is clear and strong, it is not nearly so well known as one might hope. Thus, we shall first review the literature showing the consistencies and inconsistencies in gross results and shall then examine the many limitations within which this finding can be generalized and understood. Fortunately, in view of the strength of the basic finding, the qualifications may be used for an initial conceptualization of the issues and not merely for questioning the accuracy or stability of the results. Once the facts have been reviewed and qualified, we shall consider the more difficult problem of underlying sources of the relationships, the intricacies of causal interpretation, and the implications for our understanding of mental health. Much of the more recent literature on social class and mental health or illness is filled with methodological critiques. More often than not, the very same studies that present these criticisms undo the moral position they thereby achieve by committing alternative errors in design, technique, or interpretation. We have already suggested that many of the criticisms are inappropriate in light of the cumulative impact of the findings. Since we believe that the perspicacity involved in criticism might better be devoted to unraveling the many mysteries that accompany the relationship between social class and mental illness, we shall try to eschew such methodological critiques except for generic problems of definition.

Whenever we consider the problem of mental health, we are forced into either of two contrasting and equally unsatisfactory positions. We can elect to formulate an ideal type either as a composite image of health or as a set of variables signifying attributes we regard as healthy. This is a procedure that has been used in numerous psychological studies. Some of these are based on clinical experience and represent an effort to formulate those characteristics that seem to be associated with effective performance or with some highly respected accomplishment like creativity, others are based on an analysis of data from a less highly selected population.[2] Even the proponents of this "ideal" approach often recognize the cultural, subcultural, situational, and temporal limitations of an ideal for mental health. They pursue it, however, in trying to establish a basis for evaluating the positive, healthy, competent, or creative end of a hypothetical spectrum of psychological or social accomplishments.

Another approach involves backing into the problem by delineating more clearly the more easily defined and more readily studied problem of mental illness, treating the problem of mental health as a by-product. Generally, studies in the epidemiology of mental illness do not devote much attention to mental health but focus on the more limited and more readily defined problem of illness. Indeed, this is part of the reason that a rather substantial empirical foundation exists for reviewing this interrelationship. In effect, this is the approach of the present discussion. Although we will consider primarily problems of mental illness, we shall subsequently turn to the implications of the data about social class and mental illness for the small but important contribution they make to our understanding of social class, mental health, and social process.

Indeed, the widespread use of the term mental health, in contrast to exclusive attention to mental illness, is extremely recent and implies a major reconceptualization. From the middle of the nineteenth century until the middle of the twentieth century, popular conceptions and professional judgment converged in the view that mental illness was manifested in severely disordered behavior and that this resulted from a disordered psychic state (whether developmentally, situationally, physiologically, or genetically determined). The very notion of mental illness as opposed to lunacy or madness and its acceptance by a large public are relatively recent developments and represent an effort to establish a therapeutic rather than an entirely custodial (or even punitive) orientation toward severely incapacitated and frequently hospitalized persons.

EMERGENCE OF THE CONTEMPORARY CONCEPTIONS OF MENTAL HEALTH

In recent years, the fields of mental health have developed a more substantial appreciation of the social processes that confound distinctions among a variety of forms of deviant behavior. Thus, emotional difficulties, intellectual dysfunctions and deficits, antisocial behavior, social incompetence, and other types of malfunction have frequently been clustered for study or treatment. The community mental health movement is one of the most striking examples of this trend. Coupled with this, there has been a continuous growth of a literature dealing with the social forces that influence potentials for malfunction, that define acceptable and unacceptable behavior in the community, that produce resources differentially for different communities and subpopulations, and that effect the paths to treatment and the outcome of diagnosed malfunction. Nonetheless, we are still far from an integrated understanding of malfunction, of its social origins and correlates, or of its relationships to social class differences.

In the past the social forces that affected social class differences in malfunction were all too evident. Despite differences in manifest behavior, great masses of the lowest strata experienced similar treatment or, rather, maltreatment through incarceration in punitive, custodial, and work institutions of a society on the verge of massive industrialization. Although we are most familiar with this problem through Dorothea Dix's attack on the imprisonment of lunatics and through the widespread impact of the Elizabethan Poor Laws, the use of the same institutions for a variety of forms of deviance associated with poverty was widespread. It appears to have been characteristic for most Western European countries and the United States.[3] It is hardly surprising that the vast mass of people incarcerated in asylums, workhouses, and prisons were drawn from the poverty-stricken lower classes. Alienated both from their preindustrial communities which were in the process of disintegration and from the rudimentary industrial society which could not yet provide adequate roles or opportunities for them, the poor were numerous and a potential threat to the precarious stability of rapidly changing societies. In the face of promiscuous disregard for the miseries of a large proportion of the population in Western Europe, the professionalization of psychiatry offered a new and more sensitive conception of psychopathology. By the end of the nineteenth century, the sharp distinction between mental illness and other social problems was effectively drawn, paving the way for the advances of Charcot, Janet, Kraepelin, and Freud.

During the last half of the nineteenth century, the growing field of psychiatry made several important contributions toward a reconceptualization of mental illness.

1. In providing a new system of classification, Kraepelin (and later Freud) helped to give some sense of scientific order to superficially irrational and apparently nonpatterned behaviors.

2. Charcot and Janet helped to develop a wider appreciation of the milder disorders, to reveal the compelling and involuntary character of psychological malfunctioning, and to provide a more sympathetic framework for understanding the suffering associated with psychopathology.

3. In developing a systematic etiological formulation, Freud provided both a generic and a differentiated understanding of intrapsychic and developmental forces associated with psychological disorder, and introduced an awareness of the widespread nature of psychic conflict, which could be conceived as a continuum extending from health through mild mental disorder to the most severe and bizarre forms of psychosis.

Having satisfactorily established the fundamental developmental importance of "internalization" processes relatively early in his work, Freud turned to intrapsychic processes as the focus for subsequent theoretical clarification. While his ready rejection of the importance of the social environment as a determinant of behavior (indeed, his rejection of his own prior concern with the consequences of explicit experiences and traumata) may appear cavalier, this allowed Freud to develop conceptions of human functioning and malfunctioning to which we must constantly return on the basis of expanded experiences of the effects of social structures and situations on behavior. Perhaps his single most general contribution consisted of a theoretical framework tracing neurotic and psychotic disorders of adults and children to a long, premorbid history. While psychoanalysis has never altogether succeeded in demonstrating the distinctive developmental sequences that make for symptom formation, it provides a theoretical basis for understanding important liaisons between early experience and later psychic structure. Despite the relatively meager attention Freud gave to the importance of the social environment, it is largely on the basis of his theoretical framework that we can meaningfully speak of mental illnesses as disorders of living.[4] As we pursue the association between social class position and mental illness, the appreciation of malfunctioning as disorders of living provides both a basis for more dynamic analysis of social variables and a link between social and psychological processes.

DEFINITIONS AND EMPIRICAL DATA

The most unambiguous data on mental illness and social class concern those severe psychiatric disorders which we refer to as psychosis. The data are, of course, attended by many problems of definition. Despite efforts to develop a standard nomenclature and standardized criteria for diagnosis, ambiguities are built into the total situation in which an individual comes to psychiatric notice and is diagnosed. There is an extreme view that much of the ambiguity of the term mental illness is inapplicable to the psychoses; individuals who are psychotic may remain in the community for different lengths of time but sooner or later they will come to psychiatric attention, will be properly diagnosed, and will most often be hospitalized.[5] This view is presumably based on logic and clinical impression but conceals several underlying unsubstantiated premises: that psychosis is a persistent disorder, that community tolerance operates only within a narrow range, that there is widespread agreement on diagnosis for moderate as well as for severe psychotic states.

During an era that has discovered the importance of social

factors in the "processing" of mental illness, this view is not easily acceptable. We know that (1) social factors, particularly differences in the social class position of the patient, affect diagnosis; (2) with new conceptions of a patient, many individuals diagnosed as psychotic can be maintained outside of the hospital and require minimal assistance; and (3) a great many transitory psychotic states appear among individuals with stable functioning and a great many diagnosed psychotics recover during relatively brief periods of time.[6] Of greater importance is the evidence that the ways in which people with incipient tendencies to disorganization of behavior are viewed and treated are intricate and important determinants that can modify or intensify initial behavioral (and presumably psychic) disorganization. We have witnessed a number of dramatic changes in the course of a few decades in the changing conception of hospital care, in increased concern for the role of the family, and in the increased awareness of the stabilizing potential of the natural environment of home and work. It is likely that we are still far from appreciating the full range of social influences that determine and define the phenomena we then label as psychosis.

These and many related considerations suggest that (1) communities vary considerably in their levels of tolerance and in whether or not they will view a particular behavior as severely disordered; (2) that the initial response to disordered functioning, either within the community or during early contacts with professionals, can entail either further disorganization leading to psychotic manifestations or provide support and stabilization leading to the maintenance of ego boundaries; (3) that the very path to treatment, due to availability of resources, initial professional contacts, or community and familial preferences will further serve either to disorganize or to stabilize disordered functioning and will influence the diagnosis; and (4) that whether an individual is hospitalized or not, with or without the diagnosis of psychosis, this will determine his subsequent level of organization and functioning and will vary for different patients, different professionals, and different institutional settings[7] That there may be a small proportion of extreme cases of very high vulnerability, minimally affected by current environmental transactions, negates neither these propositions nor their explanatory value for the great majority of cases.

From this point of view, the justification for considering psychosis or psychiatric hospitalization an adequate subject for empirical study is itself open to challenge. Indeed, in the absence of adequate data for extricating these variables, considerable interpretative caution is essential in dealing with data about severe psychiatric disorders. Nonetheless, there is ample justification for treating severe psychiatric disorders as a meaningful category, provided we utilize the data for continuing clarification of meaning. At the very least, within short periods of time and within similar professional environments, we can expect the differences in criteria for seeking professional assistance, in diagnosis, and in treatment to be smaller than for any other category referring to less severely disturbed behavior.

Above all else, however, the analysis of relationships between psychiatric disorders and social class are legitimate to the extent that we treat the diagnosis or treatment as a *social* fact. We do not need to concur in the diagnostic or treatment decision in order to recognize that similarities in social conditions may or may not lead to similarities in social outcome. The purpose of such study is to determine whether these similarities in social condition, in this case social class, operate to produce similar effects because of or in spite of vast differences in other variables that may also affect the outcome. This is precisely the argument Durkheim employed in his analysis of suicide.[8] He did not purport to bypass psychological processes or psychological selection in determining individual instances of suicide; he wished to focus on social conditions and social outcomes. A rate of psychiatric hospitalization or of diagnosed psychosis is precisely such an outcome. Granting the complexity of factors influencing this outcome, we want to know if there are any overriding consistencies associated with social class. If we treat this outcome as a social fact, we must still determine the ways in which other forces, psychological processes, familial relationships, community values, or professional orientations contribute to this social fact and, thereby, to the existence of the relationship itself.

PSYCHOSIS AND SOCIAL CLASS POSITION

Although only a small number of studies have been responsible for much of the public and professional awareness of the relationship between social variables and mental illness, the relationship between social class and mental illness has been studied and documented extensively.[9] The earliest studies of social class and mental illness were theoretical and were often beset with unsolved problems of epidemiological analysis. Yet the fact that the available studies go back as far as 1917 and include patient populations from several decades before, provides us with a relatively long period for analysis.[10]

From the early study by Nolan (1917) until the most recent study by Dunham (1966), the largest body of data on psychiatric disorders and social class have important similarities: they most often use records of psychiatric hospitalization and rates based on the number of patients in a given demographic category with census calculations of the population at risk in these categories as denominators; and they more often deal with occupational distributions than with any other social class indicator. On the other hand, there are also a number of important differences among them: they vary in the use of controls (or rate adjustments) for such variables as age and sex; they vary in the completeness of coverage of patients within a given geographical region; they vary from the inclusion of schizophrenia alone, to consideration of other psychoses, or of all hospitalized patients;

and they vary in the use of correlational statistics or of tests of significance. Finally, there are a large enough number of studies using variant methods to allow further comparisons: there are a number of ecological studies, using hospitalization rates and social class indices for geographical regions (generally census tracts); there are several "community" studies based either on household interviews or on selective service evaluations; there are several studies that combine psychiatric hospital information with massive efforts to obtain data about nonhospital psychiatric contacts for the population at risk; and there are a number of studies that use education, income, residential housing characteristics, and color, which provide additional comparative materials.

Nolan's study of 1917, based on 7,026 first admissions for dementia praecox (schizophrenia) to New York Civil State hospitals between 1909 and 1916, was not directly concerned with occupation as an indicator of social class.[11] He was led to examine the relationships between different aspects of occupational functioning and dementia praecox since "among the many methods of reeducation the most effectual seems to be systematic instruction in simple, interesting work" (p. 128). Although his analysis shows markedly higher rates for unskilled laborers than for any other occupational group among males (210 per 100,000 compared to 166 per 100,000 for clerical service, 149 per 100,000 for domestic and personal service, to 47 per 100,000 for trades at the low extreme), his conclusions at the end of his detailed article never mention the implicit class or status distribution of the findings.

Starting with Nolan's pioneer study and ignoring many differences in quality and methods among the available studies, there have been at least thirty-four studies that present relevant data on severe psychiatric disorders and social class indices, excluding those which deal only with Negro-white differences in severe psychiatric disorders. Limiting the first review of these data, thus, to studies based on evidence of psychosis and/or psychiatric hospitalization for mental disorder and occupational status, education, income, rental costs, or dependency as social class indicators, we shall ask three major questions: (1) What proportion of these studies provide evidence that the lowest status group or groups, by any social class indicator, have the highest rate of psychosis and/or psychiatric hospitalization? (2) What proportion of these studies provide evidence of an inverse linear relatonship of psychosis and/or psychiatric hospitalization with social class indicators? (3) Are there differences in findings associated with the different indicators used for social class or for severe psychiatric disorders? Once these issues are clarified, it will be possible to turn more systematically to several other important questions concerning differences in the findings associated with different dynamic features of social class, comparative data for Negroes and whites, variables that modify or are modified by these relationships, and causal implications. For the time being, we assume that social class differences form the independent variable and psychosis or psychiatric hospitalization the dependent variable since, in any event, we are concerned with the determinants of severe psychiatric disorders and not with the determinants of social class.

The gross question, do the lowest social class groups show the highest rates of severe psychiatric disorder, must be answered clearly in the affirmative. Indeed, among thirty-four studies that provide answers to this question, we find the following results:

	Number of studies	Proportion of studies
Lowest status group has highest rate of psychosis and/or hospitalization	29	85
Data ambiguous or contradictory findings with different indicators	4	12
Lowest status group does not have highest rates of psychosis-hospitalization	1	3
	N = 34	100 percent

Thus, using only the fairly evident social class indicators and omitting consideration of Negro-white differences and of unemployment, we find that 85 percent of the studies clearly support the proposition that rates of severe psychiatric disorder are highest among the lowest social class groups. Two of the four studies listed as ambiguous present positive support for this proposition with one social class indicator and negate the proposition with another social class indicator.[12] The two other studies, although classified as ambiguous, provide more supportive than contradictory evidence.[13]

The significance of a finding that the lowest social class group by education, occupation, income, rental, or any other characteristic has the highest rates of severe psychiatric disorder will be considerably affected by a number of other considerations. Few of the studies present statistical tests of the differences between social class groups, although inspection reveals that rates for the lowest groups are quite considerably higher than the rates for groups of a higher position. Several of the studies that do employ tests of significance reveal that the difference between the lowest status category and all others are statistically significant. Thus, the difference is not only quite pervasive; it is also quite powerful.

The other question of importance is the extent to which these differences are linear. The data for this question are more difficult to evaluate because a new judgment is required for which there is no empirical basis. We must now estimate how much linearity is linear and how many deviations justify an over-all categorization of the pattern as nonlinear. The question is complicated by other factors: the lack of clarity, in several instances, of placing different occupations along a simple scale (e.g., are agricultural laborers or unskilled workers the lowest category or how do we compare the category "trade" with the category "skilled workers"?); the different numbers and types of categories used in different studies; and the comparison of studies that use rates for different social class frequencies with those which use some measure of association. Naturally, we will get quite different results depending on how we deal with each of these issues.

The results for these thirty-four studies, while somewhat less striking than for the assessment of rates among the very lowest status groups, are quite strong:

	Number of studies	Proportion of studies
Linear trend with inverse relationship between social class and severe disorder	24	71
Data ambiguous or contradictory findings with different indicators	8	23
Nonlinear relationship between social class and severe disorder	2	6
	N = 34	100 percent

The evidence is clear that most studies show a trend toward an inverse relationship between severe psychiatric disorders and social class indicators. The greatest difference from the previous results arises in the loss of clarity and the increase in the number of reports that are ambiguous. In fact, none of the reported studies shows a perfect linear relationship either supporting or contradicting the inverse association between social class and mental illness. The evidence showing that the lowest social class groups have the highest rate of severe psychiatric disorder is highly consistent. The evidence that this inverse relationship between social class and rates of severe disorder is linear is less consistent but points quite clearly toward support of the proposition. Although these results do not allow much leeway for variations due to different methods of evaluating severe psychiatric disorders or to different social class indicators, it is useful to pose the third question about variability in the findings.

The relationships presented above hold either for a total

count of all psychotic disorders or for schizophrenia alone. The fact that schizophrenia accounts for the largest proportion of psychotic disorders means that we may get different social class patterns for other psychotic disorders, without affecting the over-all trend. The most notable deviation from this pattern is to be found for the manic-depressive or affective disorders. The eight studies that give separate rates for these disturbances are approximately evenly distributed between those that show weak positive associations with social class indicators and those that show weak inverse associations with social class indicators.[14]

We can look at the significance for these relationships of different criteria for psychosis by comparing the thirty-four studies on the basis of their method of locating patients. Most of the studies are simply based on psychiatric hospital records. However, a number of studies use other methods either to implement these data or in lieu of psychiatric records but using the same diagnostic criteria. Thus we have studies that utilize contact with psychiatric facilities other than hospitals to screen a population, studies based on selective service psycyhiatric evaluations, and a few studies using a field screening instrument for evaluating levels of psychiatric impairment. The results based on these different approaches are as follows:

Criterion employed	Linear trend	Am- biguous	Non- linear
Psychiatric hospitalization for psychosis	17	5	1
Hospitalization and diagnosis of psychosis in other facility	1	1	1
Selective service psychiatric evaluation	2	0	0
Level of psychiatric impairment from field screening instrument	4	2	0
N =	24	8	2

It is quite clear that the only two categories of criteria for severe psychiatric disorder in which a substantial proportion of the studies depart from a clear, linear trend in the relationship between social class and severe disorder are hospitalization or diagnoses of psychosis in another psychiatric facility, and level of psychiatric impairment determined through a field screening procedure. In fact, when diagnoses of psychosis from community facilities other than psychiatric hospitals are used, two of the three studies (Dunham, Jaco) fail to support the proposition. And when psychiatric screening is conducted in the field with respondents selected through some random procedure, two of the four studies (Dohrenwend and Kaplan) provide ambiguous evidence.[15]

Were it not for the two studies based on selective service evaluations, we might suggest that these results point to a differential in hospitalization rates by social class that does not correspond with an equivalent social class differential in the use of other sources of diagnosis is. Indeed, this may account for some of the relationship, a suggestion that is supported by the evidence that lower-class patients are less frequently seen in private practice, receive more severe diagnoses, and are more readily hospitalized.[16] To the extent that discriminatory diagnosis is built into psychiatric practice, it should affect psychiatric diagnoses whether established in the hospital or in other facilities. Thus, it should not account for a difference due to the source used for locating patients. The greater frequency of psychiatric hospitalization for patients from lower social class categories and the minor distortion in hospital-based studies due to a number of patients with severe psychiatric disorders from higher social class categories who are seen outside the hospital remain the major possible sources of difference in the various studies.

In spite of these qualifications, it is notable that the trend toward an inverse relationship between social class and severe psychiatric disorder remains evident. We should note, in passing, that the three ambiguous studies that go beyond hospital records of psychosis support the proposition to a considerable extent. One of them rejects the inverse linear relationships hypothesis but finds the highest rates among the lowest status groups, another one does not show the highest rates of impairment for the lowest status but the trend is clear, and a third indicates higher rates of nonhospitalized psychosis in higher status community which, however, are insufficient to compensate for the higher psychiatric hospitalization rates in the lower status community.[17]

The data for differences in results associated with different indicators of social class are interesting and suggestive but inconclusive. The table below gives these results by the major social class indicators used:

	Linear trend	Ambiguous	Nonlinear
Occupation	9	3	2
Education	4	1	0
Income-dependency	4	3	0
Rental costs	2	0	0
Multiple-item index	7	2	0
N =	26	9	2

The majority of reports support the inverse relationship between social class and severe psychiatric disorder. However, the findings are most ambiguous for occupation (5 out of 14 reports that do not support the proposition) and income-dependency (3 out of 7 reports that do not support the proposition). Although these results do not lead to any noteworthy conclusions, they do offer an interesting suggestion for subsequent consideration. Occupational achievement among adults is clearly more responsive to situational changes than educational achievement; and income or dependency status is more responsive to temporary changes in economic situation or, at least, is more immediately responsive than rental cost. Does this point to a more dynamic feature of social class position as the source of these relationships than would be indicated by a stable conception of social class status as the critical dimension? We shall address this question as we accumulate more data.

NONPSYCHOTIC DISORDERS AND SOCIAL CLASS POSITION

Many difficulties attend the study of the most severe psychiatric disorders but empirical study of the wide variety of other mental and emotional disorders is virtually impossible. Data are rarely available to permit the study of milder disorders in the entire population of a geographical region. A wider variety of resources are available for the care and treatment of milder disorders, many of which may not involve any psychiatric personnel and may not eventuate in a psychiatric diagnosis. Movement between geographical regions for treatment may lead to the disappearance of a great many cases, which means that, not only is the case count inaccurate, but there is no adequate basis for determining the appropriate population at risk. Finally, the gross behavioral criteria on which a diagnosis of psychosis or a decision for psychiatric hospitalization can be based are much clearer than the much more subjective and variable criteria for seeking evaluation or treatment in the milder disorders. For mental retardation and suicide we may approximate adequate rate analyses but for childhood or adult neuroses, psychosomatic symptoms, or behavior disorders we cannot hope to find a sufficient base for conclusions.

In spite of the many inadequacies in available sources, the data on social class and suicide are of particular interest. There is a widespread impression that suicides are most frequent among the highest status groups and least frequent among those of lowest status. Durkheim contributed to this view: "So far is the increase in poverty from causing the increase in suicide that even fortunate crises, the effect of which is abruptly to enhance a country's prosperity, affect suicide like economic disasters." [18] Dublin, moreover, suggested that a sudden loss of status and position among high status people, that is, severe relative deprivation, was one of the most frequent causes of suicide in situations of economic depression.[19] However, the facts do not consistently support the view that "more suicides occur among persons who have every financial facility to enjoy life than among those with barely enough to keep body and soul together." [20]

Following Durkheim's concept of anomie and his analysis of anomic suicide, the early sociological literature gave particular attention to social disorganization. Ecological analyses revealed a high correlation between underprivileged residential areas and suicide but this was generally interpreted as a result of social disorganization rather than of poverty or lower-class status. A more recent study tried to reformulate the problem of anomie and suicide by developing a conception of status integration. [21] Although social class position appears to play some role in the indices of status integration, they have not distinguished social class indicators for analysis. The most substantial analyses of empirical data are those by Dublin and Sainsbury. [22]

Dublin presents data from several sources. Concerning England and Wales in the years 1949–1953, he shows that the lowest social class category has the highest rates of suicide although it is closely seconded and, from ages 35 to 64, is surpassed by the highest social class. Thus, were we to formulate the proposition as we did for social class and severe psychiatric disorders, we would find support for high rates in the lower class but no evidence of a consistent inverse relationship. Recent United States data support the British results of high rates in the lowest class but reveal no differences among all the other class groups. Finally, a study covering the period 1910–1960 compares the per capita gross national product and the age-adjusted suicide rate, and despite a number of discrepancies, finds a significant negative correlation between prosperity and suicide rate. The finding provides an important clue to much of the literature on suicide and social class position. Although the literature on severe psychiatric disorders emphasizes class position per se, the literature on suicide stresses the importance of rapid and generally downward changes in position. Sainsbury's study of suicides in London points up factors of change and reveals the difficulty in assessing this from ecological correlations. His ecological analysis revealed that suicide was inversely correlated with poverty but showed little relationship with other indices of status or unemployment. A closer analysis, however, indicated that many of the higher status suicides were living in poverty, suggesting loss of status as an important factor, and showed significant correlations between suicide and unemployment. Other studies have also stressed the high correlation between unemployment and suicide.[23] The importance of the occupational role, in its social class implications and psychological ramifications, particularly when associated with downward mobility or major social transitions, has been repeatedly pointed up.[24] Clearly, however, the weight of evidence points toward the importance of loss of status or inadequacy in coping with status demands rather than poverty or stable social class positions as the critical determinants of suicide rates.

Another mental disorder in which social class differences have long been suggested is mental retardation. Despite the realization that only a relatively small proportion of retardates, generally the most severe ones, have clear evidence of organic impairment, there has been considerable reluctance to undertake large-scale epidemiological studies of mental retardation. In recent years, however, increasing attention is being devoted to social factors, and among them class differences, in the development of retardation. After reviewing the small literature relevant to this problem, Perry concludes that the vast majority of retardates present problems related to the sociocultural background of lower-class populations.[25] Similarly, Wortis points out that "by almost every available measure: correlation with family income, with social class, with parent's vocation, by comparison of white with Negro, white with Puerto Rican, white with Mexican-American, white with native Indian, we find this same marked tendency to higher concentration of the retarded in the more disadvantaged sections of our population." [26] Unfortunately, beyond so gross a statement, the data are inadequate for assessing any other features of the distribution of mental retardates.

If the data for evaluating the relationship of social class to suicide and mental retardation are inadequate, we can well anticipate the meager materials available for examining social class differences in any other form of mental disorder. Two observations stand out: the greater frequency of mild mental disorders (neuroses, personality impairments) among higher-status groups found in studies based on psychiatric treatment; and the higher rates of mild impairments along with higher rates of severe impairments among lower social class groups found in studies based on field interviews or mental health screening instruments.[27]

The existing studies, however, present no adequate empirical or rational grounds for the analysis of social class and psychiatric impairment. Under conditions of professionalization in the mental health fields of an affluent society, the difficulties that lead to psychiatric treatment for mild disturbances or to the evaluation of mild psychiatric impairments are based on complex but highly subjective and often transitory experiences. This, of course, does not rule them out as subjects for study but they present great difficulties for analysis. The significance of social class differences in mental disorder must, then, rest upon the substantial results based on severe psychiatric disorders. We have found these results to be striking both in their consistency and strength. On this basis, we can turn to a more analytic effort at extricating the components of social class position that appear to be most important in producing these relationships.

DYNAMIC RELATIONSHIPS BETWEEN POVERTY AND MENTAL ILLNESS

It is an open question whether Negro-white differences are most meaningfully treated within the social class framework or as an aspect of race relations and discrimination. On empirical grounds, it is clear that the lower social class categories are disproportionately represented by Negroes. The justification for viewing the situation of the Negro within a traditional social class framework does not lie, however, in the data on the disproportionate number of Negroes in lower social class positions but rather on whether a shift in these positions has the same consequences for Negroes as for whites. In view of the severity of discrimination and uniquely severe forms of segregation, do the factors that follow from social class positions affect the Negro in roughly comparable degrees? Even if we regard the situation of the Negro as that of an underclass or caste group, with unique experiences of degradation and relatively impermeable barriers to acceptance and absorption, the data on Negro-white differences in mental disorders are useful for clarifying the relationship between social class and severe psychiatric disorders. On the other hand, if we regard the situation of the Negro as primarily that of a newcomer to an urban lower class, we must confront similarities and differences in patterns of mental disorder as issues that help to elucidate the dynamics of social class that affect rates of psychiatric illness.

Some of the same unfamiliarity that characterizes public and professional knowledge about social class and mental illness obtains for the data concerning Negro-white differences in psychiatric disorders. There is a surprising total of twenty-one reports of Negro-white differences in rates of mental disorder.[28] The conclusions begin to become clear as soon as we look at the distribution of findings. In order to simplify some of the issues, the twenty-one studies are divided into those that are based only on psychiatric hospital data, those that include nonhospital cases but limit themselves to severe psychiatric disorders, and those that include nonhospital cases with a wider range of personality disorders:

	Negro rates higher	Differences ambiguous	White rates higher
Psychiatric hospital data only	8	0	0
Additional screening for severe cases	5	1	2
Additional screening for all disorders	2	1	2
All methods	N = 15	2	4

The results are only slightly less consistent than those for social class differences in severe psychiatric disorder; they show some striking similarities to the previous social class findings. Seventy-one percent of the studies point to higher rates among Negroes than among whites, and two ambiguous studies also point toward higher rates for Negroes. The four studies that show higher rates for whites involve locating patients in addition to or in lieu of psychiatric hospitalization for psychosis. Thus, the consistency of the results based on psychiatric hospitalization may, in part, be due to disproportionately high rates of hospitalization for Negroes relative to greater parity in levels of severe psychiatric disorder in the community. This supposition is supported by Dunham's finding of a much smaller gap between initial onset of symyptoms and the decision to seek treatment or extrusion from the community for Negroes than for whites. That is, the shorter community residence of disturbed persons implies a lower tolerance on the part of the individual or the community for Negroes than for whites with psychiatric symptoms.

The issues, however, are more complex than is suggested by the contrast between studies based on psychiatric hospitalization and those which use other means for locating patients. As Dohrenwend points out in a comparison of eight studies, three of the four studies showing higher rates for whites were done in the South and the fourth included the South; on the other hand, three of the four studies showing higher rates for Negroes were done in the North.[29] The significance of this observation can be interpreted in numerous ways but its importance is supported by several other findings which have pointed to the disproportionate increase in first admissions to psychiatric hospitals among Negroes.[30] By 1922 Negro and white rates reached parity for the United States as a whole, and this was the product of disproportionate rates for Negroes in the North along with low rates for Negroes in the South. It is concluded that "the low rates of mental disease among Negroes in the South is to be found in the lack of adequate provision for their treatment in institutions." [31]

Since 1922 Negro rates of psychiatric hospitalization have continued to increase more rapidly than white rates. A similar trend is found in the data for first admissions to psychiatric hospitals of Negroes and whites in Virginia.[32] The hypothesis of differential treatment facilities is illuminated by a comparison of patients admitted to psychiatric services in Maryland and Louisiana.[33] This study points out that in Louisiana first admission rates to all psychiatric facilities were higher for whites than for nonwhites with a major exception for schizophrenic reactions. In Maryland, however, nonwhite rates were higher than white rates for a number of conditions, including schizophrenic reactions. More generally, rates for nonwhites were consistently higher in Maryland than in Louisiana, particularly among the urban population. There are a number of possible explanations, all equally plausible and all equally consonant with these few fragments of data. Thus, it is possible that the greater opportunity for Negroes along with persistent impediments to actual achievement in the North (or in Maryland compared with Louisiana) lead to higher rates of malfunctioning.

In spite of qualifications based on the results of nonhospital psychiatric data, the findings remain quite striking for overwhelmingly higher rates of psychiatric hospitalization for severe disorders among Negroes. The weight of evidence continues to support the proposition that these high rates represent greater prevalence of severe psychiatric disorders among Negroes. It should also be noted that a number of the studies comparing psychiatric hospitalization of Negroes and whites have used extensive controls and the finding is maintained when such factors as migration, education, and occupation are taken into account. Indeed, among all the factors considered in several studies, the Negro-white difference is the largest and most consistent.[34]

If we consider only the disproportionately high rates of psychiatric hospitalization for Negroes, we are faced with the same analytic uncertainty as presented by the data on social class. We can probably account for very small portions of the difference as the result of extrinsic factors: higher rates of extrusion from the community, difficulty in access to outpatient facilities, more severe diagnoses for comparable symptoms, readier hospitalization, less adequate treatment. But there is reason to believe that intrinsic differences in the situation of lower-class groups and of Negroes compared to higher-status groups and whites could explain the differences in rates of severe psychiatric disorder. At the very least, most of the forms of situational stress, for example marital disruption, migration, and forced residential relocation, physical illness, and unemployment occur with disproportionate frequency among lower-class populations and among Negroes. If these bear any relationship to the occurrence of mental disorder, we can expect higher rates of psychiatric disorder regardless of the extrinsic influences that make them more visible or that translate malfunctioning into psychiatric disorder and hospitalization. We must now turn to these factors in an effort to extricate some of the dynamic forces that are associated with social class and color in our society and are responsible for the more striking experiences of deprivation and crisis.

Migration and Social Disruption

The earlier ecological studies of mental disorder, showing higher rates of psychiatric disorder (and particularly schizophrenia) in deteriorated central city areas, led to considerable controversy about the importance of geographical drift among schizophrenics.[35] This controversy gradually gave way to studies that implicated social isolation as a factor in the areal distribution of schizophrenics and minority group status in schizophrenia.[36] Both social isolation and minority status are, in large part, the product of geographical and social transition and can best be viewed in the context of the widespread experiences of change that characterize complex modern societies.

The most characteristic experiences of change that directly affect the lives of individuals are migration and residential displacement. The effect of migration on mental disorder has been vigorously studied and its causal implications vigorously debated.[37] We need not recapitulate the argument since there are no bases internal to the data that provide adequate grounds for discriminating between the selection hypothesis or the transition-stress hypothesis. However, the data continue to accrue revealing the persistence of a relationship between migration and severe psychiatric disorder in spite of changes in pattern from one period of study to another.

The data are remarkably consonant in showing higher rates of psychiatric disorder for migrants and for nonmigrants. As with several other variables (social class differences, Negro-white differences), Jaco's Texas data diverge from the majority of studies and, in this instance, represent the only clear negation of an association between migration and mental disorder.[38] In the recent studies of United States psychiatric hospitalization data, one of the most interesting shifts is the diminution in the differential rates of severe psychiatric disorder for the foreign-born compared to natives. By contrast, the rates of severe psychiatric disorder for interstate migrants are disproportionately high compared to nonmigrants.[39] The increased use of controls or adjustments for intercorrelated variables further reveals that the high rates of psychiatric disorder for interstate migrants hold up for Negroes and whites and within education, occupation, and age groups.

With social class variables controlled, the fact that the disproportionate rates of severe psychiatric disorder are maintained indicates that migration does not, in any simple way, explain the relationship between social class and mental illness. Although shorter range, intracommunity movements have not been adequately studied, these are unlikely to account for social class differentials. Such movement is disproportionately frequent among higher status groups, and the little evidence available suggests that short-distance moves are less clearly associated with mental disorders than large moves.[40] Lower status migrants have greater difficulty and assimilate more slowly into the new environment and this might provide a basis for linking social class, migration, and mental disorder.[41] Moreover, none of the data allow for an analysis of the level of urbanization or industrialization from which migrants derive, or of the degree of transition necessary for adaptation to the new society. It is plausible that the shift from a major difference between foreign-born and native to a major difference for interstate migrants may conceal a more dramatic change in the social background of foreign migrants than of domestic migrants but there are no data to substantiate this proposition. The effect of migration on mental disorder might account, in part, for the extremely high rates of severe psychiatric disorder among Negroes.

Another factor worthy of consideration and related to the

readier assimilation of higher status migrants is the effect of minority status on mental disorders. Faris and Dunham had originally mentioned the possible significance of minority status in pointing out the high rates of disorder for whites living in Negro areas and for Negroes living in white areas.[42] Strikingly enough, the issue received little further attention. One study implicated the factor of disparities in parental background or between parents and neighborhood mode as a determinant of schizophrenia.[43] Other studies focused attention on disparities between family and community as a factor in rates of psychiatric hospitalization. A comparison of rates of schizophrenia and manic-depressive psychosis among Italians in metropolitan Boston points quite unambiguously to the fact that the higher the proportion of Italians in a community, the lower the rates of these psychoses among Italians.[44] The use of simple demographic indices (the conceptual significance of which, as "minority status" variables, is often tenuous) finds that people with a particular personal characteristic living in communities where that characteristic is less common have disproportionately high rates of psychiatric hospitalization.[45]

These studies do not carry us very far in understanding the relationship between social class or poverty and mental illness. They do suggest that the minority status of newcomers to a community (as newcomers, as foreigners, as less urbane, as pre-industrial, as Negroes) may be the central factor in the relationship between migration and mental illness. This hypothesis receives support from a comparison of migration to different countries which suggests that the receptiveness of the host society is a major determinant of high or low rates of psychiatric disorder among migrants.[46] It may also account for the high rates of psychiatric disorder among Negroes who move to the North, not merely as members of a minority population but as strangers and aliens by virtue of unfamiliarity, less urbanized backgrounds, poverty, and low status.

Another form of social disruption, clearly correlated with

social class position, Negro status, and mental illness, is marital status. It is difficult to demonstrate its effect as an intervening variable or as a component variable in the relationship between social class and mental illness or Negro status and mental illness. Nonetheless it warrants attention as a potential basis for explaining a greater proportion of the variance than we can now achieve. The findings are, with a few minor variations, probably the most consistent in the epidemiology of mental illness.[47] The most stable finding is that married people living with spouse show by far the lowest rates of psychiatric hospitalization, while those who are divorced or separated show by far the highest rates.[48] The major variations in the data occur in the rank order of single persons and of widowed persons. Both single and widowed people have considerably higher rates than the married and considerably lower rates than the divorced or separated, but show relatively similar rates to one another and change rank positions from one set of data to another. It is of interest that, despite the very high rates of divorce and separation among Negroes, the same pattern of mental status and psychiatric disorder occurs among Negroes with only slightly smaller differences between the extremes.

Although these findings on migration, minority status, and marital disruption offer only suggestive clues to the relationship between Negro status and mental disorder, they point up some intercorrelated factors that affect the distribution of psychiatric disorders. Thus there are marked differences in the patterns, conditions, and auspices of migration for lower- and for higher-status groups which may affect the distribution of disorders.[49] Lower-status groups relatively more often leave a region because of inadequacies in the community of origin while higher-status groups more frequently seek opportunities otherwise unavailable to them. Moreover, lower-status people, Negro or white, are far less likely to have a clear idea about the work they will do, the place in which they will live, or the people with whom they will associate. At the same time, the psychological requirements of lower status people for environmental support and dependability are great. Marital disruption, more frequent among lower status people, can only intensify the need for external resources. The combination of a pervasive sense of inner uncertainty and inadequate social resources for stabilizing immediate life situations is likely to be a major factor producing the phenomena of psychiatric disorder. On this basis, migration, marital disruption or any other form of major social transition may produce differential rates of psychiatric disorder at different social class levels.

While complex theoretical considerations prove fundamental in the design of complex studies to extricate the causal sequences linking social class and mental disorder, several simpler relationships may prove more immediately useful and empirically verifiable in accounting for these associations. In most instances the studies are inadequate for providing conclusive evidence, but several investigations of the effects of employment status and of social mobility on psychiatric disorder provide a more meaningful basis for translating social class and Negro-white differences in mental illness into the dynamics of social processes.

Work and Unemployment

In view of the critical importance of occupational performance in modern societies, the large differences in the work situation of different social class levels, and the associations between occupational status and severe psychiatric disorder, the potential significance of work and unemployment for mental health and illness is apparent. Nonetheless, very few studies have examined this relationship.

Only two of the thirty-four studies dealing with social class and mental illness report rates of psychiatric disorder for the unemployed. Granting the technical difficulties of assessing unemployment for a person who is hospitalized after some period of serious malfunctioning, and the analytic difficulties of interpreting the association causally, the data are striking and warrant attention. The technical problem of assessing unemployment is minimal for the first of the two studies since it is based on selective service registrants. This study found by far the highest rates of rejection for mental and personality disorders (excluding psychoneurosis) among the category of unemployed and emergency (presumably temporary or transient) workers.[50] This category showed a rate of 84.8/1,000 compared to an over-all rate for all occupations of 50.1/1,000 and a rate of 24.7/1,000 for professional and managerial occupations. Similarly, Jaco found the extremely high rates of psychosis among the unemployed to be one of the results in his occupational analysis of three subcultural groups in Texas. Differences by employment status are also enormous although it is quite striking that among the Anglo-American group they are extremely high for both males and females but among the Spanish-American and non-white groups the disproportion for the unemployed is greater for females than for males.[51]

There is no way of extricating the different causal sequences from these data. It is equally plausible that psychiatric disorder led to unemployment or that unemployment led to psychiatric disorder. The trend data showing that increases in rates of unemployment preceded increases in rates of psychiatric hospitalization (with a lag of several years) during the great depression lend some support to the significance of unemployment as cause.[52] But they do not preclude the simultaneous operation of psychiatric disorder as a cause of unemployment. Some of the data on suicide also present evidence of the causal importance of unemployment on disordered functioning but, while suicide can hardly be a cause of unemployment (provided we maintain a labor force definition of unemployment) prior malfunctioning can be responsible for unemployment which in turn may precipitate suicide.[53] Equally inconclusive but suggestive evidence comes from a study which found a surprisingly high level of gainful employment prior to hospitalization among a sample of male schizophrenic patients.[54] On the other hand, after hospitalization there was a gradual attrition of employment rates, increasing after each subsequent hospitalization experience.

There is another way of stating these several findings. Compared to people who are gainfully employed, the unemployed have extremely high rates of psychiatric disorder. This implies the causal priority of unemployment, a suggestion that is supported by the temporal priority of increases in unemployment which parallel (with a lag) increases in rates of psychiatric hospitalization during economic depression. Among hospitalized psychiatric patients long-term rates of prehospitalization unemployment are not notably high; however, during the period immediately preceding the initial hospitalization, 38 percent had moved to continuous unemployment.[55] Moreover, there is some evidence that rates of unemployment vary inversely with occupational status level. Thus, the lowest occupational groups appear to have had the highest rates of unemployment prior to hospitalization, with lower rates for higher-status groups. These findings begin to suggest that considerable importance must be attributed to the effect of unemployment on psychiatric hospitalization although evidently it does not account for the majority of schizophrenic cases in the sample.

Of greater immediate importance is the fact that rates of unemployment begin to clarify a possible source of the relationship between social class and severe psychiatric disorder.[56] Rates of unemployment for the population of the United States as a whole increase quite markedly with decreasing occupational status. Thus, in any distribution by occupation, we can expect that the lower occupational statuses will contain higher proportions of unemployed persons. The few studies that do isolate rates of severe psychiatric disorder for the unemployed indicate their enormous preponderance over rates for the employed at any occupational level. It is quite reasonable to extrapolate from this conjunction of empirical data the likelihood that unemployment among lower occupational status groups accounts for some proportion of the high rates of severe psychiatric disorder in the same groups. The fact that there is a gradual attrition in employment among schizophrenics after hospitalization in no way belies this conclusion. Indeed, it is given some further support by the finding that, even under conditions of prior hospitalization, rates of unemployment are higher for lower-status groups and that unemployment following hospitalization tends to result in further and more frequent hospitalizations.

We can tentatively conclude that unemployment almost certainly accounts for some substantial proportion of severe psychiatric disorder; that it may well be one of the significant components linking lower social class status with high rates of psychiatric disorder; and that the very high rates of unemployment among Negroes may readily account for a significant portion of their high rates of psychiatric disorder. At the other end of the scale, a number of studies show increasing rates of work satisfaction with increasing occupational status.[57] At least one study shows an association between work satisfaction and mental health ratings.[58] In these results, therefore, we may hope that one can begin to clarify the dynamic factors in occupational position and employment status that account for a persisting but otherwise unexplained relationship.

Social Mobility

Although the potential importance of downward social mobility as a factor in explaining the relationship between social class and mental illness is self-evident, the literature in this area is particularly weak.[59] Not only are there very few studies but the samples are small and insufficient consideration is given to the population base against which mobility rates can be evaluated.

Thus, in trying to evaluate the data we are confronted with the technical difficulties of assessing social mobility: Which are the most appropriate indicators? Do we consider intergenerational or intragenerational mobility? What life-cycle status of parents or patients do we employ? How do we evaluate the social mobility status of women? Certainly of equal importance and of even greater technical difficulty is the effort to determine social mobility rates. Rates of social mobility necessitate an adequate estimate of the frequency of upward and downward mobility and of status stability in the population at risk. Even those studies that compare the occupational distribution of sons and fathers do not take account of differences in mobility rates for the population during the two periods a generation apart. Nonetheless, the issue is of such central importance that we cannot neglect it.

There are only ten studies of the relationship between social mobility and psychiatric disorder. Among these, seven suggest that there are higher proportions of downward social mobility (and/or lower proportions of upward social mobility) among the psychiatrically disturbed than are to be expected.[60] Three suggest that upward social mobility is not disproportionately low nor is downward social mobility disproportionately high among people with severe psychiatric disorders.[61] A brief review and elimination of some of these studies is necessary if we are to obtain any clarity about the cumulative impact of the findings.

We must reject two of the studies as totally inadequate for drawing conclusions about social mobility and mental illness. One study which contradicts the hypothesis warrants such rejection not only because of the great loss of cases but because of the many unjustified assumptions implicit in the use of an index based on residential changes classified according to median monthly rental.[62] Similarly, another study, supporting the hypothesis, must be excluded because of its lack of controls and its reliance on addresses and ratings of housing quality.[63] Dunham's recent analysis and support for the hypothesis cannot be included because of the absence of controls or of any other basis for comparing rates among psychiatric patients with rates for the population at risk. Clausen and Kohn's rejection of the hypothesis must be reinterpreted in light of the fact that, given the extreme categories they employ (consistent downward mobility, consistent upward mobility) their findings provide more support than contradiction for a relationship between social mobility and psychiatric disorder.[64] Thus, the percentage of consistent upward mobility among the control group is twice as great as among the schizophrenic group (16 percent vs. 8 percent) and a much smaller proportion of the controls fall into the category "fluctuation in level" than of the schizophrenics (2 percent vs. 8 percent). On the other hand, the fact that more than 50 percent of both the schizophrenic and control groups fell into the category of "all jobs—same occupational level" indicates that, at best, the relationship between psychiatric disorder and social mobility does not account for the majority of cases.

Despite reservations, we can tentatively conclude that the hypothesis that individuals with severe psychiatric disorders show either disproportionately low rates of upward mobility or disproportionately high rates of downward mobility is sustained. With the rejections of three reports and the reinterpretation of the findings in one report, there remain six instances of support for the hypothesis contrasted with one instance of rejection. There are a number of additional studies, using selected samples, which tend to give further support to the hypothesis.

A study based on earlier school records of a male schizophrenic sample and control, reveals the greater frequency, during school years, of differences and difficulties among the group who subsequently became schizophrenic, and this points toward the early development of performance failures.[65] The school staff more often perceived the boys who became schizophrenic as passive and withdrawing, and their scholastic records indicate a greater frequency of lower grades, school dropouts, and difficulties in course work. One study reports greater discrepancies between education and occupation for schizophrenic sons than for their fathers, a difference that is significantly different from the comparable ratio for nonschizophrenics and controls. It interprets these results, too unilaterally for the amount of variance it explains, to indicate that "while the schizophrenic patient may function long enough to obtain a certain level of education, the real test comes when he enters the job market. Here his traits, attitudes, mannerisms, and verbal reactions become only too obvious and operate against his securing a position in the work force and his advancement on the job." [66] The finding is supported by another study which shows that, up to the secondary school level, the school careers of schizophrenic patients compare favorably with the national average but rates of deterioration in school performance begin to increase from this time on. [67]

It is unfortunate that we try to seek in cross-sectional statistical analysis singular explanations for extremely complex phenomena. More often than not, social and psychological processes occur in spiral and mutually reinforcing or counteracting events. It is extremely rare to obtain results which are so overwhelming that they account for even the largest part of the variability in the dependent variable. There is no reason for assuming that because some proportion of the cases, even enough to effect a statistically significant difference, reveal patterns of early disorganization, this explanation precludes the existence of an alternative or opposite pattern. One clinical study of the work histories of schizophrenic patients offers greater clarity about this point with only 107 cases and no controls than do most analyses of large samples but with less detailed information and with less adequate opportunity for disaggregating their data on the basis of sequential relationships. [68] The study is particularly revealing by distinguishing four different patterns of work experience in a sample of schizophrenic patients. The distinctions indicate that less than 25 percent of the patients fall into the pattern of early onset and chronic difficulty, although for the group as a whole downward social mobility and high rates of prehospitalization unemployment were extremely frequent.

The difficulties of data interpretation are thus clearly manifest. If we accept the proposition that severe psychiatric disorder is associated with downward social mobility, to what extent does downward mobility play the critical causal role leading to psychiatric disorder? If this were the case, downward mobility as the determinant of psychiatric disorder would be an important factor in explaining the relationship between social class and mental illness. Conversely, to what extent does psychiatric disorder play a critical causal role in downward social mobility? If this were the case, it would also contribute to an explanation of the relationship between social class and mental illness. If both of these sequences operate, which we have suggested as most likely, an even greater explanatory role could be attributed to the relationship between social mobility and psychiatric disorder.

Indeed, this is the only conclusion we can draw. The data showing that psychiatric disorder is clearly associated with either high rates of downward social mobility or low rates of upward social mobility or both is, if not conclusive, quite clear. There is evidence to suggest that in some instances, probably a large minority, early signs of incipient psychiatric disorder influence subsequent mobility failures. There is also evidence to indicate that in some instances, probably something less than a majority, experiences of unemployment are significant causal factors leading to disorganization and psychiatric disorder. If the full complexity of social and psychological processes is considered, initial and quite transitory patterns of disorganization may lead to school failures or to work failures which may eventuate in further disorganization and a continuing cycle. Under these circumstances, to isolate one variable as determinant and the other as consequence is not only artificial but provides an inadequate conceptual model for finer definitions and research designs.

From the vantage point of the larger question, however, it becomes clear that disproportionately low rates of upward social mobility and disproportionately high rates of downward social mobility among persons with severe psychiatric disorders do help to account for the highly consistent and frequently powerful association between social class and mental illness. Along with such other factors as unemployment and marital disruption, which may also serve as either or both cause and effect of psychiatric disorder, the significant implication of social mobility begins to transform a static conception of the relationship of social class position to mental illness into a framework for understanding the social dynamics of this relationship.

Poverty and Powerlessness

It is hardly accidental that, although our purpose has been to discuss the relationship between poverty and mental health, we have dealt neither with poverty nor with mental health. The reasons for dealing primarily with mental illness and, within this broad category, with severe psychiatric disorders have already been mentioned. The reasons for dealing with social class rather than with poverty are not dissimilar. Poverty is an empirical category, not a conceptual entity, and it represents congeries of unrelated problems: unemployment and underemployment, the condition of the aged, the situation of the Negro, the consequences of physical illness, inadequacies in welfare policy and migration, inadequate preparation for the urban environment, changes in agriculture, and the deterioration of rural areas. The problems posed by poverty are not readily accessible for study or resolution in the name of poverty. Like psychiatric disorder, poverty is a social fact that requires explanation. It can serve as an entry into a set of issues which may be examined and changed.

The use of poverty or income levels in studies of social behavior is infrequent largely because such studies have revealed fewer uniformities than other indicators of social class.[69] Even for those forms of social behavior that presumably are most directly responsive to available financial resources, like consumer behavior or choice of housing, educational achievement, occupational status, or cultural orientation are more likely to be closely implicated than is income as such.

Some of the issues involved in the relationship of poverty as an empirical phenomenon and social class as a conceptual entity can only be clarified by extensive theoretical discussion. Even if we translate the conception of social class into empirically definable phenomena like educational attainment and occupational status, there is little enough data on which to base detailed analysis. We know that these variables show moderately high intercorrelations but not much beyond this. To a considerable extent, therefore, just as we have implied a relationship between poverty and mental illness in discussing social class and mental illness, we will base our discussion of poverty largely on what we know about low educational and occupational status.

All of the variables we have considered are objective social events. In this sense we have been dealing with objective social phenomena to explain objective social events and a straightforward association between two sets of social facts. Although it is not theoretically necessary that intervening psychological processes mediate these events, with phenomena so complex it seems essential to assume internal responses to these events, responses which affect the likelihood that particular consequent events will occur. It would be difficult to explain psychiatric disorder on the basis of prior unemployment without assuming that unemployment is experienced as a threat, a loss, a disruption, or a provocation. Similarly, in explaining the fact that unemployment sometimes leads to psychiatric disorder, other times to halfhearted job-seeking or increased determination to find a job, we imply that unemployment is experienced differently by different men and/or that the necessity, possibility, and desirability of employment are differently perceived by different men. The framework may be one of motivation, cognitive orientation, and attitudinal disposition, or it may be formulated as feedback processes in an information network. But the central importance of a psychological organism experiencing and responding to social events is common to these formulations.

From this psychological point of view, what are the components of social class generally and of poverty specifically that are likely to explain the disproportionate frequency of psychiatric disorder at lower levels of the scale? Hagstrom states the issues most cogently:

> The situation of poverty . . . is the situation of enforced dependency, giving the poor very little scope for action, in the sense of behavior under their own control which is central to their needs and values. This scope for action is supposed to be furnished by society to any person in either of two ways. First, confidence, hope, motivation, and skills for action may be provided through childhood socialization and continue as a relatively permanent aspect of the personality. Second, social positions are provided which make it easy for their occupants to be implemented in their futures. Middle class socialization and middle class social positions customarily both provide bases for effective action; lower class socialization and lower class social positions usually both fail to make it possible for the poor to act.[70]

Hagstrom stresses powerlessness as the critical factor in the psychology of poverty, mirroring the enforced dependency of the poor on the agencies of society. Powerlessness can be quite general or highly specific. Poverty as the absence of power to control goods and services represents only one form of powerlessness. For a college student, or a religious man who has taken vows of poverty, this form of powerlessness may be quite specific and limited. For those people who represent the largest proportion of the poor, powerlessness in the market is coupled with most other forms of powerlessness in society and becomes a highly general phenomenon.

Powerlessness or a sense of powerlessness may attend an individual's economic situation, his social status, or his political control. Lower class persons most frequently and quite vividly sense their powerlessness in economic choices, in social and occupational decisions, and in political access. The Negro, for whom the avenues to modest power are often closed, has given increased emphasis to "Black Power" and community-wide efforts to alter his powerlessness in all these spheres. Strikingly, however, the emergence of lower status groups as "countervailing powers" does not readily alter the widespread sense of powerlessness among the rank and file who now must deal with a new, if more responsive and more closely identified, bureaucracy or leadership. Perhaps the reason for this lies in the immediacy and urgency of economic powerlessness which, even if welfare agencies are available to stave off starvation, allows virtually no options and no sense of self-esteem and participation in one's own fate. It is an ultimate form of enforced situational dependency.

It seems reasonable to link the sense of powerlessness to the development of psychiatric disorder. Most of the social factors which help to explain the association of social class and psychiatric disorder can readily be understood as stimuli to an increased sense of powerlessess. Whether this is the single most general and useful conceptual formulation is not altogether clear. However, the sense of powerlessness does have this high degree of generality; it can potentially include these diverse social events, and there are few alternative psychological variables that meet these qualifications. In the absence of relevant data we can try to examine the adequacy of this variable by simulating imaginary data. Let us consider, for example, a situation in which unemployment leads to psychiatric disorder. For the person who is unemployed, a number of options exist. In order to accept the precarious and threatening option of psychological and behavioral disorganization leading to psychiatric disorder, he would have to find other options completely intolerable and feel powerless either to expand the range of options or to alter the definition of the situation which makes other options intolerable. Alternatively, we might say that he feels hopeless rather than powerless. He might, of course, be hostile or diffident but these appear to lead to determined or sporadic efforts to find another job. Hopelessness, we may note, implies the expectation that no external change will occur; powerlessness implies the expectation that one has no control over his own destiny.

Another conjectured situation may help to discriminate between these conceptions. Let us imagine a case in which, with no prior evidence of malfunctioning, the incompatibility of two marital partners leads to divorce, which eventuates in psychiatric disorder for one of the partners. As the statistical findings indicate, this is considerably more likely to occur to husbands than to wives. Hostility or diffidence are likely to be frequent responses but would not account for increasing disorganization. Hopelessness is certainly a possibility assuming the man's thoughts tend toward remarriage coupled with feelings of inadequacy. With these feelings of inadequacy, of course, we approach a sense of powerlessness. But why is psychiatric disorder associated with marital disruption more frequently for women than for men? Are men more likely to feel hopeless in response to marital disruption than women? This seems unreasonable, particularly since the realistic situation of the divorced or separated women, who most often maintain the children, is more complex, more difficult, and more realistically hopeless. It is not obvious that men are more likely to feel powerless than are women in this situation except for the fact that, in our society, divorce or separation implies that the man has not maintained adequate control over the marriage even if the immediate cause is the wife's dissatisfaction, her sexual inadequacy or infidelity, or her desire to attain greater independence and freedom. And this conception of the man's responsibility for the inviolability of the marriage is more frequently at lower social class levels.

It would be pointless to carry this imaginary simulation beyond these few examples. Clearly, we cannot expect to obtain conclusive evidence nor even a clear delineation of the alternative psychological processes that might intervene between social disruption and psychiatric disorder. In the absence of virtually any effort to link a relationship between social class factors and psychiatric disorder through intervening psychological processes, and in view of the lack of any attempt, in the data on psychological processes in psychiatric malfunctioning, to tie these processes to antecedent social events, some initial formulation seems essential. The sense of powerlessness appears to be a potentially important psychological variable that is meaningfully tied to social class position and to social disruptions and transitions that are frequent among lower social class people. At the same time, it provides a useful bridge to the development of psychiatric disorder. The primary purpose of this imaginary simulation, however, is as much methodological as substantive. It serves to indicate the ways in which psychological processes can implement and further clarify the analysis of relationships between an antecedent and a consequent social event.

Even assuming the substantive importance of a sense of powerlessness as a consequence of lower social class position and as a determinant of psychiatric disorder, there is no reason to believe that the form of powerlessness associated with poverty is of any greater significance in this sequence than the forms of powerlessness associated with deprivations of social position and opportunity. On the one hand, as our review of the data has indicated, the relationship between income variables and psychiatric disorder is, if anything, more tenuous than the relationship of psychiatric disorder to other social class factors. On the other hand, there is a wider variety of resources available for emergency and longer-term assistance with poverty than for other forms of deprivation. One of the merits of the conception of sense of powerlessness is that it provides a common psychological base for the impact of different forms of deprivation. In the light of current data, one can only conclude that if poverty per se is closely linked to psychiatric disorder, it must be through some intervening psychological mechanism which also bears the burden of other forms of deprivation.

Psychiatric Disorder and Hospitalization

We have devoted considerably more attention to those variables we have regarded as independent or antecedent than to those we have viewed as dependent or consequent. Apart from an initial formulation posing a social view of psychiatric disorder, we have not dealt with class differences in the manifestations, the processing, or the consequences of psychiatric malfunctioning. While this is a large and complex subject for review in its own right, it is essential that we consider at least some of the more promising directions of current investigation.

Relatively little attention has been devoted to social class differences in the phenomenology of psychiatric disorder. Two major contributions to the literature devote most of their analysis to early experience and precipitating events that distinguish people with effective functioning from those with psychiatric impairments.[71] One of the few findings that is beginning to emerge with some degree of consistency is the emphasis on physical symptoms, physical interpretations of psychological symptoms, and an organic conception of psychiatric disorder and treatment among lower class patients. This difference appears to be quite general and holds for different degrees of psychiatric impairment.[72]

The explanation for this finding is not clear. To what extent is there a difference in organic symptomatology, in preimpairment experiences of organic illness, in understanding and conceptualization of psychological processes, in the forms of defense and the denial of mental illness, in the bases for legitimizing sick roles? Some data from Puerto Rico point to striking differences between schizophrenic and control families in physical illness, hospitalization for physical illness, and experiences of illness and death in the family.[73] It is reasonable to interpret these findings to suggest that recent histories of severe or protracted illness, more frequent among the lowest-status groups, color the experience of mental illness and may more often initiate psychological disorganization among lower-class people. Unfortunately, there is nothing in the available data to preclude the opposite interpretations: that early signs of psychological disorganization are viewed as physical illness and that psychosomatic pathways for the expression of malfunctioning are more readily available to lower-class people.

Class differences in psychiatric disorder may be affected by social and professional responses to malfunctioning. The data concerning social class differences in response to disordered behavior suggest that, whatever the intrinsic differentials in rates of disordered behavior, individuals from the lower social classes are more likely to be extruded and hospitalized, and more likely to receive more serious diagnoses and inadequate treatment. Several studies suggest that lower-class families and communities have lower levels of tolerance for disordered behavior and more readily seek hospitalization for malfunctioning family or community members.[74] In view of results indicating minimal class differentials in tolerance and different paths to treatment in different social classes, we may wonder whether the fairly evident difference in extrusion is due to different tolerances in family and community or, rather, to the different role of public representatives and professionals in encouraging higher rates of psychiatric hospitalization.[75]

Differences in diagnosis due to implicit or explicit social class characteristics have only recently become evident. Hollingshead and Redlich hypothesized and several studies demonstrated this effect. Thus, Haase has shown remarkable discrepancies in the interpretation of paired examiner-constructed Rorschach protocols when these were associated with different social histories stressing the different social class background for each pair of protocols.[76] A careful analysis of casework records similarly reveals that social workers' evaluations of the treatability of clients is inversely related to the social class position of clients.[77] Perhaps the most striking finding was that the lower the social class of patients coming to the emergency ward of a general hospital, the more likely he was to be diagnosed as alcoholic even when identical signs and symptoms of alcoholism were reported by the intake physician for people in other social class positions.[78] Differences in treatment-experience by social class were also first reported systematically by Hollingshead and Redlich. Although this issue has been accorded little replication, several studies agree with their data in showing the diminished expectations of treatability for lower class patients, a lower rate of acceptance for treatment, and a higher dropout rate from treatment.[79]

The data are clearly inadequate for allowing us to discriminate between the social events surrounding psychiatric malfunctioning which may lead to psychiatric hospitalization and the social factors antecedent to malfunctioning in accounting for the observed relationship between social class and mental disorder. They are, however, sufficiently striking to warrant greater attention and encourage more carefully designed studies in which several explanatory variables can be examined simultaneously.

Interrelationships Between Forms of Disordered Functioning

As we move from relatively simple efforts to study the relationship between two variables such as social class and mental illness to more complex relationships that not only deal with a large number of variables, but attempt to delineate sequences of determinism and directions of interaction, the theoretical formulation begins to approximate the reasonably life-sized conceptualization but the methodological and analytic problems become enormous. Indeed, only in passing have we suggested some of the complexities that go far beyond any we have discussed in detail. Some of these, however, are worthy of discussion if only to point up the great need for recursive analytic models that more closely approximate, not merely our theoretical wisdom, but some self-evident aspects of the processes in the development of illness and disorder. Two of the most critical of these issues are: (1) the interrelationship between different types of pathology and disordered functioning and the different patterns of health and welfare services associated with them; and (2) the cumulative and spiraling effects of deprivations, problems, stresses, and crises which culminate in the situation of families with multiple, chronic problems.

Little research has been done on the interrelationships between different types of disordered functioning or on the interrelationships between different patterns of health and welfare agency usage. The literature is barren and leaves the issue open to wholly unsupported conjectures. Indeed, not only are these interrelationships important in their own right but the absence of information raises serious questions about any study in which the dependent variable is either some form of malfunctioning or some form of contact with professional health and welfare resources. If we make several conventional and unsubstantiated assumptions about malfunctioning and the use of professional services, of course, this problem does not arise. These assumptions are that (1) different forms of malfunctioning like mental disorder, physical illness, drug addiction, alcoholism, delinquency, and social problems are discrete, conceptually unrelated to one another, and technically distinguishable one from the other; and (2) specialized professional health and welfare services are designed to deal with specific forms of malfunctioning and, through distinguishable paths to treatment and proper diagnosis, an accurate sort is made between the form of malfunction and the service specialty. These assumptions are probably more widespread among professionals working in the health and welfare fields than most social scientists are wont to imagine and enter into the scientific study of these problems.

If one makes these assumptions, some contrary evidence invariably intrudes itself. Over the past few decades it has gradually come to be accepted that a very large proportion, probably more than half, of the persons coming for medical assistance have no physical illness or disability but show signs of emotional impairment or behavioral malfunction. For the most part, juvenile courts have accepted the necessity of having a court psychiatrist who could distinguish the psychiatric case from the delinquent. Most social agencies maintain an extensive roster of medical and psychiatric consultants, not merely for general consultation but quite specifically for help with cases in which the predominant form of malfunction is physical or psychological. Similarly, social workers in psychiatric services have long served multiple functions, including greater attention to the social background of mental illness. One could continue to expand this list but there is, to our knowledge, not a single piece of research that carefully documents this problem with respect to multiple forms of malfunctioning and multiple forms of services used or to the relationship between paths to treatment and characteristics other than intrinsic features of the disordered functioning.

If it is the case, however, that many individuals show multiple forms of disordered functioning, and there is a great likelihood that any one form of disordered functioning will show up in individuals who already show other forms of disordered functioning, then our empirical and analytic categories for disordered functioning must be revised. If a large proportion of the population falls either into the "no professional services" category or into the "multiple professional services" category, and relatively few in the "one professional service" category, then our conceptions of health and welfare services have to be reviewed.

If most professional services deal with a multitude of different problems, many of which might be more appropriate to another service, then studying a particular form of disorder through any case count based on a discrete conception of disorders or on discrete services is bound to commit serious miscalculations due both to false positives (cases counted which do not properly belong) and to false negatives (cases uncounted). If any of these contentions is correct, it suggests that, in addition to independent estimates of disorder and of health or welfare agency contact, we must take account of the potential "false negatives" —those individuals who might have been counted but are using a different kind of service. This means that most of our estimates of the relationship between social or psychological variables and disordered functioning should be made against a background of all forms of disordered functioning or all forms of health and welfare service contact.

For purposes of understanding the relationship of social class and mental illness, these considerations provide us only with suggestive clues. Most forms of disordered functioning show some relationship to social class differences. The lowest social class groups have the highest proportions of disorder for suicide and mental retardation, while delinquency, crime alcoholism, drug addiction, and other social problems show some association with social class. Kadushin argues that this inverse relationship no longer holds in modern societies but the data he presents are ambiguous, and important technical questions raise doubts about his argument.[80] He questions the accuracy of disability days lost as indicators of physical illness but accepts the data for chronic illness as an accurate count of illness. Is the diagnosis of chronic illness completely independent of reactions to illness and disability days lost solely a consequence of such reactions? It may be that low status people more readily stay away from work on minimal physical grounds, as Kadushin implies, and, at the very same time, fail to recognize, and come to professional attention for, chronic illness they suffer. If this is so, the data on chronic illness are subject to as many questions as are the data on time lost due to illness. Indeed, more recent statistics from the National Health Survey indicate that the social class (income) difference for disability days is far greater for the categories "restricted activity" and "bed disability" than for "work loss," and the category "hospital" shows almost no class difference (and, we might add, includes an extremely small proportion of the cases in any income group).[81]

On this basis, it seems quite reasonable to include physical illness among the list of disorders which show the highest rates among the lowest social class groups. The essential point is that the congruence of these findings necessarily implies either or both of two conclusions: that the over-all relationship between social class and any single form of disordered functioning is far greater than the relationship between social class and any single form of disordered functioning, and/or that the likelihood of multiple contacts with professional services is disproportionately high among lower social class groups.

Cumulative Impact in the Determinants
of Psychiatric Disorder

These considerations lead quite naturally to the problem of the multiple or cumulative effects of diverse forms of deprivation, disruption, and difficulty of disordered functioning. If we were to read the literature on disordered functioning and were to record all the factors that have been implicated for that form of disordered functioning, we might well collect a volume of substantial size. Undoubtedly a large proportion of these factors would disappear with a few careful studies devoted to the exclusion rather than the inclusion of variables. Nonetheless, even those studies which control for a modest number of variables rarely emerge with single variables that would account for most of the variance. But it seems that a large number of theoretically independent but empirically intercorrelated forms of deprivation and disruption during all phases of the life cycle contribute to psychiatric disorder and that, in turn, psychiatric disorder contributes to or exacerbates many different situations of deprivation and disruption.

The Midtown study is one empirical examination that presents controlled analyses of a wide variety of deprivations and disruptions during childhood and adulthood.[82] While it could dismiss many variables as spurious, there remained a huge number of variables which separately bore modest relationships to impairment ratings, and a fairly large number showed strong, independent relationships to psychiatric impairment. In addition to age, socio-economic status, and marital status, there were eight composite childhood factors and six composite adult factors. Of greatest interest is the fact that the sheer number of negative sociocultural background factors (mainly deprivations and disruptions) reported by individuals showed the strongest relationship to mental health risk. No single experience was implicated either as a primary cause or as a uniquely important precipitating event. It may be, therefore, that our usual expectation that a single major factor will account for a large part of the variance is inappropriate for the investigation of psychiatric disorder, that many diverse factors have minor and independent determining effects and that only their cumulative effect serves as a potent and highly general determinant of mental illness.

Although experiences of deprivation and disruption were more frequent among the lower socio-economic status groups, these differences were not sufficient to account for the great differences in mental health risk. With the number of stressful experiences held constant, the lower socio-economic status groups showed much higher mental health risks. At the low stress extreme, where there were virtually no reported experiences of deprivation or disruption, the different social class groups showed almost identical (and low) mental health risks, but at the other extreme of high stress, the mental health risk among the lower social class groups was disproportionately higher than among the higher social class groups. Langner points to three alternative hypotheses that might account for these findings: (1) social class differences in inner personality resources with greater resilience and resistance to impairment among higher-status groups; (2) social class differences in external resources which are less frequently available to lower-status groups for helping in stress; and (3) differences in meaning of the same reported experience for different class groups with higher thresholds among lower-status people who might report only more pathogenic experiences.

It is not possible to discriminate among these hypotheses from the available data nor to support or reject several other relevant hypotheses. Three other hypotheses in particular warrant consideration in trying to interpose dynamic sequences in the relationship between social class and mental illness: the role of selective (pathological) factors in producing lower social class status as opposed to social class as a source of frequent pathogenic influences; the cumulative impact of disruptions and deprivations; and the more complex formulation of converging psychological and social forces in producing psychopathology. We have already shown that many of the reported findings can be interpreted as consequences of pathological influences in producing lower social class status or as the particularly severe and pathogenic effects of deprivation and disruption on lower-class people. The evidence is quite unambiguous that selective factors cannot possibly account for all of the findings but, beyond this, the issue remains open. The most reasonable hypothesis is that both types of relationships operate. However, even if the alternatives can be stated in the form of a critical test, there remain serious problems in the differential definition and conception of symptoms and disorder in different social class and subcultural groups that lead to difficulties in the very categorization of the dependent variable, psychiatric disorder.[83]

The hypothesis that gives importance to cumulative effects of disruption and deprivation involves two components: that deprivation and disruption are more frequent among people in lower social class positions; and that these deprivations and disruptions are not merely additive but each additional stress has increasingly greater impact among lower-status people. Indeed, this is one way of interpreting Langner's data, which show a steeper curve of increasing mental health risk with increasing numbers of stress factors among lower than among higher-status people. Clinical and participant observation reveal that, in addition to the generic importance of a sense of powerlessness associated with social class position itself, experiences of deprivation and disruption tend to intensify feelings that the total situation has gone beyond the point of control. Is there a point, differing by social class positions, at which this sense of powerlessness frequently becomes overwhelming and results in disorganized behavior? This seems to be a reasonable conjecture that bears closer examination in empirical study.

Closely related to the cumulative stress hypothesis but theoretically more complex is the formulation derived from a principle of psychosocial complementarity.[84] In an application to the development of psychiatric disorder, this formulation would hold the following:

1. Among adults, reliance on personality resources and on social resources tend to be mutually exclusive, a pattern that results from structural features both of personality and of social roles.

2. Such predominance and acceptance of either role-determination or of personality-determination are complementary patterns and allow for modest, progressive change within a relatively stable context.

3. The simultaneous absence of opportunities for clear role-determination and for clear personality-determination or the simultaneous presence of powerful inner and outer resources are noncomplementary patterns which are inherently unstable and facilitate either uncertainty and withdrawal or anxiety-laden and nonrational actions.

4. Deprivation and disruption exacerbate rapid changes in role-demands and role-expectations and place increased burdens on either the supportive functions of external resources or the coping functions of internal resources.

5. People of lower social class backgrounds and statuses less frequently have developed the inner resources for rapid adaptation to changes in role-demands and, under conditions of severe stress, go beyond the resources of informal or formal social networks, organizations, and agencies in their needs for support and assistance.

6. Under these circumstances, given identical phenomena of deprivation and disruption, people in lower social class positions

readily develop noncomplementary patterns while people in higher social class positions can maintain themselves at a more modest level of disorganization in relatively complementary patterns.

This formulation implies that the situation of lower social class groups is more vulnerable by virtue of their intrinsic dependence on external support under conditions in which, at best, such support can be provided for short periods of time and quite conditionally. At the same time, the pace of modern social change frequently places large lower-class populations in situations which exacerbate the need for coping with changing role-expectations without preparation for the internal demands involved and without appropriate external facilities for assistance in adaptation. Most of the social factors that have been implicated as components or intervening factors in the relationship between social class and psychiatric disorder can be seen as precisely such forms of deprivation or disruption, changes that can be conceived as opportunities or threats depending on the inner preparedness and the external resources to facilitate their definition as meaningful options rather than as disorganizing threats.

We are far from an adequate theoretical or empirical appreciation of the complex processes that might meaningfully account for the persistent finding that lower social class groups show the highest rates of psychiatric disorder. At the same time, the meaning of mental health cannot adequately be understood as a set of traits, competences, or achievements independent of the social matrix in which they function. The effort to develop a reasonable nosology and a fund of information concerning the attributes and consequences of those phenomena labeled physical or mental illness was a great achievement for the nineteenth and the early twentieth century. By the middle of the twentieth century, it became increasingly evident that social factors were of such great importance in the definition, conception, symptomatology, visibility, diagnosis, and response to treatment that a fuller examination of the host of problems was essential.

The relationship between social class and mental illness is only one special case of this more general issue, of particular practical and theoretical importance because of the needs of the population involved and because of the relative clarity of the relationship. But further development of our understanding demands a far more open conception and far greater challenge to existing conceptual investments. We have yet to learn about the dynamics of social class positions and their psychological implications and about the dynamics of psychological disorganization and its interrelationships with social processes in order to account more fully for massive findings that are all too often massively denied.

V · Prevention of Illness
and Maintenance of Health

by Irwin M. Rosenstock

This chapter will explore the problem of whether the seeking of preventive or diagnostic services is associated with income, and if so, why the association exists. In the present context poverty will be considered, insofar as possible, in its literal sense of paucity of money. Thus, the effects of low income upon behavior will be separated from the effects of educational status upon behavior. But it is perfectly apparent that in reality income is not disassociated from other characteristics. The socio-economic and racial characteristics are usually found in combination and it is only on the analytic level that they can be separated.

It will be shown that there are striking correlations between poverty and health behavior as defined below. It will be of importance, however, to go beyond a mere description of the associations and consider whether income itself accounts for differential responses or whether personal and social factors related to income are also involved in the causal sequence. To the extent that the former is true, social policy in the health area could be based on the effort to make services available at ever decreasing financial costs in the confident expectation that this approach alone would be effective in stimulating the poor to obtain the needed health services. On the other hand, if it should be found that health behavior cannot be explained entirely by income, the social policy issues would be much more complex because they would necessitate identifying the factors associated with income which help to account for public response to health services, and the development of intervention strategies which either alter these factors or obviate their role.

INCOME AND PREVENTIVE BEHAVIOR

Kasl and Cobb have distinguished among health behavior, illness behavior and sick-role behavior.[1] The latter two refer respectively to behavior undertaken by persons who feel ill, for the purpose of defining the state of their health, or activities undertaken by persons who consider themselves ill, for the purpose of getting well. Health behavior, however, is defined as the activity undertaken by persons who believe themselves to be healthy, for the purpose of preventing or detecting disease in an asymptomatic stage. Although the distinctions among the three forms of behavior are not perfect, the intent in the present chapter is to focus principally upon health behavior.

Unfortunately, most of the relevant studies have focused on illness behavior or sick-role behavior.[2] They are either frankly restricted to the behavior of persons who believe themselves to be ill, or they include composite data on all three classes of health-related behavior. Thus, generalizations drawn from such studies cannot be readily applied to the description and understanding of the key questions in this chapter: do relatively poor people take asymptomatic health action less often than those who are less poor, and, if so, why?

A small number of studies have focused specifically and exclusively on such preventive or diagnostic health behavior.[3] But even these studies of preventive behavior are of limited value since they were performed on relatively small samples or in highly restricted geographic regions. Moreover, most of them obtained measures at only one point in time, precluding the analysis of behavioral consistency over time, and they dealt with responses to a single health condition, eliminating the possibility of assessing the consistency of behavior for several health conditions.

One study has attempted to overcome such limitations.[4] A nationwide study of health beliefs and health behavior was undertaken with a probability sample of the adult United States population living in private households. The interview focused on beliefs and actions concerning dental disease, tuberculosis, and cancer—diseases selected to provide a range of clinical severity. The respondents were questioned about visits to physicians during the preceding five years for medical checkups or tests; visits to dentists during the preceding three years for prophylactic purposes in the absence of symptoms; frequency of toothbrushing practices; and frequency of examinations or tests for detection of tuberculosis or cancer during the preceding ten years.

Fifteen months later, a resurvey of half of the sample was taken, inquiring about the same aspects of behavior during the fifteen-month interval. The findings provide information on the extent of preventive actions, the consistency of preventive behavior, and the personal factors associated with taking such actions.

It was found that about one third of the eligible public had not visited physicians for checkups during the previous five years, about half had not made a prophylactic visit to the dentist within the last three years, and nearly half had failed to brush their teeth after a single meal on the day preceding the interview. Nearly half who could have taken voluntary tuberculosis tests in the absence of symptoms failed to take a single test in the past ten years, and only about one in twenty who could have taken a voluntary test for cancer while asymptomatic had received any such test in the same period. It is thus clear that though each of the preventive health actions, except screening tests for cancer, was taken by a substantial proportion of the public, a sizable number who could have taken each of the preventive actions did not do so.

The issue of the consistency of health behavior was subdivided into two questions: did members of the sample display consistency of behavior across the different health actions, and did they behave consistently with respect to given actions over time? To answer these questions, persons who had taken and those who had failed to take a given action on a voluntary, asymptomatic basis were compared to determine the extent to which they had taken a combination of the other three actions. For example, those who had visited their physicians for a checkup and those who had not were compared for the total number of other actions they had taken. In each instance, those who took a particular action had significantly higher scores on a combination of other behaviors than those who failed to take the action, though the differences were modest in size. The fact that behavior in the various preventive actions was consistent beyond chance expectations can be regarded as supporting the idea that people displayed a generalized pattern of response concerning preventive health action. However, such consistency was present only to a moderate degree.

To determine whether people behaved consistently over time, voluntary actions reported in the original survey were compared with those reported in the resurvey. For one analysis, the four separate actions were combined into an over-all index of preventive behavior with each action given equal weight. When the index scores of individual respondents on the two occasions were compared, a marked consistency of behavior was observed. In other analyses, a non-chance consistency of behavior over time for each of the four separate actions studied was found; that is, persons who reported in the original survey that they took an action also tended in the resurvey to report having taken that action again. Similarly, those who reportedly failed to take an action when originally questioned subsequently tended to report a similar failure. These data and those cited earlier support the tenability of the idea of a general behavioral orientation, although the strength of that orientation is limited.

As for differences associated with income and socio-economic status, the data indicate that there is a strong association between income level, other personal characteristics, and the proportion of persons visiting the physician for checkups, visiting the dentist for prophylaxis, and obtaining chest X-rays. However, the association between income and reported frequency of brushing one's teeth "yesterday after one or more meals," though statistically significant, was much smaller than the former associations. It seems reasonable to conclude from these data that where substantial cost is involved, those with more income are far more likely to use the service than those in poorer financial circumstances. But where the action in question, i.e., tooth-brushing, involves only minimal or no cost, such differences are greatly reduced though still present. This finding is consistent with the observation noted by Kadushin that, while there are consistent income-related differences in the obtaining of medical care in the United States, such differences occur less often in the United Kingdom, where care is available through the National Health Service.[5]

A number of studies of more limited scope, investigating the association between income and the acceptance of preventive and/or screening services, support the above findings consistently and to a remarkable extent. Level of income is positively associated with the proportion of persons seeking each of the several tests. It should be noted that educational level is also correlated with the frequency of taking preventive and diagnostic actions. Although it is difficult to separate the effects of education from those of income, nevertheless there is good basis for believing that the effects of education and of income upon preventive health behavior are at least partly independent. Two bases for this connection can be provided. One of these is found in the Kegeles study which shows that income accounts for a larger proportion of the variation in taking a Papanicolaou test than does education.[6] If the correlation between income and behavior were wholly or largely attributable to education, one would not expect the income association to be greater than the educational association. A second basis is the earlier mentioned finding that income appears to make more difference for behaviors that usually entail expense. Again, if the income-behavior correlation were spurious and attributable to education, then the failure to show a high correlation between income and engaging in cost-free actions is more difficult to explain.

In summary, virtually all relevant studies lead to the conclusion that income and preventive behavior are positively related. The higher the income level of a group, the more will they follow recommended preventive or diagnostic recommendations. However, it has been noted that the correlation is drastically reduced for tooth-brushing, an item entailing minimal expense, although it remains statistically significant. The bulk of the studies also show that even when direct cost is minimized or removed, as in the case of inexpensive or free chest X-rays or inoculations, income is still associated with health behavior. But it would be too simple to assume that cost has been removed in such cases, for there may be greater costs associated with taking inexpensive or even "free" actions than middle-class persons can readily appreciate. A one-dollar charge for a polio inoculation may seem small but, when multiplied by six children for four inoculations, it may represent one half to one percent of a family's annual income. The seemingly small cost of public transportation may impose considerable financial burden on the poor, and where paid baby-sitting is required, this also adds to the financial burden. Systematic studies have not been made of all of the costs of obtaining a so-called free service, but they exist in most circumstances where individuals desiring a service are required to obtain it at a facility some distance from their homes. It is thus by no means certain that economic factors do not play a significant role even where direct cost has been removed.

It would seem fair to conclude that removal of all financial barriers to health service might immediately lead to an increase in the proportion of poor people who use such service, but the result would fall far short of what is usually desired because large numbers of people would still refrain from taking the recommended action. Even at the highest levels of income large numbers of people, in one study as many as 37 percent, still fail to take the recommended action.[7] According to another study, as many as 40 percent of the highest income population failed to brush their teeth after one or more meals.[8] Thus, while income does provide a barrier to obtaining health services, the elimination of that barrier would by no means insure the desired response. It is necessary to look at the correlates of the decision to seek or not to seek a particular health service in the absence of symptoms.

HEALTH BELIEFS AND BEHAVIOR

Although research demonstrates that those with lower income are less likely to accept or seek preventive or diagnostic health services than those with higher income, it does not provide a simple explanation of why this is so. The cost of the service does not wholly account for the response of those at lower income levels since they are also more prone to avoid presumably free services and refrain to a greater extent from personal health practices which can be undertaken at nominal cost. We are thus left with a perplexing problem of explaining why poorer people are less likely than richer people to take inexpensive or free health services.

Several efforts to explain the phenomenon have been made.

One of the most comprehensive attempts proposes a model for explaining health behavior in individuals who believe themselves to be free of symptoms or illnesses. The major variables in the model are drawn and adapted from general social-psychological theory, notably from the work of Lewin.[9] The explanatory model links current subjective states of the individual with current health behavior.

It has become a truism in social psychology that motivation is required for perception and action. Thus, people who are unconcerned with a particular aspect of their health are not likely to perceive any material that bears on that aspect of their health; even, if through accidental circumstances, they do perceive such material, they will fail to learn, accept, or use the information. Not only is such concern or motivation a necessary condition for action; motives also determine the particular ways in which the environment will be perceived. That a motivated person perceives selectively in accordance with his motives has been verified in many laboratory studies as well as in field settings.[10]

The proposed model used to explain health behavior grows out of such evidence. Specifically, it includes two classes of variables: (1) the psychological state of readiness to take specific action, and (2) the extent to which a particular course of action is believed, on the whole, to be beneficial in reducing the threat. Two principal dimensions are presumed to define whether a state of readiness to act exists. They include the degree to which an individual feels vulnerable or susceptible to a particular health condition and the extent to which he feels that contracting that condition would have serious consequences in his case. Readiness to act is defined in terms of the individual's points of view about susceptibility and seriousness rather than the professional's view of reality. The model does not require that individuals be continuously or consciously aware of the relevant beliefs. Evidence suggests that the beliefs that define readiness have both cognitive (i.e., intellectual) and emotional elements.

Perceived susceptibility. There is a wide individual variation in the acceptance of personal susceptibility to a medical condition. At one extreme is the individual who during an interview may deny that there is any possibility of his contracting a given condition. In a more moderate position is the person who may admit to the possibility of the occurrence but who does not really believe it will happen to him. Finally, a person may express a feeling that he is in real danger of contracting the condition. In short, susceptibility refers to the subjective risks of contracting a condition.

Perceived seriousness. Convictions concerning the seriousness of a given health problem may also vary. There is reason to believe that the degree of seriousness may be judged both by the degree of emotional arousal created by the thought of a disease as well as by the kinds of difficulties the individual believes a given health condition will create for him.[11]

A person may, of course, see a health problem in terms of its medical or clinical consequences. He would thus be concerned with such questions as whether a disease could lead to death, or reduce his physical or mental functioning, or disable him permanently. However, the perceived seriousness of a condition may, for a given individual, include such broader and more complex implications as the effects of the disease on his job, family life, and social relations. A person may not believe that tuberculosis is medically serious, but may nevertheless believe that its occurrence would be serious by creating important psychological and economic tensions within his family.

Perceived benefits of taking action. The acceptance of one's susceptibility to a disease that is believed to be serious provides a force leading to action, but it does not define the particular course of action that is likely to be taken. The direction of the action is influenced by beliefs regarding the relative effectiveness of known available alternatives in reducing the disease threat. His behavior will depend on how beneficial he thinks the various alternatives would be. An alternative is likely to be seen as beneficial if it relates subjectively to the reduction of one's susceptibility to, or seriousness of, an illness. Again, it is the person's belief about the availability and effectiveness of various courses of action that determine the course taken.

Perceived barriers to taking action. An individual may believe that a given action will be effective in reducing the threat of disease but at the same time he may see that action as expensive, inconvenient, unpleasant, painful, or upsetting. Such negative aspects of health action arouse conflicting motives of avoidance. Several resolutions of the conflict are possible. If the readiness to act is high and the negative aspects are seen as relatively weak, an action is likely to be taken. If, on the other hand, the readiness is low while the potential negative aspects are seen as strong, they function as barriers to prevent action.

Where readiness and perceived barriers to action are great, the conflict is more difficult to resolve. The individual is highly oriented toward acting to reduce the likelihood of the perceived health danger. He is equally highly motivated to avoid action since he sees it as highly unpleasant. Sometimes, alternative actions of nearly equal efficacy may be available. For example, the person who feels threatened by tuberculosis but fears the potential hazards of X-rays, may choose to obtain a tuberculin test for initial screening.

But what can he do if the situation does not provide such alternative means to resolve his conflicts? Experimental evidence obtained outside the health area suggests that one of two reactions occur. First, the person may attempt to remove himself psychologically from the conflict situation by engaging in activities which do not really reduce the threat. Vacillating (without decision) between choices may be an example. Consider the individual who feels threatened by lung cancer and believes that stopping cigarette-smoking will reduce the risk, but for whom smoking serves important needs. He may constantly commit himself to give up smoking soon and thereby relieve, if only momentarily, the pressure imposed by the discrepancy between the barriers and the perceived benefits. A second possible reaction is a marked increase in fear or anxiety. If the anxiety or fear become strong enough, the individual may be rendered incapable of thinking objectively and behaving rationally about the problem. Even if he is subsequently offered a more effective means of handling the situation, he may not accept it simply because he can no longer think constructively about the matter.

Cues to action. The variables which constitute readiness to act (perceived susceptibility and severity), as well as the variables that define perceived benefits and barriers to taking action, have all been subjected to research that will be reviewed subsequently. One additional variable is believed to be necessary to complete the model but it has not been subjected to careful study.

It appears essential to include a factor that serves as a cue or a trigger to set off appropriate action. The level of readiness provides the energy to act and the perception of benefits (fewer barriers) provides a preferred path of action. However, the combination of these could reach quite considerable levels of intensity without resulting in overt action unless some instigating event sets the process in motion. In the health area, such events or cues may be internal (e.g., perception of bodily states) or external (e.g., interpersonal interactions, the impact of media of communication, knowledge).

The required intensity of a cue that is sufficient to trigger behavior presumably varies with differences in the level of readiness. With relatively low psychological readiness (i.e., little acceptance of susceptibility to, or severity of, a disease) rather intense stimuli will be needed to trigger a response. On the other hand, with relatively high levels of readiness even slight stimuli may be adequate. For example, other things being equal, the person who barely accepts his susceptibility to tuberculosis will be unlikely to check upon his health until he experiences rather intense symptoms (e.g., spitting blood). At the same time, the person who readily accepts his constant susceptibility to the disease may be spurred into action by the mere sight of a mobile X-ray unit or a relevant poster.

Unfortunately, the settings for most of the research on the model have precluded obtaining an adequate measure of the role of cues. Since the kinds of cues that have been hypothesized may be quite fleeting and of little intrinsic significance (e.g., a casual view of a poster urging chest X-ray), they may easily be forgotten with the passage of time. An interview taken months or years later could not adequately identify the cues. Freidson has described the difficulties in attempting to assess interpersonal influences as cues.[12] Furthermore, it seems reasonable to expect that respondents who have taken a recommended action in the past will be more likely to remember preceding events as relevant than will respondents who were exposed to the same events but never took the action. These problems make it most difficult to test the role of cues in any retrospective setting. It would seem that a prospective design, perhaps a panel study, will be required to assess properly how various stimuli serve as cues to trigger action in an individual who is psychologically ready to act.

EMPIRICAL EVIDENCE AND THE MODEL

Evidence for the importance of the variables described is considerable. Hochbaum studied more than one thousand adults in an attempt to identify factors underlying the decision to obtain a chest X-ray for the detection of tuberculosis.[13] He tapped beliefs in susceptibility to tuberculosis and beliefs in the benefits of early detection. Perceived susceptibility to tuberculosis contained two elements, the respondent's beliefs about the real possibility of tuberculosis in his case, and the extent of his accepting the fact that one may have tuberculosis in the absence of all symptoms. On the group of persons that exhibited both beliefs (that is, beliefs in their own susceptibility to tuberculosis and in the over-all benefits accruing from early detection), 82 percent had had at least one voluntary chest X-ray during a specified period preceding the interview. In the group exhibiting neither of these beliefs, only 21 percent had obtained a voluntary X-ray during the criterion period. It appears that a particular action is a function of the two interacting variables—perceived susceptibility and perceived benefits.

The belief in one's susceptibility to tuberculosis appeared to be the more powerful variable studied. For the individuals who exhibited this belief without accepting the benefits of early detection, 64 percent had obtained prior voluntary X-rays. Of the individuals accepting the benefits of early detection without accepting their susceptibility to the disease, only 29 percent had had prior voluntary X-rays. Hochbaum failed to show that perceived severity plays a role in the decision-making process. This may be due to the fact that his measures of severity proved not to be sensitive, thus precluding the possibility of obtaining definitive data.

Another study dealt with the conditions under which members of a prepaid dental care plan will come in for preventive dental checkups or for prophylaxis in the absence of symptoms.[14] While the findings generally support the importance of the model variables, an unusually large loss in the sample limits the general applicability of the study. Within the major limitations implied by a small sample, it was found that with successive increases in the number of beliefs exhibited by respondents from none to all three, the frequency of making preventive dental visits also increased. The actual findings show that (1) of three persons who were low on all three variables none made such preventive visits; (2) 61 percent of 18 who were high on any one variable but low on the other two made such visits; (3) 66 percent of 38 persons high on two beliefs and low on one, made preventive visits; and, finally, (4) 78 percent of 18 persons who were high on all three variables made preventive dental visits.

While none of the studies reviewed provides convincing confirmation for all of the variables, each has produced consistent findings in the predicted direction which, when taken together, provide strong support for the model. Any interpretations are based on an assumption. The hypothesis that behavior is determined by a particular constellation of beliefs can only be adequately tested where it is established that the beliefs existed prior to the behavior that they are supposed to determine. However, the studies reviewed have been undertaken in situations which necessitated identifying the beliefs and behavior at the same point in time. It had always been clear that this approach was quite dangerous. Work on cognitive dissonance supported these suspicions and suggested that the decision to accept or reject a health service may in itself modify the individual's perceptions in areas relevant to that health action.[15] Obviously, what was needed was a two-phase study in which beliefs would be identified at one point in time, and behavior measured later.

Such a study was undertaken in the fall of 1957 on the impact of Asian influenza on American community life.[16] Its design called for the first interview to be made before most people had the opportunity to seek vaccination or take other preventive action, and before much influenza-like illness had occurred in the communities; the second interview was to be made after all available evidence indicated that the epidemic had subsided. In fact, only partial success was achieved in satisfying these conditions because community vaccination programs as well as the spread of the epidemic moved much faster than had been anticipated. For these reasons the sample on which the test could be made was reduced to eighty-six. This sample had, at the time of initial interview, neither taken preventive action relative to influenza nor had they experienced influenza-like illness in themselves or in other members of their families. Of the twelve respondents who scored relatively high on a combination of beliefs in their own susceptibility to influenza and the severity of the disease, five subsequently made preventive preparations relative to influenza. On the other hand, of the remaining seventy-four persons (who were unmotivated in the sense of rejecting either their own susceptibility to the disease or its severity or both), only eight made subsequently preparations relative to influenza. The data thus suggest that prior beliefs are instrumental in determining subsequent action.

A second prospective study aimed to determine whether the beliefs identified during the original study were associated with behavior during the subsequent three-year period.[17] It found that neither perceptions of seriousness, whether considered independently or together with other variables, nor perceptions of benefits, taken alone, were related to subsequent behavior. However, the perception of susceptibility did show a correlation with making subsequent preventive dental visits. Fifty-eight percent of those who had earlier seen themselves as susceptible made subsequent preventive dental visits, but only 42 percent of those who had not accepted their susceptibility made such visits. When beliefs about susceptibility and benefits were combined, a more accurate prediction was possible. Considering only those who scored high on susceptibility, and cross-tabulating against beliefs in benefits, 67 percent of those high on both beliefs made subsequent preventive visits while only 38 percent low in benefits made such visits. Thus, the combination of susceptibility and benefits is demonstrated to be important in predicting behavior.

The results of the studies cited above lend support to the importance of several variables in the model as explanatory or predictive variables. However, another major investigation conflicts in most respects with the findings of earlier studies.[18] This study analyzes the beliefs and behavior of a probability sample of nearly 1500 American adults studied in 1963 and the subsequent behavior of a 40 percent subsample studied fifteen months later. Perceived susceptibility and severity, whether taken singly or in combination, did not account for a major portion of the variance in subsequent preventive and diagnostic behavior, although predictions based on the belief in benefits (and barriers) taken alone was significant. The findings did not disclose any explanation for the failure to obtain results similar to those of the earlier studies, but the national study was conducted in a setting which distinguished it from all the other reported studies. In the earlier studies, the settings had been such that the population in each case had been offered opportunity to take action through directed messages and circumstances that could have served as cues to stimulate action. In contrast, no such condition obtained for the national sample. With respect to the several health problems covered in the study, neither the sample nor the United States adult population, which it represents, had been uniformly exposed to intensive information campaigns about available services and persuaded to use such services.

It is not reasonable to assume that preventive and diagnostic services were equally available to all. It may well be that the absence of clear-cut cues to stimulate action as well as unequal opportunity to act may account in large measure for the failure to replicate the earlier results. However, those possibilities must be treated as hypotheses which need to be tested in new research.

It is beyond the scope of this chapter to provide a critique of the explanatory model. Such a critique is available elsewhere.[19] It is clear, however, that the bulk of evidence pertinent to the model supports the view that perceptions of susceptibility to, and the severity of, a health problem, perceptions about the benefits of taking preventive actions, and perceptions about the barriers standing in the way of the action are generally associated with decisions to accept or not a particular preventive or diagnostic service. It is suggested that where the applied constellation of beliefs exist, the presence of a situational cue, trigger, or critical incident is likely to trip off the desired response.[20] Where such cues are not present, the individual is presumed to be in a state of readiness without necessarily engaging in the appropriate behavior.

Health Beliefs and Income

It is appropriate now to turn to the question of the relationship between health beliefs and demographic factors. One study investigated the relationships among the use of Papanicolaou tests, demographic factors, and beliefs in the benefits of early detection of cancer.[21] Beliefs in benefits were measured by responses to questions on the perceived importance of early versus delayed treatment for cancer and on opinions as to whether medical checkups or tests could detect cancer before the appearance of symptoms. The findings disclose that personal characteristics and beliefs are highly correlated, with each of them making independent contributions to the understanding of behavior. Tests were much more likely to have been taken by women of higher income, who were relatively young, white, married, well educated, and of higher occupational levels. It was also shown that acceptance of the benefits of early professional detection and treatment was highly associated with having taken the test. However, it is the joint analysis that is of most interest. Within every demographic grouping, those who held a belief in benefits were much more likely to have taken the test than those not holding that belief. Similarly, within each of the belief categories, those with the appropriate demographic characteristics were much more likely to have taken the action than those who did not. It is clear that the joint effect of the beliefs and the personal characteristics is much greater than the effects of either alone.

Hochbaum's earlier study obtained similar findings. Socio-economic status (education and income) and the combination of beliefs in susceptibility and benefits were associated independently with having taken voluntary chest X-rays in the absence of symptoms. Within each socio-economic category, however, those who scored high on the combination of beliefs were much more likely to have taken the X-ray than those scoring low.

An interpretation of the two studies suggests that certain beliefs may be necessary for taking preventive or screening tests, but that they are unevenly distributed in the population and tend to be more prevalent among the higher-income females, the whites, the better educated, and the relatively young. It would thus appear that part of the association between income and the use of free preventive health actions is accounted for by an association between health beliefs and taking health actions. In short, poor people tend to exhibit the necessary constellation of beliefs far less often than people of higher income. Little evidence is available to indicate why this should be so although a number of variables seem particularly relevant to any effort to account for the findings.

The taking of a preventive or presymptomatic health action on a voluntary, health-motivated basis presumes both knowledge of disease processes and a value for, and interest in, planning for the future. To what extent are these characteristics related to differences in income? It has generally been shown that those with low income possess less information about health and disease than those with high income.[22] Even when educational attainment is controlled, a marked association has been found between income and the possession of correct information about health effects of insect and plant sprays, radioactive fallout and fatty foods.[23]

Studies of the mass communication media have long demonstrated that those lower on the economic scale fail to obtain health and science information from the mass media to the same extent as do those of higher income, although in terms of exposure the poor attend to health information transmitted via radio and television to about the same extent as the financially better off.[24] The previously established relationships, however, hold for exposure to the print media.[25] In short, nearly all available evidence supports the proposition that knowledge of health matters and exposure to health information is associated with income even when educational attainment is controlled.

There is some evidence that health is more salient to individuals of higher social status than those of lower socio-economic status. For example, when presented with a list of seventeen medically recognized danger signals, more than three quarters of the highest-class respondents checked all but two as requiring the attention of a doctor, while the lowest socio-economic group displayed a marked indifference to most signals, with 50 percent checking only three.[26] Two points are worthy of note. First, the salience of health is quite different in the several socio-economic groups and, second, the scale of values reflected in the findings may be quite functional. For people at subsistence levels the expenditure of money to ward off disease or check on symptoms that are not disabling may be a luxury which must be foregone in preference to providing food, clothing, and shelter. It cannot be surprising that many people who reported being unable to go to a dentist also owned television sets. Kadushin and Levine question whether health is less salient for the poor than for the rich, but the bulk of evidence supports the conclusion that middle and higher economic groups value health more than those in the lower economic groups.[27]

It has been noted that persons of lower status accord greater priority to immediate rewards than to the achievement of long-range goals.[28] Yet the system of health beliefs that has been described earlier requires an orientation toward the future, toward planning, and toward deferment of immediate gratification in the interest of long-range goals.

The data concerning salience of health and subjective time horizons are associated with the well-known finding that there is a high correlation between income and the extent of hospital and surgical insurance coverage.[29] Even with education held constant, the marked correlation between income and insurance status holds; those who need insurance the most, possess it to the least extent. Once again one may ask whether that finding reflects a rather rational assessment on the part of those who must choose between the necessities of today and the contingencies of tomorrow.

Another factor that generally distinguishes the poor from the economically more advantaged concerns their feelings of helplessness and psychological inability to cope with a hostile environment. It has been shown that such feelings tend to characterize the lower-economic group's response to local government and to social welfare.[30] We do not yet know whether and to what extent the concept of anomie carries over into one's responses to health matters, but it would seem reasonable to expect such a relationship.

A consideration of the institutional settings in which most health actions are taken may throw further light on the association of income and preventive action. It is clear that most preventive actions require the individual to enter into a professional health system. Yet, it has been noted that those lower on the socio-economic scale are more prone to use a lay referral system than a professional referral system, at least in the early stages of symptomatology.[31] If those of low income who experience symptoms are less likely to go to the physician than to friends and family, and will enter into the professional referral system only when they have exhausted lay remedies, they must be even more reluctant to enter the professional referral system when they are feeling reasonably well.

It would be well to recognize that the professional referral and care systems are middle-class institutions conceived by middle-class planners, oriented toward rationality in health matters, generally staffed by representatives of the middle class and, in the United States at least, involving a system of financial arrangements that are more feasible for the middle class to manage than for the lower classes. It does not seem surprising that members of the non-middle class may be reluctant to enter this foreign world.

The findings of research on health behavior support the conclusion that there is a culture of poverty that helps to explain the health behavior of the poor. The culture of poverty may originally be based on a history of economic deprivation, but it seems to be a culture exhibiting its own rationale, and structure, and reflecting a way of life that is transmitted to new generations. It is therefore suggested that while financial costs may serve as barriers to obtaining health services, their removal would probably not have the effect of creating widespread changes in the health behavior of the poor, at least not in the forseeable future. The values for knowledge and for health exhibited by the poor, their tendency to use a shorter time horizon as a framework for planning, their reluctance to use professional referral and service systems, perhaps guided by a general feeling of powerlessness in the face of a hostile environment, all suggest that the problem of altering their behavior will prove to be highly complex and not susceptible of simple remedy.

There is much knowledge about the health behavior of the poor and the non-poor that can be stated with confidence and there is much that is still unknown. Among those items that may now be regarded as factual are the following:

1. There is a marked association between income level and the proportion of persons seeking preventive or diagnostic health services in the absence of symptoms.

2. The observed association remains statistically significant, though it is much less marked in connection with tooth-brushing, an action that is both relatively inexpensive and can be undertaken without entry into a professional referral system.

3. There is a marked association between income and the possession of correct knowledge about a wide variety of health-related matters.

4. There is a marked association between income and the extent of belief in the efficacy of alternative procedures for preventing or controlling various health conditions.

5. It is suggested, though by no means demonstrated, that the behavior of the poor may be in part attributable to their beliefs about their susceptibility to, and severity of, various health conditions and the perceived benefits of taking associated professional health action.

6. The associations between income and behavior and between income and knowledge are related to educational attainment but are not wholly explained by educational attainment.

7. The professional referral and health system tends to be used relatively infrequently by those low on the economic scale; the preference seems to be for a lay referral system.

The foregoing evidence supports the concept of a culture of poverty with its own structure, rationale, and values. However, any effort to explain the dimensions of the culture of poverty as it relates to health matters must currently be based on less certain knowledge than that which demonstrates that such a culture exists. Even more hypothetical must be any explanation of why that culture contains specific characteristics and how an intervention may modify it in a professionally desired direction. Among the issues that need to be resolved are those concerning the extent to which health behavior, knowledge and attitude are explainable by such factors as subjective time horizons, values for rationality and planning, feelings of powerlessness, salience of health and the extent to which such factors overlap each other. A rational approach to the development of intervention strategies must await more information on these issues, although it must be confessed that the very desire for rationality in developing an intervention strategy in itself reflects a middle-class value. It is not necessary to await the data that would permit such a rational development before attempting intervention and, in fact, that is what many health workers are currently doing.

VI · Illness and Cure

by David Mechanic

The concept of illness behavior refers to the ways in which given symptoms are perceived, evaluated, and acted (or not acted) upon by different people.[1] Behavioral scientists have been concerned with studying illness behavior in two ways. First, they have investigated a variety of factors (such as social class, ethnicity, urban residence, sex, reference group, stress, and social values) which distinguish among persons with different patterns of illness behavior. Second, using some measure of illness behavior as an independent variable (for example, a tendency to adopt the sick role), they have tried to account for differences in the actual use of health facilities.[2]

Illness behavior is important in at least three different ways. Since different illness behavior patterns in part determine how a diseased person selects himself for treatment, they in various ways bias the samples of some illnesses that medical researchers study. Unless the nature of such selective biases on the basis of illness behavior factors is recognized, serious errors may occur in medical investigations that use samples from clinics, private practitioners, and even hospitals.[3] Second, since medical diagnosis is often achieved on the basis of a medical history in which the patient provides the information, the diagnostic process can be biased by different respondent tendencies that are characteristic of the person's illness behavior patterns.[4] Such respondent tendencies are particularly important in many psychiatric and some nonpsychiatric conditions where it becomes difficult for the clinician to distinguish between the symptoms and the typical behavioral and expressive patterns of the subgroup. Finally, since illness behavior patterns influence patients' responses to treatment, taking account of such influences often facilitates the management of the patient.[5]

Illness behavior is a general rubric encompassing complex patterns of responses that are determined by different social processes and a wide variety of variables. Socio-economic levels are related to illness behavior patterns both directly and indirectly. For example, there is a substantial literature demonstrating that low socio-economic status is associated with a lower level of utilization of medical services based on consumer decisions when the consumer must pay for the services himself.[6] Income is a relevant factor because persons with higher incomes have more money to invest in such services without sacrificing other family needs and priorities. However important the income factor may be, it is possible that the indirect influences of socio-economic level on illness behavior in the long run will be of greater analytic significance than its more direct effects. As more liberal definitions of medical indigence are formulated within various government programs, services will be available to persons who have ordinarily lacked funds to buy such services, and thus the relationship between income and utilization of services will have to be explained by factors other than income. Although inadequate income probably explains in part the relative failure of the lowest income groups to buy medical and other health services, it does not explain this failure in full.

Indirectly, socio-economic level is an important variable in accounting for response to illness because in a very gross way differences in socio-economic level encompass differences in health values, understanding and information concerning disease, future and preventive planning, cultural expectations concerning health services, feelings of social distance between oneself and health practitioners, and so on.[7] Thus, impoverished persons tend to know less about disease than more affluent members of our society, and they engage less in preventive planning, accept discomfort more routinely, and feel less at ease in medical settings.[8]

One must be particularly careful in using the concepts of socio-economic level and poverty, since these are crude social rubrics and encompass a very wide variety of groups and social characteristics. There is no such thing as the illness behavior of the poor or the illness behavior of the affluent. One may find differences on the basis of the socio-economic variables because the poor, on the average, tend to have a higher concentration of people with particular cultural and social characteristics relevant to health than the rich. In the long run, it is more illuminating to learn the precise factors that account for differences in illness behavior than it is to note some gross variations between socio-economic levels. Most of the discussion that follows will be an attempt to specify in detail the underlying variables that explain differences in illness behavior rather than a summary of the gross, and frequently unilluminating, differences of varying socio-economic levels.

One further caution. The relationship noted between socio-economic indicators and illness behavior is usually of a descriptive rather than an analytical kind. Thus, a relationship between socio-economic level and illness behavior found in 1958 does not imply such a relationship in 1968. The entire population, including the poor, is better informed about health matters today than ten years ago, and different levels of knowledge among the poor may vastly affect illness behavior patterns. In contrast, we may find growing gaps between the rich and the poor resulting from different rates of adaptation to medical innovations. All too frequently, the data cited in support of illness behavior differences by socio-economic status are very much dated and may not characterize accurately the period of time we are most concerned with. The most widely quoted study, that of a New York State community, was carried out in the early 1950's.[9] One seriously wonders if a group comparable to Koos's class III would respond today as it did then.

For the most part, adequate data linking socio-economic factors to illness behavior are extremely limited. Most such information of an intensive sort is based on small samples unrepresentative of the general population. Often the group of poor people studied is very much biased in terms of ethnicity or some other factor, and it is not clear when the differences noted are products of socio-economic differences or of any of the other variables characteristic of the samples used.

If we are to make progress in the study of illness behavior, it becomes necessary to move beyond gross cultural and social differences in illness behavior patterns toward the development of a social-psychological model which gives a clearer conception of how people come to the realization that they are ill and how they decide that some form of help is necessary. In recent years, there have been several attempts to do this. Rosenstock has suggested that preventive health behavior relevant to a given problem is determined by the extent to which a person sees the problem as having both serious consequences and a high probability of occurrence.[10] He believes that behavior emerges from conflicting goals and motives, and that action will follow those motives which are most salient and those goals which are perceived as most valuable. Zola, approaching the problem from another perspective, has attempted to delineate five timing "triggers" in patients' decisions to seek medical care.[11] The first pattern he calls "interpersonal crisis," in which the situation calls attention to the symptoms and causes the patient to dwell on them. The second trigger he calls "social interference." Here, the symptoms do not change but come to threaten a valued social activity. The third trigger, "the presence of sanctioning," involves others telling him to seek care; the fourth trigger implies "perceived threat," and the fifth, "nature and equality of the symptoms," involves similarity of symptoms to previous ones or to those of friends. Zola reports that these triggers appear to have different degrees of importance in varying social strata and ethnic groups. He suggests that "interpersonal crisis" and "social interference" were used more often by Italians, while "sanctioning" was the predominant Irish pattern. The Anglo-Saxon group, he reports, responded most to the "nature and quality of their symptoms."

If one considers the range of factors discussed in relation to varying patterns of responses to symptoms, it appears that they fall into one of ten possible sets:

1. Visibility, recognizability, or perceptual salience of deviant signs and symptoms.

2. The extent to which the symptoms are perceived as serious (that is, the person's estimate of the present and future probabilities of danger).

3. The extent to which symptoms disrupt family, work, and other social activities.

4. The frequency of the appearance of deviant signs or symptoms, their persistence, or their frequency of reoccurrence.

5. The tolerance threshold of those who are exposed to and evaluate the deviant signs and symptoms.

6. Available information, knowledge, and cultural assumptions and understandings of the evaluator.

7. Basic needs which lead to autistic psychological processes (i.e., perceptual processes that distort reality).

8. Needs competing with illness responses.

9. Competing possible interpretations that can be assigned to the symptoms once they are recognized.

10. Availability of treatment resources, physical proximity, and psychological and monetary costs of taking action, including physical distance and costs of time, money, and effort, as well as such costs as stigma, social distance, and feelings of humiliation.

Since these categories and their relevance are reviewed in

some detail elsewhere, I shall not attempt to justify them here.[12] Instead, I wish to analyze how socio-economic factors relate to these correlates of illness behavior. Before undertaking this task, it is necessary to consider some special issues that bear on the later discussion.

THE UNITARY THEORY OF ILLNESS BEHAVIOR

The character of mental illnesses appears so different from that of physical conditions that, on first consideration, it is difficult to see how a unitary theory of illness behavior can be applied to both. However, when the dimensions of illness and the factors affecting its definition are made explicit, it becomes apparent that the differences between various illnesses can be managed within the framework of a single model. Illness as a social phenomenon depends upon the assertion by someone that some deviation from normality has taken place. There are varying definitions of normality; the concepts held by lay persons may vary from the conceptions held by medical practitioners, and the concepts held by practitioners may vary among themselves depending on the state of medical knowledge and scientific information. In one pattern, the individual views himself as sick on the basis of his own norms of functioning and in the light of his knowledge and experience, and then seeks medical confirmation of this situation. On other occasions, the individual does not recognize himself as sick, but comes to accept this definition when some other person defines him as ill; this is the case of a person who is informed that he has hypertension or tuberculosis although he does not feel sick. Finally, there are occasions when others define a person as sick, but he vigorously resists this definition—as frequently happens in the case of persons with psychiatric conditions. A basic difference between psychiatric and nonpsychiatric conditions is that resistance to being defined as "sick" is much more common in the former than in the latter. One should not forget, however, that there is a considerable overlap between psychiatric and non-psychiatric conditions in this respect.

Since pathology frequently becomes manifest through visible signs and aberrations in feelings or behavior, these manifestations may be disruptive of social life and associated with stigma. In general, psychiatric conditions are more disruptive and generate greater stigma than nonpsychiatric ones, but once again there is an overlap between the psychiatric and nonpsychiatric categories. Thus, there is no need to consider psychiatric and nonpsychiatric conditions separately as long as we give due attention to such factors as social disruption, stigma, and resistance to accepting a definition of illness as appropriate.

In applying the ten categories discussed previously, it should be clear that they pertain equally to situations where an individual defines himself as ill and to those where others in association with an individual come to regard him as sick or deviant. For example, let us consider how these categories would apply to a man who has a stomach ulcer and to one who becomes an alcoholic. The recognition of a stomach ulcer depends on the extent to which it becomes evident through pain and discomfort. There are many people with ulcers who do not become aware of pain and only seek medical attention after the ulcer begins to bleed. Similarly, the recognition of a problem and willingness to seek help for it would depend on the extent to which the symptoms are perceived as serious, that is, the extent to which they disrupt activities (work, sleep), the frequency or persistence of the pain and discomfort, and the person's tolerance for pain. These categories apply equally well to community definitions of alcoholics. Individuals are more likely to be defined by others as alcoholic when their drinking is visible than when it is private. Similarly, the definition and response will depend on how serious the person's drinking is regarded; the extent to which his drinking disrupts work, family, and other community activities;

the frequency with which he becomes drunk; and the community's tolerance for drinking and drunkenness. From a theoretical point of view, there is no need to maintain a separate theory of illness behavior for self-defined and other-defined conditions.

A final issue which bears on the illness behavior problem involves the contention that the behavior disorders are not illnesses. Although there is a large polemical literature on whether mental illnesses are "illnesses" in the usual sense, the answer to this dilemma lies not in the intrinsic nature of these conditions but, rather, in the manner in which the question is formulated.[13] If one considers medical models of disease, it is apparent that, in one sense, medical diagnoses are hypotheses based on some underlying theory. A given theory at a given time may be fully confirmed, partially confirmed, or unconfirmed. The various physical conditions that doctors deal with today vary from those whose underlying theories have been confirmed (such as pernicious anemia) to those that are unconfirmed (such as sarcoidosis). Most disease entities fall within the partially confirmed classification (heart disease, cancer, and so on). Psychiatric diagnoses derive from theories which, on the whole, have a lower level of confirmation than many medical conditions, but psychiatric disorders need not be seen as qualitatively different from nonpsychiatric ones. The usefulness of a theory will depend on its level of confirmation, which in turn depends on the reliability of the diagnoses which it leads to and the utility of the diagnoses for predicting the course, etiology, and successful treatment of the patient's condition.[14]

In sum, the psychiatric conditions need not be treated as fundamentally different from nonpsychiatric disorders, and each does not require a separate theory of illness behavior. However, psychiatric conditions as compared to nonpsychiatric ones are more likely to be defined by persons other than the ones affected, are likely to be more disruptive to social situations, and are likely to be associated with greater social stigma.

THE NATURE AND QUALITY OF SYMPTOMS AND THE LAY REFERRAL PROCESS

As Freidson has pointed out, responses to illness, once defined, may involve widely differing attempts to deal with the problem.[15] The person may first try home remedies; he may discuss his troubles with neighbors, friends, and fellow workers in a casual way and explore various alternative explanations for the way he is feeling. He may ask the advice of others as to whether he should seek the care of a physician and which one; he may go to the doctor on a trial visit, comparing the diagnosis with his own conceptions and diagnoses made by friends and acquaintances. In short, professional help-seeking may occur through a lay referral process. In most situations of serious illness, the sick person consults others before seeking care. Suchman found that three quarters of his respondents reported having discussed their symptoms with some other person, usually a relative, before seeking care.[16] Such discussions are believed to result in a "provisional validation" for the sick person to release himself from responsibilities and to seek medical care. The literature suggests that lay referral systems are much more elaborate and important among the poor than among those who are more conversant with the medical-scientific culture.

Before elaborating on the influences of social processes on care-seeking, it is essential that this concern be seen in proper perspective. One must not forget that probably the most important determinant of care-seeking is the character of the symptoms themselves. Much of the behavior of sick persons is a direct product of the specific symptoms they experience: their intensity, the quality of discomfort they cause, their persistence.

It is as misleading to exaggerate the social influences on definitions of illness as it is to ignore them. Many symptoms leave the person little alternative but to recognize that he has a medical condition and that medical care is essential. It is unlikely that a person experiencing a temperature of 105 degrees will find alternative definitions as compared with the idea that he is sick. And no matter how stoical a person is, or how extreme his attitudes toward symptoms may be, a fractured leg, a broken back, a severe heart attack, an extreme psychosis, or any of a variety of other conditions is likely to bring him into professional care.

Suchman has provided some evidence involving the influence of disturbing symptoms.[17] He selected 137 cases from his larger survey of 5,340 persons in the Washington Heights community of New York City. This subsample included adults who had a specific, relatively serious illness episode during the two months previous to the interview which required three or more visits to the physician and incapacitated the person for five or more consecutive days, or which required hospitalization for a day or more. Pain was clearly the most important initial sign that something was wrong, and pain was mentioned by two thirds of the respondents. Considerably less important were fever and chills (mentioned by 17 percent) and shortness of breath (10 percent). These symptoms were "usually severe, continuous, incapacitating, and unalleviated," and approximately three quarters of the respondents reported that they immediately saw the symptoms as indicative of illness. Although we do not know from this study how symptoms were perceived by those who did not seek medical care, this investigation does confirm that many of those who turned to professional help were motivated by the manner in which their symptoms developed and became evident.

Every investigation this author is aware of, that considers the severity, seriousness, or nature of the perceived symptom, has found that social factors are considerably less important in help-seeking among those who have severe symptoms than among those who have lesser symptoms. This fact appears to be as relevant to the mental disorders as to the physical disorders.[18] Although there are vast differences in willingness to tolerate bizarre and difficult behavior, few relatives apppear willing to house a patient who is suicidal, homicidal, incontinent, hallucinatory, delusional, or disoriented.[19] In short, if the patient is sufficiently bizarre and disruptive, the probability is extremely high that he will come into care in one way or another. Social definitions of illness are relevant because many serious illnesses develop so that they are not particularly striking in their impact. It is this ambiguity surrounding the occurrence and severity of pathology that makes the sociological concern useful.[20] But we must not forget that the nature of symptoms is the most powerful factor influencing the definition of illness and the seeking of care.

Illness Behavior and Socio-economic Status

A few studies allow for the assessment of the influence of socio-economic factors on variables relevant to illness behavior in specific terms. In general terms there is much evidence that socio-economic factors are related to knowledge about disease, use of medical and dental services, acceptance of preventive health practices, purchase of voluntary health insurance, delay in seeking treatment, use of folk remedies and self-medications. From the studies available, however, it is extremely difficult to assess the relative importance of economic means, knowledge, attitudes and beliefs, cultural values, life situations, and fear and anxiety—all of which may be distributed somewhat differently among the various social strata. Moreover, available studies make it impossible to assess the direction of various influences. Is the lack of knowledge about medical affairs, for example, in part the consequence of the fact that doctors do not take the same pains to inform and instruct working-class patients as compared with higher status patients or is this finding solely the result of different educational levels? [21]

For our purpose, the most useful reports come from a study by Suchman which found that the more ethnocentric and socially cohesive groups included more persons who knew little about disease, who were skeptical toward professional medical care, and who reported a dependent pattern of response to illness.[22] When measures were constructed of individual medical orientation (an index based on knowledge about disease, skepticism about medical care, and dependency in illness) and social group organization (an index based on ethnic exclusiveness, friendship solidarity, and family orientation to tradition and authority), it was found that low socio-economic status was substantially associated with a "parochial" as compared with a "cosmopolitan" social structure and with a "popular" as compared with a "scientific" orientation to medicine. The relationships between socio-economic status and "social organizaton" and "medical orientation" were consistent for each of the ethnic groups included in the study (Puerto Ricans, Negroes, Irish, Jews, white Protestants, and Catholics). Finally, controlling for socio-economic status, a clear relationship was observed between a "parochial" form of social organization and a "popular" health orientation in each socio-economic grouping.

Although the data are interesting, we must face the difficult question of what meaning should be attributed to the various attitudinal responses. Some further data from the same study suggest the difficulty. Although Suchman had no behavioral data, he did include items dealing with reports of behavior. He found that persons of higher socio-economic status were more likely to report that they buy health insurance, get a periodic medical checkup, receive polio immunizations, eat a balanced diet, and have more frequent eye examinations and dental care.

The data suggest that socio-economic status is the most important indicator of these behaviors since there is no relationship between "group organization" or "medical orientation" and such behaviors once socio-economic status is controlled. Moreover, the relationship between social "group organization" and "medical orientation" to health status was slight and variable. Thus, we are left with the possibility that the relationships among the various attitudinal scales reflect little of behavioral significance.

Unfortunately, there are few studies that allow us to assess the influence of illness attitudes and social patterns on important behavioral factors except those which deal in a gross fashion with socio-economic differences. Various data from the National Health Survey show that for various consumer health decisions (such as buying health insurance or using physician or dental services) income and education each contribute independently in explaining variations in behavior.[23] One of the few studies that has attempted to go beyond such factors, using a behavioral indicator as the dependent variable, was carried out within the context of a private university setting and, therefore, cannot very effectively be generalized to lower socio-economic groups. This study suggests, however, a frame of reference which might be relevant for understanding some of the motivational patterns underlying the use of medical services.

Mechanic and Volkart, in a study of six hundred students at a major university, investigated the relationship between "stress" and a measure of "illness behavior." [24] Perceived stress (as measured by indices of loneliness and nervousness) and illness behavior (as measured by several hypothetical items concerning the use of medical facilities) were clearly related to the use of a college health service during the one-year period. Among students with high stress and a high inclination to use medical facilities, 73 percent were frequent users of medical services, while among the low inclination-low stress group, only 30 percent were frequent users of such services. Attention was focused on the interaction between stress and illness behavior in encouraging a person to present a complaint. When illness behavior patterns were controlled, it was found that the influence of stress was somewhat different in the two inclination groups. In the high inclination group, stress was a rather significant influence in bringing people to physicians: among those with high stress, 73 percent used health facilities frequently, while only 46 percent did so among those with low stress. Although the same trend was observed among those who were less inclined to use the health service, the relationship was substantially smaller and not statistically significant.

In a very tentative way, these data reflect an underlying coping process. Persons who are distressed seek some way of dealing with it, and it has been argued that the use of medical services is frequently motivated by emotional needs and problems not necessarily related to the physical symptoms presented to the doctor.[25] The data from the study discussed above suggest that the process is probably more subtle and complicated than observers have indicated. There are various alternatives for dealing with stress, and it is not clear why people choose the doctor. The results suggest that persons under stress choose to bring their problem to the doctor primarily when they start out with a high receptivity to medical services. Those under stress who have a low receptivity to medical services presumably try to deal with their difficulties in other ways. Thus, the data support the interpretation that stress leads to an attempt to cope, and those who are receptive to adopting the patient role tend to use this method of coping more frequently than those who are less receptive.

Receptivity to health care and general response to illness depend on a wide range of factors. Only some of these factors appear to be affected by socio-economic status, although adequate data on many relevant points are not available. We shall now consider those findings that have relevance for understanding the relationships between socio-economic status and some of these variables.

TOLERANCE OF SYMPTOMS AND SOCIAL CLASS

Investigators in the mental health field have suggested that socio-economic status is related to the perceived seriousness of symptoms, i.e., the person's estimate of the present and future possibilities of danger associated with a condition.[26] There are reports that aggressiveness, excessive drinking, and social withdrawal are seen as less serious indications among lower-class persons than among higher status persons. However, the extent to which cultural patterns, lack of knowledge and tolerance confound such relationships is not fully clear. In the area of physical illness, Suchman found little difference among socio-economic groups in the interpretation of symptoms as illness: both higher and lower socio-economic groups indicated about the same amount of concern about their symptoms.[27] Although lower-class persons are more likely to delay seeking treatment than higher-status persons, it is not clear precisely which factors lead to delay: differential perception of symptoms, knowledge, fear, cost of care, access to health services.[28]

Levine presents some survey data indicating that persons of limited education report that they fear certain diseases (cancer, polio, cerebral palsy, arthritis, tuberculosis, birth defects) more than those with higher education.[29] Knowledge about these diseases and acquaintance with someone who has had them increases the level of fear, and fear is also related to income and the perceived expense of treatment. Moreover, low-income persons were somewhat more likely to fear these conditions than persons with higher income, but in both groups, persons who viewed treatment as expensive feared these conditions substantially more than those who did not. The interaction of variables is complex because knowledge and limited education are both related to degree of reported fear, but these variables are themselves inversely related. The data are not sufficiently detailed to clarify the nature of these interactions.

Although it is difficult to find definitive data concerning tolerance of symptoms, some studies show that lower-class people are more likely to "put up" with a variety of symptoms than higher-status persons.[30] Once again, the data do not demonstrate clearly that differences exist in perception of such behavior, and the unwillingness of lower-status persons to seek help may be a consequence of many other factors. In the area of psychiatric disorders, however, there is fairly strong evidence that social class is related to expectations concerning performance.[31] Working-class persons are more likely to tolerate a low level of performance than higher-status persons, but ineffective performance does not appear to be directly linked to hospitalization for a psychiatric condition. Although there are many observations that working-class persons are more willing to tolerate a variety of disruptive symptoms than higher-status people, it is not clear to what extent this denotes a differential level of real tolerance or different expectations and values as to what should be tolerated. Moreover, we have little knowledge concerning the range of toleration for various conditions in different social strata.

Most studies that purport to show a relationship between social class and tolerance pertain more to the manner in which symptoms are defined than to the extent to which they are tolerated.[32] The Hollingshead and Redlich's study, *Social Class and Mental Illness*, typifies the literature that presently exists concerning tolerance. Through the citation of various case examples, they argue that persons in the lower social strata, and especially the lowest one, tolerate more abnormal behavior. It is clear that their definition of tolerance encompasses the failure to see the motivation underlying the behavior as pathological, and has little bearing on the extent to which lower-class persons find the symptoms and behavior troublesome. In short, their observations really bear on differences in cultural definition and response and do not illuminate the issue of tolerance per se. Although there are several studies showing ethnic differences in willingness to tolerate discomfort, the data available in the area of pain response provide little support for the conclusion that there are significant differences among various socio-economic groups.[33]

The tendency to view aberrant symptoms within a framework of normality is a typical response, but this does not suggest that the symptoms are not disturbing or disruptive. Indeed, a study of definitions of mental illness in the family suggests that the family suffers considerable pain and discomfort before accepting a definition of illness.[34] Although the symptoms are disruptive, the wife attempts to explain or justify them within a context of normality. She mobilizes her defenses in various ways so as to handle the disruptive behavior without resorting to a psychiatric frame of reference.[35] One should not imply that there are no significant differences in people's tolerance for a wide variety of deviance, but there is little real evidence for the claim that these differences occur on a systematic basis.

The most consistent and abundant finding in the literature of illness behavior is that lower-class persons have less information and knowledge about disease, and have different cultural assumptions, beliefs, and understandings concerning symptoms and disease processes. Lower-class people are less likely than persons in higher social strata to recognize the signs of major illnesses, to understand body functioning, to use preventive health services, but are more likely to hold irrational ideas about illness, rely on folk medicine and fringe practitioners, and delay seeking medical treatment.[36] As noted earlier, except for the consistent evidence on different degrees of knowledge by socio-economic status, it is difficult to unravel the influence of beliefs and cultural assumptions from other social and psychological factors affecting illness behavior.

Perhaps the greatest difference in beliefs about illness among the various socio-economic groups relates to psychiatric disorders. It is frequently observed that lower-class persons are more likely to see emotional disturbance in somatic terms than higher-status persons and do not seem to be receptive to a psychological approach to their problems.[37] They also apparently are less able or willing to see various disruptive patterns of behavior within a psychiatric frame of reference. They less readily seek help for psychiatric problems, and when they come into psychiatric care, they come through different routes. Hollingshead and Redlich, for example, found that persons from the higher-status groups came into treatment largely through referrals of private physicians, family, friends, and through self-referral, while persons in the lowest class came into treatment involuntarily, largely through the police, courts, and other social agencies. Although there are a variety of ways to interpret the findings, it seems reasonable to believe that there were at least two processes at work. First, it is likely that upper- and middle-class persons are more inclined than working-class persons to perceive particular indications as symptoms of psychiatric disorder. Second, it is probable that once having defined the need for treatment, patients in the various class groups have different information and knowledge about arrangements for help. While middle-class persons are more likely to call their personal doctor when difficulties develop, working-class people are probably more likely to seek help from the police in handling the disruptive behavior of a psychotic person.

There are some indications that working-class persons are more likely to respond to illness with fear, anxiety, and denial than are higher-status persons. Since autistic defense processes are poorly defined in discussions of illness, it is not clear what psychological processes are really involved. Much of the discussion concerning the denial of illness among the working class fits as readily within the conception of competing needs. Illness is more threatening to the lowest socio-economic segments because they less frequently have insurance to pay for the costs and savings to sustain the family during the period of illness. Moreover, working-class people have less knowledge about medical settings and may feel less comfortable and more threatened than higher-status persons within such settings. As Rosenstock has noted, behavior takes place within a context where motives are frequently competing or in conflict.[38] Health motives are not always the most central ones, especially when people are healthy or suffer little incapacity. One of Koos's respondents posed the conflicting interest issue clearly: "I wish I could get it fixed up, but we've just got some other things that are more important first. Our car's a wreck, and we're going to get another one. We need a radio, too, and some other things . . . But it's got to wait for now—there's always something more important." [39]

Whether or not symptoms are defined as illness also depends on competing definitions of the symptom. Laborers are probably more likely to accept certain aches and pains as normal than are persons in less active occupations. Fatigue and other diffuse symptoms may be attributed more to general conditions in life than to an illness. In any case, there is very little data that allow us to ascertain if there is a relationship between socio-economic status and the opportunities for competing definitions of symptoms.

Whether a person decides to seek help, and the form of help he seeks, depends on the availability of treatment resources, their physical proximity, and the psychological and monetary costs of seeking assistance. There is no question that cost is a significant barrier to seeking care among those with limited economic means. The differential utilization of medical and dental services by socio-economic status disappears in large part, if not completely, when medical services are made available to those with limited means. Socio-economic differences in the use of medical services comparable to those found in the United States do not exist in Great Britain, where services are provided without cost on the basis of need.[40] It is significant that in the United States, when public health and research programs offer free services to a particular population, such as in the National Health Examination Survey or in the Baltimore Morbidity Survey, persons of lower socio-economic status and nonwhites (the two groups with the lowest level of utilization of services on a national basis) are usually overrepresented in their participation as compared with other population groups.[41] Although receptivity to medical care may depend on various aspects of the person and the structure of the medical service itself, socio-economic differences in utilization can be reduced significantly by providing free services in a manner which is sensitive to the cultural and social needs of people.

There is a considerable anecdotal literature which supports the conclusion that working-class persons feel more uncomfortable and embarrassed in dealing with middle- and upper-status professionals than do persons who have higher status.[42] Moreover, within the psychiatric area, it is generally recognized that therapists prefer to work with patients who share their cultural and social values and orientations.[43]

CULTURAL FACTORS AND ILLNESS BEHAVIOR

Most data concerning illness behavior deal with cultural characteristics such as ethnicity and religion rather than with socio-economic factors. These studies of ethnicity, however, are frequently concerned with the ethnicity of lower social status and, thus, they have some bearing on the issue at hand. The classic study in this area observed that while Jewish and Italian patients responded to pain in an emotional fashion—tending to exaggerate pain experiences—"Old Americans" tended to be more stoical and objective, while the Irish more frequently denied pain.[44] It also noted the difference in the attitudes under-lying Italian and Jewish concern about pain. While the Italian subjects primarily sought relief from pain and were relatively satisfied when such relief was obtained, the Jewish subjects were mainly concerned with the meaning and significance of their pain and the consequences for their future welfare and health. Although the data do not bear on socio-economic charac-teristics, they offer some observations. Manual workers with herniated discs were more disturbed by their pain than profes-sional or business people with a similar disease, a difference presumably due to the significance of the pain to their abilities to earn a living. In the same vein, intellectuals were more con-cerned by headaches than manual workers.

Zborowski suggested that the more educated patients are more conscious of their health and more aware of pain as a possible symptom of a serious disease. He indicated some doubt, however, about the influence of socio-economic factors:

> The education of the patient seems to be an important fac-tor in fostering specific reactive patterns. The more educated patient, who may have more anxiety with regard to illness, may be more reserved in specific reactions to pain than an unsophisticated individual, who feels free to ex-press his feelings and emotions. In interpreting the differ-ences which may be attributed to different socio-economic and educational backgrounds there is enough evidence to conclude that these differences appear mainly on the mani-fest and behavioral level, whereas attitudinal patterns toward pain tend to be more uniform and to be common to most of the members of the group regardless of their spe-cific backgrounds.[45]

Ethnic attitudes toward medical institutions and equipment in controlling pain were most characteristic of immigrants while later generations approximated the American pattern more closely. This, however, appeared to be less true for attitudes toward pain "which seem to persist to a great extent even among members of the third generation and even though the reactive patterns are radically changed." American-born Jewish or Italian patients behave like Old Americans but express typical ethnic attitudes.

A later study brought Irish, Jewish, Italian, and Yankee housewives into a psycho-physiological laboratory, where they administered pain by electric shock, recording skin potential responses.[46] The findings tended to be consistent with some of Zborowski's observations. They found, for example, that Italian women showed significantly lower upper thresholds for shock, and fewer of them would accept the full range of shock stimulation used in the experiment. Their response is consistent with the Italian tendency to focus on the immediacy of the pain itself as compared with the future orientation of the Jewish response tendency. Similarly, the finding that Yankee housewives had faster and more complete adaptation of the diphasic palmar skin potential has an attitudinal correlate to their "matter-of-fact" orientation to pain. The authors argue that socio-economic differences did not affect the findings, since the groups most different on the dependent measures were most similar on the social status measures.

A few other studies provide some data on the relationships between ethnicity and socio-economic indicators in relation to illness behavior. Croog, administering the Cornell Medical Index to two thousand randomly chosen army inductees, found that Italian and Jewish respondents reported the greatest number of symptoms of illness.[47] Although the Italian response was associated with low educational status, reports of symptoms among Jewish respondents were not affected by the educational variable. Mechanic, studying 1,300 students at two American universities, found that Jewish students reported higher illness behavior patterns than either Protestant or Catholic students.[48] Since income was also found to be related to reports on illness behavior, and since Jewish students were more likely to be of higher income groups, the analysis was repeated controlling income. The differences in illness behavior reports between Jewish and other students were only significant for the high income group. Several other studies show that Jewish students and those with high social status are more receptive to the use of psychiatric facilities than non-Jewish students and those with lower social status. Receptivity to psychiatric services has been interpreted by various analysts to be relevant to a theory of "social circles." [49]

In general, the studies of ethnicity and illness behavior suggest that ethnicity exerts a more powerful effect than socio-economic status in illness behavior. Indeed, useful health patterns may exist among groups that are of low socio-economic status and undesirable ones may exist among some subgroups of higher status. For example, an early study of infant mortality in the United States found that the Jewish immigrant group, although it had as many children and an income which was much lower than that of the native-born whites, had the lowest rate of infant mortality of all the groups studied. Apparently, these immigrants were able to sustain a high level of infant-rearing and caring despite their poor socio-economic status.[50]

We must be careful, however, to separate analytic distinctions from descriptive ones. Although the evidence suggests that poverty and a harmful health culture need not go together, the fact is that dysfunctional health attitudes and lack of useful knowledge are more likely to occur among ethnic groups that are of relatively low socio-economic status. The Puerto Rican and Negro groups in New York City are particular examples of subgroups which deviate substantially from a "desirable" level of sociomedical knowledge, attitudes, and responses to illnesses.[51] Since these groups also appear to have very substantial health problems as well as social problems, the best way of bringing better medical and other social services to these populations deserves considerable attention.

Having reviewed various factors affecting illness behavior—the manner in which people differentially perceive, evaluate, and respond to symptoms—we found considerable evidence that socio-economic factors influence the utilization of medical care and the receptivity to preventive health practices. From the research point of view, however, many uncertainties remain. The data which would allow a clear resolution of important theoretical and practical issues are often either unavailable or are in a form unsuitable to answer the questions. The literature on illness behavior contains an abundance of hypotheses and impressions, and perhaps we should attempt to clarify some of these before we go on to construct too many more.

VII · The Treatment of the Sick

by Julius A. Roth

When considering kind of medical care available to the poor and the way they obtain the needed medical care, one must keep in mind that the private physician-patient relationship on a fee-for-service basis is regarded as a basic condition of American medical practice.* This assumption is held by the majority of the country's physicians and, especially, by organized medicine. A recent publication of the American Medical Association, issued as a teaching outline for medical students, states: "The physician's fee should be commensurate with the service rendered and the patient's ability to pay . . . Both physician and patient are free to seek care or not, or to accept a particular individual as a patient or not." [1] This formulation, which sums up the traditional usage of the majority of the country's practicing physicians, clearly determines the practical accessibility of physicians in private practice for patients in different income classes.

In our affluent society, where the conspicuous consumption of necessary and unnecessary services is a characteristic mark of the life of broad masses, a great many people do not see any reason to question, or seek an alternative for, the traditional principle of rendering medical services. Those who would have a good reason to do so are likely to be poor, uninformed, and perhaps even apathetic. Thus, the discussion of the basic principles of financing medical care has been, at least until quite

* The criticism of an earlier draft of this chapter by Dorothy J. Douglas helped the author to avoid some errors of fact and forced him to face some questions of interpretation.

recently, restricted to a small circle of intellectuals. Although a fair number of physicians, those who have been generally opposing the policies of the American Medical Association, have been constructively participating in this discussion, the public at large knows very little about, and has a very small interest in, the whole problem.

Although a substantial amount of medical care is delivered by full-time salaried physicians working mainly in governmental and academic settings, this care is commonly regarded within the profession as contrary to the ideal patient-doctor relationship, and—except for the leading medical schools—the institutions providing this care are likely to suffer in their recruiting from the resistance and criticism of the rest of the medical world which portrays their services as inferior and almost bordering on the unethical.[2]

In the present context we do not aim to discuss the just and equitable ways of paying for medical services or the possible alternatives to the principle of fee-for-service. But we intend to assess, insofar as possible within the limitations of the available knowledge, the differences that exist in obtaining medical care among the socio-economic classes and, particularly, between the poor and the more affluent segments of the population.

THE UTILIZATION OF PRIVATE PHYSICIANS

It is often said two distinct kinds of medical service exist in the United States. The middle class uses physicians in private practice and the low-income class uses the public clinics.[3] The general validity of this statement cannot be contested, but one has to realize that patients use a variety of medical services, and for each type of service the differential utilization by social classes yields a different pattern. Consider, for example, the common utilization type of having a family doctor, an ideal type that is generally recommended by medical authorities. The actual services delivered by the family doctor greatly vary from one family to the next; he may give total or partial care to one or all members of the family in all kinds of combinations (care for acute illnesses only or for chronic illnesses only, general-practice care only or with surgical, pediatric, and obstetrical care); he may have a paramount or a subordinate role when compared to the various specialists that the family uses simultaneously. But in any case, having a family doctor means a stable relationship with one doctor in which the effectiveness of the more-or-less systematic consultations is well supported by the benefits arising from the fact that physician and patient know each other.

The utilization of a family doctor is the function of income. When 4320 families with children in the pediatric age group were asked whether they had a doctor who usually looked after the children, the proportion of affirmative answers increased dramatically from the lowest to the highest income group (see Table VII–1). Only 16 percent of the families on welfare had a doctor; 85 percent of the families with an income of more than $10,000 did. In the steady increase of the percentages two breaking points should be noted: under an income of $4,500 only a minority of the families have a usual physician; beyond that income, the majority of them have a family physician. Furthermore, above an income of $10,000 practically all families have such a doctor.

The other indices of socio-economic status (occupation and education) show a similar, although weaker, correlation with the frequency of having a "usual physician." At the same time, the effect of two intervening variables—race and rural-urban residence—must also be considered. Negroes at any income and occupational level are less likely to have a continuing relationship with a physician than whites of the same income and occupational level.[4] Several explanations may account for this finding. The utilization of a family doctor may depend on cul-

Table VII–1. Relationship between income and having a physician.

Family income	Number of families	Percent of families having a physician who usually looks after the children
welfare	621	16
less than $3,000	333	24
$3,000–$4,500	1369	38
$4,500–$6,000	1009	55
$6,000–$7,500	452	62
$7,500–$10,000	191	63
more than $10,000	75	85

Source: Joel J. Alpert *et al.*, "Types of Families That Use an Emergency Clinic," *Medical Care*, 7 (Jan.–Feb., 1969), 57.

tural traits such as patterns of consumption and spending in which the white and Negro populations are known to differ. Again, it may depend on the somewhat elusive psychological factor of social distance: the Negro at any income level may feel more distant from the white, upper-class physician than the white of the same income level; hence, the Negro tends to eschew the offices of private-practice physicians and instead prefers the public clinics where the institutional setting works to protect against the feeling of social distance. This explanation is supported by a study of the physicians' knowledge of their patients which found that, in addition to the frequency of contacts, the social class and race of the patient were factors and that the physicians seemed to know the lower-class Negro patient the least.[5]

Most of the studies on medical care have been conducted in urban areas and relatively little is known about the delivery of such care in rural America. However, we have every reason to believe that because of the relative unavailability of physicians in rural areas any segment of the rural population is less likely to have a family physician than a comparable segment of the urban population. Physicians tend to settle in urban areas, and this trend has been increasing since World War II; in addition, it is often noted that within the urban areas physicians tend to move into the suburbs and other high-income areas, and their number is decreasing in the low-income neighborhoods of the core cities. A study of the ecology of primary-care physicians (general practitioners, pediatricians, internists) in Boston does not fully bear out this latter observation. General practitioners were slightly more often found in the lower socio-economic areas ($r = -.20$) but there was no correlation between the socio-economic status of the city's census tracts and the distribution of the offices of internists and pediatricians. Furthermore, there was no relationship between the distribution of physicians and the distribution of the nonwhite population.[6]

It might very well be that the situation in New York or Chicago is different from that in Boston; but, generally speaking, the availability of private-practice physicians in the cities, even to the poor, is favorable when compared to their availability in the rural areas. In spite of many national and local campaigns, the rural areas have not been able to attract sufficient number of practicing physicians, and many of those who have been attracted are foreign-trained physicians who are more likely to take the less desirable positions avoided by their American-trained colleagues.[7] Moreover, the location of physicians in the commercial centers of the urban areas makes any access to them difficult for those residing in the remote parts and makes access extremely difficult for the rural poor who do not have cars. A study of the ambulance services in North Carolina concluded that ambulances are used in a disproportionate degree to transport the poor, mainly Negro and aged, to hospitals and physicians' offices for routine treatment involving no emergency.[8]

For the rural population the accessibility of the physician is further hampered by the relative lack of health insurance which would help to pay for the medical expenses. The most popular health insurance plans recruit the participants at their places of employment and labor unions, and such an arrangement puts the farming population at a disadvantage. A study carried out in North Carolina found that coverage by health insurance was more common among urban people, white families, and those with higher incomes and education than among their counterparts; moreover, it found that those who had dropped their insurance and had not re-enrolled, had the greatest unmet medical needs.[9] Another study put the conclusions in more general terms: "Subscription to health insurance is more a function of ability to pay than of health needs." [10]

The facts—that the rural poor have to summon the ambulance to get to a doctor and that they are least likely to be covered by health insurance—call attention to an often neglected point: that the lack of medical services is greatest in the rural areas and that the effective organization of medical services for the rural poor is one of our most pressing tasks—if not the most pressing one—in the health policy of the nation.

THE UTILIZATION OF PUBLIC CLINICS

Those who do not use private practitioners have to turn to the public clinics, and public clinics represent the main sources of medical care for the country's poor. In every group, as the income decreases more families use the public clinics (see Table VII–1), and the families use the public clinics more frequently. When more than 4000 families who used the Boston Children's Hospital Emergency Clinic were followed up for a period of six months, the welfare patients were most likely to return for one or more visits to the same clinic, while the group with the highest income was least likely to do so (see Table VII–2). The proportionally greatest decline by income groups appears for those making two or more repeat visits to the clinic, suggesting that the low-income groups are more likely than the high-income groups to rely on the services of the emergency clinic. They tend to return to the same clinic with another complaint or use the clinic for the treatment of prolonged and perhaps chronic ailments.

Table VII–2. Repeated utilization of a pediatric emergency clinic during a six-month period.

Family income	Number of families	Percent with no repeat visits	Percent with one repeat visit	Percent with two or more repeat visits
welfare	601	71	21	8
less than $4,500	1705	79	16	5
$4,500–$7,500	1439	86	12	2
more than $7,500	263	91	8	1

Source: Personal communication from John Kosa, based on the Harvard Study of Health Care Among Low-Income Families.

As some other observations also indicate, the middle-class family tends to use the public-clinic occasionally, for accidents and other emergencies, in times when the family doctor is not available or as a checkup in times when the family is not fully satisfied with the usual doctor. (In addition, the middle-class family is likely to take to a selected public clinic certain chronic diseases requiring prolonged treatment.) The low-income family, on the other hand, relies on the public clinic as the main source of care. This does not mean that the low-income family receives its total care from public clinics, let alone from one clinic. One study found that 57 percent of clinic users also had a private physician and for certain disorders they would contact their regular physician or arrange for an office visit with a recommended doctor, but in other situations they would consider the clinic as the best source of care.[11]

A more detailed study actually distinguishes four typical utilization patterns. (1) A stable relationship with a private-practice physician implies that such a physician is used for total primary care and that the public clinic is visited only at the recommendation of the usual physician or when the latter is unavailable. (2) An unstable relationship with a private-practice physician implies that such a physician is named and from time to time is used as the regular physician, but on other occasions the family freely uses the public clinics without contacting the regular physician. (3) A stable relationship with a clinic implies that the family uses one public clinic at least for one kind of service and approaches other sources of medical care only occasionally or rarely. (4), Finally, the unstable relationship with a clinic implies that the family uses several public clinics, indiscriminately, without any discernible system, and presumably in accordance with the momentary convenience. The four typical utilization patterns are conspicuously differentiated by the socioeconomic status of the users. The group having stable relationships with a private-practice physician is characterized by the highest socio-economic status, the status of the group decreases for each following type and reaches the lowest level among those who have unstable relationships with a clinic. In the Boston sample studied, more than half of the Negro families and families with Spanish surnames (mainly Puerto Ricans) belonged to the fourth type.[12]

It is impossible to compare the middle-class pattern of private-practice care with the lower-class pattern of public clinic use without inquiring into the differences in the quality of care. Popular statements on this issue are numerous beyond count, and even medical authorities are wont to issue impressionistic judgments under the claim of general validity. Objective assessments of the issue are not available and mainly so because there is no simple over-all index measuring the quality of health care which would compare one complex system of care to another vastly different but equally complex system. As for the complexity of the system it is useful to realize that there are numberless public clinics in this country which differ not only in their organization, affiliation, program and policies but also in their quality of care. While many of them (and particularly those affiliated with medical schools) have a long tradition of competence and social consciousness, others (and mainly the municipal and church-affiliated institutions) have been established for the purpose of caring for the poor, adjusted themselves to this limited aim and have made less than the desired efforts toward improving the quality of the care.[13]

At present, instead of making an over-all comparison, we shall take up certain aspects of the qualitative differences. One of the outstanding features of private-practice primary care is that it offers personal, systematic, and total care as against the impersonal, episodic, and fragmented care given in public clinics.[14] In private practice the physician, aided by his personal relations with the patient, can exert what Kosa called charismatic medicine, i.e., the assumption of a leadership role in times of distress and the personal intervention of the physician in family problems surrounding the illness.[15] In the public clinics, however, there are practically no chances to establish personal relations between the physician and the patient; accordingly, all those aspects of the treatment process which deal with the personal and emotional problems of the patient are likely to remain unattended. To be sure, the public clinics tend to give competent diagnoses and equally competent symptomatic treatment, but their impersonal atmosphere, time schedule, and lack of privacy discourage—or outright impede—any treatment going beyond the management of a specific complaint.

A number of specialty clinics, and particularly those dedicated to the concept of community psychiatry, aim to deal with the psychiatric problems of those patients who do not use private-practice specialists. But there is a broad range of symptoms

—psychosomatic as well as emotional and social problems—which are often described as "normal problems" and are treated by a primary physician in private practice but seldom receive attention and adequate response in public clinics. A study of a low-income group, representing the users of a large public clinic, pointed out the emotional and social problems (marital difficulties, school problems of children) as the most conspicuous unmet medical need of the group. This unmet medical need could not be fully attributed to the lack of clinical facilities: even when certain specialty clinics (e.g., those dealing with alcoholism) were available in the community, they were not used by the families in the sample.[16]

One may assume that the very structure of the public clinics, denying intimacy between doctor and patient, militates against the treatment of all those problems which do not fall into one clearly defined diagnostic category and is less than efficient in recognizing those problems which patients are reluctant to bring to medical attention.[17] It is reasonable to add that the reluctance of the patient to bring up personally related problems increases with the size of the clinic and with the impersonal, bureaucratic structure of its organization. But, whatever size and structure might be present, the public clinic is rather unlikely to offer charismatic medicine, leadership in times of distress, or personal intervention of the physician.

A combination of convenience, easy availability, and efficiency characterizes the usual middle-class utilization of private-practice physicians, and the frequent use of the telephone in the communication between doctor and patient is a case in point.[18] A telephone call saves time and often saves the inconvenience of visiting the physician's office; moreover, it serves to give psychological support to the patient and to resolve his anxiety. In public clinics, however, telephone calls as means of communication between patient and physician are usually not used and for any problem the patient has to visit the clinic. Although a group of low-income mothers with relatively low education, when given an opportunity within a demonstration project, could make good use of telephone communication and could enjoy the resulting convenience and efficiency of medical services, the bureaucratic, impersonal setting of the public clinics militates against the general adoption of this communication pattern.[19]

Altogether considerable differences undoubtedly exist between private practice and public clinics in the quality of the care given; the human aspect of the differences as they affect the poor will be discussed below. Before considering the human aspects of the dual standards in the existing system of health care, it is necessary to point out that many attempts are being made to improve the services in the public clinics. Among the various reform movements the comprehensive care programs appear to be most important in promising personalized, nonfragmented, and systematic care to the users of public clinics.[20] One experimental study has furnished rather convincing evidence that a properly conducted comprehensive care program is able to overcome the usual shortcomings of the public clinics and provide a system of care for a low-income population that is near to the care given in the private practice of medicine. In the sample receiving comprehensive care the rate of hospitalization and operations became lower and the rate of health visits became higher than in the control group; while the rates of more than twenty categories of morbidity were about the same for both groups, the mothers receiving comprehensive care judged the general health of their families in more favorable terms than the mothers in the control group.[21]

Encouraging as such findings are, one has to question whether the dedication shown by a group of physicians at Harvard Medical School, participating in the above experiment, can be duplicated on a nationwide basis in the other public clinics of the country. It is another question whether the methods used in the small population of a demonstration project can be applied to the masses of poor in the urban centers, let alone the rural areas, of the country. It might very well be that the idea of comprehensive care is a luxury that the country as a whole cannot afford. Seeing the paucity and variety of the comprehensive care programs it is reasonable to believe that the dual medical care system—private practice versus public clinics—is a stable institution that is likely to stay with us for the foreseeable future.

The Case of the Poor Patient

So far we have attempted to investigate health care as an ongoing system, and such an approach hardly needs any justification. Yet system analysis as a method of investigation often implies the danger of forgetting the human element involved. An analysis of the health care system has made it sufficiently clear that the patient of the poor class cannot fare as well as the well-to-do patient. The human element of this difference has to be investigated from a psychological point of view by asking the question: What does it mean to be a poverty-stricken patient? Rather few empirical data are available to answer the question. After all, research is usually carried out by health care systems and institutions, and the patient from the poor class is seldom able to convey his experiences to interested professionals. Thus, the present answer will be essentially impressionistic in an attempt to outline the experiences of the patient from the poor class.

As we have seen, the use of a family doctor may encompass a variety of utilization patterns, and over several years many families receive care from a number of general practitioners and/or internists and pediatricians as well as from many other specialists. Such families may call upon any one of these physicians in an emergency (that is, a complaint which they believe cannot wait until the regular office hours), depending on their conception of the current medical need, the availability of physicians, and the personal preferences of the family.[22] Families that commonly use a private practitioner, and can pay his fees either directly or through insurance coverage, can usually call upon a private physician, but the impoverished family, having made no recent use of private practitioners, finds it difficult to obtain private services and, very often, does not even try to obtain it.

It is difficult for an indigent person to show up at a physician's office and ask to be treated for a routine illness. The old medical practice of carrying some "charity cases" is still maintained by physicians, but the actual impact of charity medicine upon the health status of the poor must be rather small.[23] The private practitioner may apply differential charges based on his concept of the patient's ability to pay, and this is particularly frequent in case of the more expensive services such as major surgery. Again, some poor patients may be on government programs (federal Medicare or state Medicaid) or on the Blue Cross-Blue Shield minimum payment provision, in which case the established fee schedules limit the charges, and the physician is likely to collect less from such persons than from the regular patients. Thus, he tends to classify such persons as less desirable patients whom he may refuse to accept entirely, or more often, tries to pass on to a colleague with a less thriving practice.

Aside from the ability to pay, people coming from a recognizable poverty subculture are likely to have less access to private physicians. They are considered the least desirable patients. The doctor has probably dealt with "their kind" during his years as a student and resident on outpatient and emergency clinics, and he has concluded that they are often dirty and smelly, follow poor health practices, fail to observe directions or meet appointments, and live in a situation which makes it impossible to establish appropriate health regimens. As one resident put it, this offers "a less pleasurable way to practice medicine." [24]

People who are blocked in their access to private physicians tend to visit other healers. Limited evidence indicates that osteopaths, chiropractors, and naturopaths are used to a progressively greater degree as one moves down the socio-economic scale, especially by persons with racial or ethnic stigma. Calling on the advice of druggists and using patent medicines also seems to be more common at the lower socio-economic levels. Such treatment is not only less costly but the lower-class person is less likely to feel rejected by a druggist and is more likely to be given the treatment he wants than if he were to visit a physician.[25]

The major point of contact with the orthodox medical world for the urban poor has been through the outpatient clinic. In such settings there is typically no continuity of care, although it is commonly assumed that continuity of care by the same physician is desirable and that the care given in outpatient and emergency clinics is inferior. But a few data from observations on emergency wards suggests that from the viewpoint of the patient, continuity is not always the desired form of care.[26] Some patients prefer using medical professionals on an episodic basis and to dispense with their help, and with their potential control as well, between these episodes. This is particularly clear in case of patients who have been involved in fights, suspicious accidents, and of women who have attempted abortion. In addition, some patients who do not have such obviously compelling reasons prefer to present themselves to a new physician each time; they would just as soon not have somebody reconstructing their past history from a cumulative chart and basing the treatment on what went before, rather than on the story the patient is presenting at the moment.

In public hospital outpatient clinics there is no question about admitting the poor. The care these clinics provide has commonly been labeled as inferior by private medical practice, although for expert attention private practitioners may refer their patients to clinics associated with medical schools. The care is provided largely by the staff of house officers-in-training. The equipment for diagnosis and treatment is usually more readily available in a clinic than in a private doctor's office, as some patients point out when claiming that they receive better treatment at outpatient clinics than in doctor's offices.

From the viewpoint of the staff, the outpatient clinics are medical Siberia. House officers tend to dislike the kind of people they come to meet in the clinics. The clientele is often seen as desirable only insofar as the doctors-in-training can learn more about medicine by treating them.[27] With medical students and interns the patient is likely to receive careful (and often slow) attention with a risk that mistakes will be made because of the student's inexperience. The more advanced resident, having seen many cases of the common conditions, will be interested in the less common disorders and in disorders of his area of specialization. Patients falling into the right categories will be treated as "interesting cases" and will receive exceptional attention.

One may assume that the alienation of the poverty patient from private-practice medicine has its origin in the usages of the public outpatient clinic. Here the neophyte doctor learns that these people are unwanted as private clientele. His later decisions about where to practice and what kind of practice to establish are affected by what he learns in this setting.

THE SOCIAL ATMOSPHERE OF THE EMERGENCY CLINICS

In city and county hospitals the emergency ward serves mainly as an unscheduled clinic of the poor for accidents and acute illnesses, as well as a clinic for those patients who cannot obtain medical service elsewhere during off hours.[28] It is a rule of public hospital emergency clinics that everyone should be seen by a doctor, and everyone is if he waits it out. The nature of the medical service provided is, in some ways, similar to those of the outpatient clinics, although more episodic. Usually there is no follow-up and at each visit a different physician treats the patient.

The workers on emergency wards with large slum-area clienteles develop a negative conception of their patients. They seek to establish a defensive position against the lower depths of our society. They often exchange stories demonstrating how unintelligent, untrustworthy, and immoral the patients are. New clerks, aides, nurses, and doctors are instructed by the older hands not to tolerate any abuse or disobedience from the clientele, not to accede to their demands, or do burdensome favors for them. Of course, such talk does not closely represent the actual behavior of the personnel; the clerk who states categorically that most patients are "garbage," in fact treats most of them with a fair degree of politeness. However, the patient entering an emergency clinic is not likely to find himself in a friendly comforting atmosphere. He will often wait until employees get around to him, be made to stand while questioned even if ill or aged, notified peremptorily about the rules and procedures ("Sit down over there"; "Put out the cigarette"; "You can't go back there") and subjected to questioning which would be considered impertinent by middle-class people ("Are you on welfare?"; "Is there a father in the home?"; "Are you able to pay for this visit?").

The regulars—patients who receive much of their care at the emergency ward—expect long waits and little concern for their comfort or self-respect, they "roll with the punches" more than the newcomer. They are not entirely helpless in the hands of the hospital personnel and have their techniques for obtaining prompt and effective treatment. They know the best times to come; they know when to remain silent and when to assert themselves in order to be assigned to an appropriate treatment area; they know what symptoms to dramatize to get priority, and what persons to approach for the needed information.

Of course, the staff does not treat all patients the same way.

Some patients are seen as urgent emergencies who deserve all the assistance that the personnel can give them ("That's what we are really set up to do"). Other patients are clearly respectable middle-class persons or fall into some favored category (for example, city employees, policemen, friends of staff members), and are treated with special consideration. The common stance of emergency personnel is, however, that a patient is a "welfare case" unless there is evidence to the contrary.

On the other hand, certain categories receive the brunt of staff hostility and these tend to come from the impoverished and disreputable segments of our society. There is an almost universal hatred of drunks. If they have to be transported, they will be treated like baggage. Their stories are not believed, and they are frequently insulted or treated with a deriding jocularity. They are kept for a long time without examination and then given only cursory attention even when they have sustained an obvious injury. Serious disorders producing neurological malfunction (epilepsy, diabetic coma) are sometimes missed because of the assumption that a dirty ragged man smelling of alcohol is "just a drunk."

Abdominal pain among unmarried young women is often labeled "pelvic inflammatory disease" (PID) before examination and is associated with a dissolute sex life or attempted abortion. Patients with suspected venereal disease are occasionally rejected by clerks and even physicians who establish their own moral barriers. Psychiatric cases are commonly regarded as nuisances, and the tendency is to get rid of them quickly, either to the psychiatric ward or to the outside world. (However, psychiatric patients and children who cause trouble often get quick treatment because they are considered uncontrollable.)

A patient who does not like the way he is treated can always leave (except for a small number of police holds), and in fact, "elopement" is common, running as high as 5 to 10 percent in some emergency clinics. If a person has a private physician, he can contact him; the private-doctor system and the public-clinic system can be used interchangeably. However, precisely those who are treated with hostility by the clinic personnel are least likely to have ready access to a private physician. Their rejection of clinic care may mean that they deprive themselves of all possibilities of care, although in large cities a patient may move from one clinic to the other.

The employees of the emergency clinics cannot overlook the fact that the vast majority of patients coming for care do not have a real emergency and, in the view of the employees, are "abusing" the clinic. They mention, for example, the patient who had a sore throat for two weeks and showed up in the emergency room on Sunday at 3:00 A.M. for immediate treatment. Welfare cases are more likely to be denigrated than patients of private physicians. "They're getting free care, so they think they can take up the valuable time of doctors and nurses any time they please." Thus, if the patient has no problem which is "real emergency" by the definition of the staff, he is more likely to be given short shrift, superficial diagnosis, and careless treatment.

Smaller private hospitals without training programs usually have no house staff and operate limited emergency services. Their standard way of dealing with emergencies is to have one physician on call (with members of the staff taking turns in rotation), who must be summoned from his home or office by a nurse after assessing the situation, collecting information, and deciding what should be done. A number of hospitals are experimenting with a contract physician plan which has a doctor in the hospital available for emergency care. In practice, this service is limited by an adherence to the norms of the private medical system. Thus, it requires that each patient first declare his private physician and that the private physician should be contacted before referring the case to the contract physician. Nurses often insist on notifying the patient's family doctor even when the patient would prefer the doctor on call. Patients who persist in trying to bypass their own doctor are told that "the system doesn't work that way." And indeed it does not. In such a case, the patient can gain his preference only by denying that he has a family doctor. Poor persons without private physicians are even less welcome in such hospitals than in public institutions.

The clerks or nurses ask the patient about insurance, employment, responsibility for payment, and other matters of bill collection. Obviously the poor are at a severe disadvantage at this point since the picture they present of themselves does not make them readily acceptable to the hospital. It is noteworthy that in presenting one's ability to pay, a good insurance policy is frequently better than income and wealth, unless the latter are so conspicuous that they are matters of public knowledge. However, an offer to pay cash is not likely to be refused and may even be encouraged. If the patient is on a state or local medical aid program, he is tabbed as "welfare" with the discriminatory behavior that goes with the label. He is likely to get relatively superficial treatment and discouraged from becoming a regular patient.

INPATIENT CARE

Almost everyone receives some medical attention on an emergency ward, but when it comes to inpatient service, the private hospitals are restrictive. The hospital administration wants payment guaranteed before admission, and sometimes a deposit is required for as much as one week's room and board. The usual way of handling the indigent person who requires admission is to transfer him to the appropriate city or county hospital. The question of finances may occupy the major attention of the nurses and physicians involved in the case. In one case of a private hospital the diagnosis of acute appendicitis requiring surgery was quickly established, but most of the time was spent with patient and physicians discussing the patient's ability to pay. The doctors' notations in the chart were concerned in large part with financial matters.

Because of the complexities of the means tests and residence requirements stipulated by state and local governments for welfare eligibility, a great many patients do not qualify for welfare aid but are unable to meet their medical expenses. These people are the men without a country in the medical world: they are unacceptable to the private medical system and face serious obstacles when trying to obtain care in public hospitals and clinics. The teaching hospitals need indigent patients as teaching material and admit such patients to service wards. Here they are treated by the house officers with the attending physicians supervising. Costs on such wards are held down by having somewhat less nursing coverage, using less floor space per patient, and doing without amenities such as television sets in each room. It is usually more difficult to get admitted to a service ward than to a private room; service wards are more crowded and may specifically exclude patients with given conditions which are not considered sufficiently serious or important to the training program. The indigent patient with a given condition is less likely to be admitted than a private patient with the same condition.

Thus, the poor are taken out of the private medical-care system and relegated to the care of public hospitals. In New York City, for example, about 90 percent of the patients in municipal hospitals are public charges. The municipal hospitals of New York have substantially larger proportions of poor, old, minority-group patients as well as long-stay patients than the service wards of the voluntary hospitals.[29]

Some of the government medical care programs have intended to change the categories of indigents to groups of deserving people and encourage private doctors and hospitals to accept them. Thus, Medicare makes an effort to define its beneficiaries as similar to those who have acquired a Blue Cross-Blue Shield contract or some commercial insurance plan. It is still too early to tell just how this attempt at redefinition will work out, but the present information available indicates that so far it has not been completely successful. One hospital, for example, had an old geriatric building with large open wards with no partitions except pull curtains. Since the local Medicare administration required units with no more than four beds to qualify for payment, the hospital administration erected partitions within the large wards of the geriatric building and divided the open units into four-bed cubicles; the building was then assigned to Medicare patients. Whether this meant that Medicare patients would be treated in the way the old welfare cases had been treated we do not know; but it certainly suggests that the Medicare program has not led the hospital administrators to abandon the old welfare category.

Another private hospital changed the label "Ward Service" to "Chief of Medicine Service" (or "Chief of Surgery Service"), but in other respects seemed to leave the operation of these floors unchanged. Altogether the innovations in these hospitals seemed to be purely nominal. The fact is that many elderly people under the Medicare program are not able to afford the co-insurance part (Medicare pays only 80 percent of the costs over a deductible of $50) and must apply for welfare to cover the rest of the costs. This promptly causes them to be labeled as welfare cases.

CHRONIC PATIENTS

Chronic diseases requiring long-term care give the poor person a greater claim on public treatment facilities than acute disorders. If the chronic ailment poses danger or inconvenience to the public, special facilities are likely to be provided (tuberculosis or mental hospital, nursing home, home for the crippled and disabled, school for the mentally retarded).

Long-term treatment institutions are largely government-operated and publicly financed. This is a matter of default. The private medical system has shown little interest in populations which are difficult to treat in the medical as well as the social sense and are also in a very poor financial state; it has been quite willing to leave such institutions to socialized medicine. It is instructive to consider why public chronic-disease institutions have populations which are heavily overrepresented at the lower socio-economic levels.

Studies of tuberculars have repeatedly pointed out that in the tubercular population the income and occupational levels are relatively low, with single (unmarried) status, separation and divorce, transient life, unemployment before hospitalization, and drinking or alcoholism more common than in the general population. A sizeable portion of the tuberculars are on welfare.[30] However, a study of tuberculosis clinics found considerable evidence that many tuberculosis patients were unknown to public health authorities because they were being treated by private physicians.[31] There is no way of getting accurate data on the size of this group but their numbers may be a significant ratio of those hospitalized for tuberculosis treatment in the same area. Such nonreporting has been recognized as a serious problem by the National Tuberculosis Association.[32] These patients have never been included in the tuberculosis populations on which the reports of social characteristics have been based. There is every reason to believe that patients who have private doctors and thus manage to avoid public hospitals and clinics are of a higher socio-economic status and are likely to have a stable family life and stable employment. This throws considerable doubt on the reports of the common social characteristics of tuberculosis populations and makes one wonder whether there are similar biases among other patient populations also.

Now that effective drug treatment for tuberculosis is available, a poor person usually has no difficulty getting into a hospital. His problem is more likely to be one of getting out and having some choice in entering or leaving a hospital.[33] The patient of higher social status, receiving treatments from a private physician, never becomes entangled with public health officials. If he does enter a hospital, he is likely to get out earlier than others because he is trusted to take care of himself. The poor patient especially with a history of being transient, unemployed, or alcoholic, tends to be regarded by the medical staff as irresponsible and requiring additional hospitalization "to be on the safe side." Many hospitals keep those labeled as alcoholic substantially longer than other patients in the same condition. In one hospital Negroes were explicitly kept longer (and also more often given chest surgery) on the grounds that they led a "harder life" on the outside and required more treatment.

A patient may leave against advice. In tuberculosis hospitals this happens frequently; in some hospitals 50 percent or more of the discharges may be against medical advice. The hospital staff has ways of discouraging discharge against advice and applies these methods primarily to those in a weak social position. If the latter leave the hospital, they may be harrassed by the representatives of the health department and may be threatened with eviction from their living quarters, loss of jobs, or with having their welfare aid discontinued. Frequently the public agencies within an area establish a blacklist of patients who have left one facility against advice and make sure that the patient does not receive treatment during a certain period of time.

Some communities enforce laws against patients who leave against advice or refuse hospitalization. The laws are backed by the argument that tuberculosis is an infectious disease and patients must be isolated to protect others. There is a considerable disagreement among medical authorities concerning the virtue of this argument. It is clear, however, that these laws are applied differentially by social status. Persons prosecuted and jailed (or placed in a locked ward) are almost entirely those of unmistakably lower socio-economic status—largely transients, alcoholics, and persons with limited education and without influential allies. In one area where incarceration for tuberculosis has a long history, I once inquired whether anybody from the middle classes had ever been placed in the locked ward. Three different persons interviewed mentioned the same dentist who had consistently refused treatment even though he had positive sputum, and who was finally locked up under court order for violating the health code; this was the only example they had. As it turned out, this dentist had received special consideration and given repeated chances to institute private treatment on his own, but continued to practice his profession for months in spite of warnings about the danger to his clientele. When action was finally taken against him, his lawyer got him released within three months, while other patients spent six to twelve months in the locked unit before being released.

The Unwanted Patient

In mental disorders we have a similar picture on a larger scale. While the diagnostic category might be the same for patients with different social backgrounds, the received treatment is certainly different. Persons of low socio-economic status are less likely to be able to put up an effective defense in commitment procedures.[34] They are much more likely to end up on the wards of a state mental hospital rather than at a private hospital or with a private practitioner; they are more likely to be institutionalized in a home for the retarded than kept at home; they are more likely to be treated in public clinics than in private clinics. They are more likely to be given custodial care than therapy, organic therapy rather than psychotherapy, and directive psychotherapy rather than analytic psychotherapy. Even when financial ability is not directly concerned, such as in free public clinics, their treatment is more likely to be relegated to medical students and social workers, while those of higher status receive the services of established psychiatrists.[35]

If the tuberculosis patient finds it difficult to leave the hospital, the difficulties are compounded for the mental patient whose admission is often tied to legal commitment and whose release is subject to reviews and hearings. In other cases it is a lack of suitable living arrangements after hospitalization that keeps many patients institutionalized for an unduly long time, and the arrangements for suitable living are closely associated with the patient's socio-economic status. Altogether it is generally recognized the patients of low socio-economic status find it more difficult to leave a treatment institution, and they stay institutionalized longer than patients of higher socio-economic status.[36]

The problem of the differential treatment of the chronically ill is best illuminated by the large chronic-disease hospitals that are becoming increasingly common features of metropolitan areas. Their many inmates have some specific chronic ailment or disability, but so have many people on the outside who manage to keep out of public institutions. Indeed, these chronic-disease hospitals, instead of being primary treatment institutions, serve mainly as the dumping grounds for the unwanted such as the aged. Most of their patients have no families or friends or are not wanted by them. Most of them were economically marginal before entering the institution, and the welfare policy of seizing any of their assets in payment for hospitalization, destroys whatever financial independence they had.[37] The practice of stripping patients of their assets and blocking them from any income while hospitalized (even Social Security checks are seized by the welfare agencies) tends to perpetuate their residential and economic dependency. Their indigency becomes a sentence of enforced institutionalization.

Such patients are forced to depend on institutions although not all of them spend the rest of their lives there. Some are able to take advantage of the treatment services offered and gain release, and those with family ties, with money, or outside support are more likely to escape. In a sample of sixty cases, it was found that only one fourth of those who had been impoverished when entering the hospital returned to community living; about one third of those whose income was markedly reduced during hospitalization returned to the community; but all those who continued to be financially independent left the hospital. In this selective process the financial ability to live outside the hospital appears to be more important than the actual physical condition.[38]

The mental hospitals, chronic disease hospitals, homes for the mentally retarded, nursing homes, or training schools serve ostensibly different purposes; yet, any description of their operations makes it sufficiently clear that they fulfill the same function in our society. They are intended to remove those who have proved nuisances to others in more advantageous social positions. They give a chance to remove unwanted people from the midst of the communities and their mere existence, as a psychological solution of a disturbing problem, blocks any efforts toward finding viable ways of accommodating the aged, the disabled, the poor, and the other unwanted.

It is essential to realize that medical care in the United States is not generally regarded as the right of an individual. Each person or family must demonstrate in what way he deserves medical attention. Because of the widely accepted primacy of the private fee-for-service medical care system, one can most readily show that he is deserving by establishing an ongoing relationship with a private physician. If one is poor, the chances of establishing oneself in a deserving category is difficult.

Of course, the identification of "deserving" and "undeserving" patients is not a simple matter. If the patient has not been labeled from a previous contact, physicians and hospitals use a combination of clues (dress, cleanliness, residence, employment, education) to place him and such clues will influence the immediate response that he will receive. Even among welfare patients there is a clear discrimination by levels of deservingness. Those on Aid to the Totally Disabled (if it is not their own fault) are rated more deserving than those on Aid to Dependent Children (result of a life of sin). In any given welfare category, a patient is likely to be treated as more deserving at a public clinic than at a private hospital.

The definition of what constitutes a deserving applicant for medical care has changed and presumably will continue to change; Medicare is a recent example of organized official effort to change. The Medicare program was intended not simply as a means of paying medical bills, but also of placing a category of persons, the aged, into the "deserving" class much the same way as Social Security, retirement pay, and the Blue Cross refund are regarded as deserved compensations rather than doles.

It is clear, however, that the state medical-aid programs have not succeeded in defining their beneficiaries as deserving. Our society is so lacking in clear-cut indicators of one's station of life that it is often difficult to tell the deserving from the undeserving. The Medicare system applies without discrimination to an ascriptive class and does not provide categorical indicators within that class. The state aid programs provide an indicator, the means test; by virtue of being on a state program, a person has placed himself in the class of indigency or poor risk. He becomes classified as a welfare case and his unacceptability becomes pronounced if the state aid program is poorly financed and the doctor or hospital are uncertain about receiving payment for their services. Generally speaking, medical-care programs have no chance of getting their beneficiaries accepted as deserving unless they are applied in a categorical manner to all persons in an ascriptive class without regard to income or assets. Such a principle, although it would not remove all the differentials among socio-economic groups in medical care, is the basic precondition to a greater acceptance of the poor by the private medical system.

There are, of course, other possibilities. The private-practice view of the welfare patient is much less pronounced among the physicians and administrators of medical schools. Through a variety of programs, medical schools are gradually spreading their influence and control over an increasing portion of medical care in this country. Along with this increasing influence we might expect a broadening of the concept of the deserving patient in more and more areas of private medical practice, and a redefinition of the concept that will be less closely tied to economic status.

Still another approach is to place more medical-care resources in publicly operated organizations under conditions which attract physicians. Such a move would make publicly sponsored medicine the norm rather than the deviation which it now is. But at this point in history, this seems to entail an even greater task of redefinition than getting private practitioners and private hospitals to accept the poor as deserving.

We have argued that, given the currently dominant nature of American medical practice and, in particular, its failure to include competent medical care in the broadest sense as an inalienable right of all, the poor person who becomes sick is subject, at every stage and in every way, to inferior medical care and to human indignity. In large measure barred from access to private physicians, he must turn—if indeed he does turn—to other, largely inferior, treatment frameworks. Over and above the more strictly medical criteria, the sick person who is poor and turns to the outpatient clinic or the emergency ward, suffers indignity, abuse, and disregard. Nor, with few exceptions, is his fate any better when hospitalized. But if he can opt out or be opted out of outpatient treatment or inpatient care for acute disorders, chronic illness presents a different picture. Chances are that the tubercular, the mentally ill, and other chronic sufferers are more likely to be hospitalized and kept incarcerated for reasons which have little to do with medical criteria.

We are aware that the picture we have painted derives, to some extent, from experiences and impressions, although the studies of the problems have been cited above. If the reader prefers to regard our account as tentative, subject to correction, so it be. This account is certainly testable.

VIII · Readjustment and Rehabilitation of Patients

by Marvin B. Sussman

We know very little about what happens to patients after they have gone through a hospital, medical-care or rehabilitation institution, and a number of factors have inhibited research in this area.* First, not enough investigators have found it sufficiently rewarding to undertake costly longitudinal studies and follow up patients after their discharge from a rehabilitation setting. It is difficult indeed to deal with the problems related to the design of such studies in view of the limitations of current methodological techniques, the persistence, motivation, and longevity of investigators and subjects, the cost of such studies, and finally the inherent biases in studying institutional populations.[1]

A second inhibitor has been the posture of the institutional system regarding follow-up studies and evaluations of service. Most of these institutions require a form of evaluation which will indicate that the services offered have beneficial consequences for the patient population and promote convalescence, recovery, and eventual restoration as a working member of the community. The very nature of the institutional system requires that it produce successful cases in order to obtain funds from the public or government. A number of investigators have pointed

* I wish to express appreciation for the assistance of Kim Siegel, research assistant, Department of Sociology, Case Western Reserve University, in the preparation of this chapter.

out that any agency must justify its existence by translating the services it performs quantitatively in terms of dollars per person served.[2] The agency is forced to function with a marketplace ideology while espousing humanitarian concerns and maintaining an other-oriented posture. In the case of rehabilitation, success is measured by the expected contribution the handicapped person will make to the gross national product after he is restored to the community. This type of orientation, attempting to satisfy the demands of other institutional systems upon which health systems are dependent, requires a biased evaluation. It begins with the selection of cases which are "good" from the standpoint of consequences of treatment, and this selection usually takes place when the patient is admitted. Institutional systems, being evaluated by lay boards and other groups that furnish financial support, tend to select clients who will optimize their success rates in terms of client economic productivity after treatment.[3]

A third inhibiting factor has been the lack of conceptual clarity concerning such terms as illness, disease, social class, and the deployment of social class in studies regarding differential morbidity. It is obvious that each of these phenomena require different structures, mechanisms, and processes for proper handling; yet they are treated as being identical, and the consequence is terminological confusion. The recent spirited debate between Kadushin and Antonovsky makes it clear that, in the development of concepts such as social class in relation to illness, we have tended to ignore the meaning of illness, the setting in which it occurs, and the relationship of illness to other problems the individual must learn to handle.[4]

Part of the cause of the conceptual ambiguity surrounding social class is that most research using socio-economic status as an independent or explanatory variable employs ordinal rather than interval scaling methods for indexing class status. Ordinal scales are prone to produce variable conclusions over observed class differences depending upon the cutting points used by the researcher in scoring class position. There is some advantage to consider such variables as education, income, or occupation as independent measures of socio-economic status because each of these vary from one another in their power of association with dependent variables.[5] It is generally difficult to use the social class concept as currently formulated when occupation and education are employed as the two main indicators.[6] The limitations in the indicators of social class can be overcome by methodological techniques which compensate for lower occupational placement of Negroes, higher occupational status of wives in some family units, and by updating the occupational classification system. All these changes do not rectify our neglect of such factors as poor sanitation, overcrowding, and dietary practices, all of which place limitations upon the individual's life style and contribute to poor health and achieved levels of rehabilitation.

Poverty stands out as a major factor associated with disability. Dishart documented this relationship in a comprehensive study of disability in the state of Maryland, where he found 300 percent more disability among the very poor. While there was a generally higher incidence of disability among Negroes than among whites, this difference disappeared among the poor. Negroes, however, had higher incidence rates than whites in certain disability categories, seven times as much blindness, and twice as much diabetes.[7]

Rehabilitative Hospitalization Among the Poor

One may speculate whether the need for rehabilitative treatment is more pressing among the poor than among the non-poor, but, in any case, the availability and utility of such treatments show conspicuous variations by income classes. Getting into a hospital or other rehabilitative institution poses different problems for members of different classes because there is more than one path to medical care. Individuals of different economic levels enter at various stages of illness and vary in their experiences with medical care systems, particularly with their getting discharged from a hospital or rehabilitation setting. There appears to be an interrelationship between gaining entrance to, and obtaining discharge from, a medical care institution.

In the field of mental health, studies indicate an under-utilization of medical facilities by the poor because of their negative attitudes toward mental illness, the middle-class character of mental health rehabilitation, and their limited knowledge of the routes to medical care systems. The poor as a rule "get in" when they come to the attention of social and welfare agencies.

Most lower-class individuals view mental illness as the opposite of "normality," and they equate mental disease with one of the severest forms of disorder, namely, being "crazy." [8] They avoid voluntary hospitalization and regard any institutional treatment as involuntary. Those in control of mental-care institutions look at this orientation as being basically primitive and backward but accept it; as a consequence, lower-class individuals with disturbed behavior are not only institutionalized but, unless they respond quickly to treatment, are relegated to custodial care. As a result, as one study found, within the surviving population of a state hospital, 93 percent of the lowest income group were still in the state hospital ten years later, while almost all patients in the middle- and upper-income groups had been released.[9] According to another study, the functionally psychotic individuals of the lowest socio-economic group stay in the hospital longer than other groups.[10]

Social marginality appears to lead to a prolonged stay in mental hospitals. Aged, divorced, or single patients, those in unskilled occupations and of low education and social class have the longest hospital stay.[11] Such indicators of social conditions evidently enter into the hospital staff's decision to discharge or retain a patient. The lack of family pressures for discharge, the absence of an appropriate home for the patient after discharge, difficulty in obtaining work, marital status, race, and many related factors lower the probability of a discharge and tend to produce that residue population which fills the back wards of our mental hospitals.

A study of an experimental home care program of schizophrenics reported that better-educated and higher-status persons were more successful in home treatment than lower-status persons.[12] This study was not measuring specifically post-hospital performance but was concerned with the consequences of treatment of schizophrenia in the hospital or in the community. Nevertheless, its finding substantiates the notion that less-educated and lower-status persons do less well in handling their illnesses at home, while higher success rates in maintaining rehabilitation gains are positively related to social class status.[13]

Another variable seems to obscure the effect of socio-economic differences upon the length of hospitalization for physical illnesses. One study which compared three hospitals obtained an estimate of the average duration of hospitalization for common operations and found that, regardless of the treatment, patients remained longer in teaching than nonteaching institutions.[14] In addition to this institutional factor, the methods of paying for hospital care—an indicator of socio-economic status—also marked considerable differences. Private patients and those with voluntary commercial insurance had slightly shorter hospitalization periods than patients with Blue Cross, while patients who had "other" methods of payment, such as welfare, government funding, or industrial compensation, stayed in hospitals the longest. Another study, concerned with the ability of the patient to maintain rehabilitation gains after discharge from a chronic disease hospital, found that the patient is likely to arrive at his maximum hospital benefits about the same time his hospitalization insurance expires.[15] The underlying logic of this situation is the high cost of medical care: in the hospital concerned, the average cost for care had risen to fifty dollars per day in 1967. As a consequence, great pressure is placed on public officials in the case of welfare patients and on family members in the case of private patients to make arrangements for a discharge about the time the hospitalization benefits expire.

There is other evidence that the economic factor is related to length of stay in the hospital. Investigating the efficacy of the kin network in providing adjunct support and therapy to the disabled individual during and after discharge from the rehabilitation hospital, the patients were categorized as to whether they were in functioning family and kin networks or whether they were relatively isolated. The differences were insignificant between those who were isolated and those who were in active kin networks in receiving financial support from family members to pay for their illness; both groups paid about the same amount of money for their illness and relied largely on nonfamily sources of payment. There were, however, significant differences in the amount of emotional support given to the individual—a support vital for effective rehabilitation. It appeared that chronically ill individuals and their responsible others were willing to accept financial support from established sources such as government pension plans, insurance programs, and prepaid hospital insurance. They accepted a third party for the support of illness, and this had a very specific relationship to the length of stay in the hospital.

REDUCED REHABILITATION POTENTIAL

Social group identification, membership in a family, active work, and social life are important factors in a study concerned with predicting the vocational and economic status of patients after their discharge from a tuberculosis hospital.[16] Three types of patients had markedly reduced rehabilitation potentials, and they were designated as "family isolates," "anomic," and "otherwise ill" (see Table VIII–1). The family isolates, i.e., individuals found to be living alone, were classified in light of the notion that living alone can bring forth by-products of isolation that militate against rehabilitation. Patients classified as anomic not only lived apart from family members but in addition had unstable work records for five years prior to diagnosis of tuberculosis. The "otherwise ill" were those individuals whose tuberculosis was complicated by other medical conditions. It was found that those living alone suffered disproportionately from other illnesses compared with those living with family members. Each of these "problem types" was more likely to suffer medical relapse, fail to find steady employment, or have economic difficulties than the "normal" group. In short, they were least able to shake off the effects of the illness.

Table VIII–1. Tuberculosis patients with reduced rehabilitation potentials.

Patient sample	Number	Percent
Total medical register sample	384	100
Never hospitalized	79	20
Hospitalized	305	80
Total hospitalized sample	305	100
Normals	115	38
Types with reduced rehabilitation potentials [a]	190	62
Family isolates	108	35
Anomics	65	21
Otherwise ill	154	51

Source: Marvin Sussman, Marie R. Haug, and Marjorie R. Lamport, "Rehabilitation Problems Among Special Types of Tuberculosis Patients," American Review of Respiratory Diseases, 92 (August 1965), 262.

[a] Because of overlapping, patients were categorized in more than one type. Numbers and percentages of types add up to more than the total with reduced rehabilitation potentials.

Concerning the severity of illness at time of diagnosis and ultimate hospitalization, most patients were already infected with active tuberculosis when originally diagnosed and were promptly hospitalized. Among the others (N=86), whose first diagnosis showed a nonactive and noninfectious state, those whose disease remained in the minimal stage were compared with those whose disease progressed until hospitalization became necessary. The two groups showed clear differences in family living arrangements. More than two thirds of the family isolates were eventually hospitalized due to exacerbation of the disease, while of those living with family members, two thirds maintained a dormantly stable disease without hospitalization.

The finding that isolation is a condition related to progressing disease supports Kissen's research in Scotland, where he found significant relationships between "broken love links" and the onset or relapse of tuberculosis.[17] Love links are ties that provide identification, security, affection, attention, and other conditions necessary for the individual's psychological well-being. A break in a love link, such as the end of a love affair or marital separation, may create a crisis with such effects that the individual is unable to cope either with long-range problems or those of everydyay life. It could be argued that in a medical sense the individual's resistance to disease decreases, the loss of the love link triggers an onset of tuberculosis, and the latent or inactive infection now becomes manifest.

Hospital admittance itself seems to be related to both isolation and socio-economic status. One might rightly assume that persons living within family networks are subject to family pressures to "take care of themselves" and thus tend to seek medical advice sooner than persons living alone. At the same time, it is generally observed that persons of higher socio-economic groups are likely to obtain medical help at an earlier stage of illness and thus often manage to avoid hospitalization.

In the tuberculosis study just described, the higher-income patients were more apt to receive drug treatment at home or in a general hospital, while patients of the lower socio-economic level, with their tendency to defer treatment until a severe stage of the illness, were likely to be admitted immediately into a tuberculosis hospital.

REHABILITATION PERFORMANCE AND SOCIAL CLASS

The ways in which the patient with a chronic disease enters a rehabilitation hospital differs markedly from the pattern of hospital entry associated with acute illness. In one rehabilitation center of Maryland, a study of 612 patients with cerebrovascular accidents showed that socio-economic conditions rather than the desire for rehabilitation appeared to be the major reasons for seeking hospitalization with minimal delay.[18] Patients who were seventy-five years and older, females, nonwhites, and without spouses, showed a short delay, perhaps because such "down and outers" had fewer of those obstacles in their paths to rehabilitation which are presented by anxious family members and physicians. It is probable that patients used to having "troubles" can perceive of rehabilitation as improving their current level of minimal functioning.

A pattern of exchanging noninstitutional for institutional living conditions may be emerging among the disabled poor. Potentially the patient may profit from this exchange because, in long-term medical care, he receives social services and vocational retraining also. Support for this notion comes from the five-year follow-up study of the maintenance of rehabilitation gains after discharge from a rehabilitation hospital.[19] Table VIII–2 sums up the data on patients discharged over a five-year period who did not participate in follow-up observations after discharge. It indicates a tendency on the part of the lower-class patients to maintain contact with the hospital personnel and use them as consultants for their problems. For such patients, the long-term experience in the hospital might have created "dependency longings" and a desire to return; thus, they are likely to respond with a willingness to cooperate to the interest shown by the medical staff. Successful post-hospital care appears to be the result of hospital personnel interest and the poor patient's needs and longings.

Table VIII–2. Rehabilitation patients (by social class) failing to participate in follow-up observations.

Social Class	Number	Failed to Participate [a]	
		Number	Percent
I	3	0	0
II	5	1	20
III	23	4	17
IV	58	10	17
V	64	5	8
Underclassed	24	1	4

Source: Morris W. Stroud, III, *et al.*, "Rehabilitation Patient's Needs: A Five-Year Follow-Up Study" (in process).

[a] Includes those who could not be located as well as those who refused to participate.

Leaving the hospital against medical advice (AMA) has grave implications for the patient's post-hospital functioning and eventual rehospitalization. Reports that every year almost half of all tuberculosis patients leave the hospital against the advice of their physicians do not appear to stimulate research in this area.[20] To be sure, such studies might make visible what appears to be an institutional failure.

One study of AMA used a stay-response or quit-response dichotomy among patients of a Veteran's Administration hospital.[21] The probability of the quit-response was highest for the unemployed (.83), followed by the laborers (.64) and other physical workers (.62), while white-collar people scored .51, and students only .27. These data indicate some relationship between economic-work status and use of hospital facilities.

It would be erroneous, however, to assume that poverty in itself increases the incidence of AMA. It is rather the conditions surrounding poverty and the medical resources available to the poor that are more specifically related to AMA. In looking at our rehospitalized group, a marked relationship appeared between rehospitalization and AMA discharges. Over half the patients hospitalized more than once had left against medical advice. The chances were almost two out of three that, if the patient left the hospital before the physician considered him ready, he would be back for another stay. Most of the AMA cases came from the isolated and anomic groups.[22]

Longitudinal studies on the post-hospital performance of patients with severe physical disabilities and from different socio-economic strata are limited in number. The data of one study, however, indicate that deterioration in activities of daily living or early death in the post-hospital period is associated with economic dependence. The economic dependence scale is composed of evaluations in four areas: (1) receiving or not receiving agency support for maintenance; (2) ownership or nonownership of residence; (3) employed or not employed; and (4) independent living without personal assistance, or living in a protected environment such as a boarding home. The index of Independence in Activities of Daily Living (ADL) is based on an evaluation of the functional independence of patients in bathing, dressing, using toilet, transferring from bed to chair, continence, and feeding.[23] The data show that higher economic dependence is associated with higher rate of ADL deterioration and early death (see Tables VIII–3 and VIII–4). Class I is of low economic dependence and Class V is of high economic dependence. ADL evaluations were made one, two, and five years after discharge from hospital. For both hip fracture and stroke patients the higher economic dependence was associated with a faster rate of deterioration or early death.

Table VIII–3. Economic dependence and deterioration of activities among patients with fracture of the hip.

Level of Economic Dependence	Percent deteriorated in activities of daily living or dead		
	One year	Two years	Five years
I (N = 5)	20.0	20.0	20.0
II (N = 52)	46.2	57.7	71.1
III (N = 71)	66.2	71.9	84.5
IV (N = 15)	80.0	93.4	100.0
V (N = 4)	75.0	100.0	100.0

Source: Sidney Katz *et al.*, "Continuing Care Project," unpublished manuscript, Benjamin Rose Institute and Case Western Reserve Medical School.

Table VIII–4. Economic dependence and deterioration of activities among patients with first stroke.

Level of Economic Dependence	Percent deteriorated in activities of daily living or dead		
	One year	Two years	Five years
I (N = 17)	76.4	76.4	82.3
II (N = 54)	68.5	75.9	90.8
III (N = 39)	89.8	92.3	100.0
IV (N = 15)	93.3	80.0	100.0
V (N = 2)	100.0	100.0	100.0

Source: Ibid.

The data on post-hospital performance and AMA behavior unequivocally indicate a relationship between socio-economic status, morbidity, mortality, and maintenance of rehabilitation gains. Causation between poverty and these factors has not been established, but the correlation is sufficiently high to suggest collective efforts to modify this association and devise new approaches to dispense medical care.

The Medical Care System
and the Rehabilitation of the Poor

Contemporary patterns of medical care and the demands placed upon the health institutions mean that follow-up of patients is rarely accomplished by the medical institution alone and is much more a function of the patient's willingness to maintain a relationship with the health-care system. We have to make the assumption that the conditions which lead individuals to seek medical care and to utilize medical-care systems at the onset of illness are the same which motivate them to use such facilities after parenthood. The few modifying variables would be their experiences with the medical-care system as well as their acceptance of, and identification with, the medical-care system.

The principal factors in the under-utilization of medical-care facilities by the poor are the bureaucratic structure of medical care, the value orientations dominating the medical-care system, the differential assessment by health organizations of the desirability of clients, the potential outcome of treatment, the economic costs, and the family responses to discharge.

Medical-care systems are bureaucratic organized according to specialization of functions. It was found that under-utilization of medical care by New York City blue-collar workers was related to the fact that the poor had little contact with professional members of medical-care specialties and turned first to a "lay referral network of immediate friends and relatives." [24] They were ignorant of the services available, especially preventive services, and were unprepared to cope with the bureaucratic structure of medical care. Medical-care systems operate on principles of scientism and rationality. They believe in performing a service and assume that a person coming to them is willing to have his problem solved and permit the system to operate fully. In other words, they expect the patient to assume the traditional sick role and allow the medical system to work out the solution. In this sense the health enterprises are culture-bound, basically directed by middle-class-oriented technology which severely limits their availability to impoverished individuals.[25]

Bureaucratic health systems consist of specialized professional and occupational systems, each possessing a theoretical stance in regard to illness, treatment, and rehabilitation. The separate systems are more or less integrated into a complex system of work in which there is constant competition and struggle for status and power. Each occupational system has its own needs, and much of the behavior in an occupational system is found to be consistent with these occupational values and goals.[26] These occupational systems make demands on their co-workers as well as on their patients, and these demands may not be in consonance with the demands of the recipients of medical care.

This last point is illustrated by a study on the expressed satisfactions and dissatisfactions of givers and receivers of outpatient care, namely, staff and patients, in a large university hospital.[27] One important finding related to the variability and ambivalence expressed by different occupational groups composing the hospital staff. They differed greatly in value systems, perceptions, and definitions of the ideal and real clinical situation; they varied in satisfactions and especially in their concern for the patient. All stated a concern for good outpatient care, but manifested occupational variations as to whether their primary interest in the patient was for purposes of teaching or research. Members of the paramedical staff indicated a greater concern with deficiencies in patient care, whereas the medical-clinical staff felt that patient care was adequate but deficiencies existed concerning teaching and research.

One can interpolate from these findings that the patient is

viewed as a subject who fits into the rest of the institutional system. The patient is confronted with a bureaucratic system which adapts his interests to its own. If there is a happy coincidence of interests, the patient will gain in treatment and care. Patients who do not fit the model, either in terms of diagnosis or the role of the good patient, find the system too formidable to handle, especially for post-hospital treatment.

The effects of victimization of the poor client by powerful bureaucratic systems may be mitigated by actions of another and contending bureaucracy, the welfare system. The lengthy stay of poor patients in hospitals, the high cost of therapy and inadequate service in meeting patient needs may result in tension and hostile action by the welfare system, which is legally required to pay the bills of the indigent. Complaining in order to initiate investigation and organizing indigent groups to support change in institutional policies are two devices increasingly used by the underclassed.

The association of certain types of illnesses with deviance is another factor explaining the small amount of follow-up in the post-hospital period.[28] Lower-class patients are more sensitive and defenseless to the public's labeling of their illnesses as deviance. This holds whether or not a stigma (such as the stigma of irresponsibility) is attached to the particular illness. Because of the many psychological and economic losses that may arise as a consequence of a deviant label, the lower-class patient is reluctant to participate in follow-up programs unless they are offered in a discrete unobtrusive way.[29]

Let us consider a patient with a relatively favorable condition, i.e., one which is curable and free from the stigma of irresponsibility. Such a patient, if he is from the lower class, can ill afford to participate in follow-up programs because participation implies absence from work and loss of income. While one cannot fully agree with the statement that, "the poor person actually cannot afford to recover from illness," the major point is well stated.[30]

Tuberculosis is a disease which arouses loathing, for which the individual is often held responsible, and which has a prognosis of possibly being improved and controlled but not cured. The public response of fear, disgust, or loathing produces for the individual a barrier to normal social interaction and, as Goffman has indicated, makes him feel isolated.[31] A high percentage of tuberculosis patients, like alcoholics, deny that they have the disease. Streeter, investigating the fantasies of tuberculosis patients, found that one third of them denied that they had the disease or that the disease was caused by tuberculosis bacillus.[32] Even after a lengthy hospitalization and successful treatment, our post-hospital study found that many tuberculosis patients refused to be interviewed, claiming that they never had been in the hospital; some of them undertook elaborate steps to avoid the interviewer and refused to be followed.

All treatment control and welfare agencies use diagnostic stereotypes. What may start initially as diagnostic hypotheses usually persist, and all cases are fitted into these stereotyped descriptions. The consequence is a scientific model of diseases relying on the notion of "normal cases with standardized treatment, prognosis and diagnosis." [33] Each practitioner attempts to utilize these diagnostic categories in handling the illnesses of clients and attempts to convince the patient that his stereotype is the correct one. The patient in turn may have his own, but the physician to some degree proselytizes the patient into believing that he has the type of disease that the physician perceives according to the symptoms.[34] The physician "sells" the patient on this diagnosis and the appropriate behavior which will enhance recovery. It is obvious that if the patient does not agree with the physician, he is apt to go elsewhere or disregard the medical regimen. Consequently, if the patient feels that he has been mislabeled, he will avoid involvement in any post-patienthood program. In case of mental illness where the lower-class patient is forceably detained in an institution, the chances of his entering and staying in a post-hospital treatment program are practically nil. In case of physical illness and disability, the same patient is likely to delay rehospitalization in the hope that he may enter a preferred institution or service which has a diagnostic model closer to his perceived condition.

LENGTH OF HOSPITALIZATION

The economic costs of medical care and convalescence are factors impeding follow-up after discharge from a hospital or rehabilitation center. They deter institutional systems from expending effort in follow-up programs, especially for the poor. At the same time, the lengthy hospitalization with often insignificant improvement in the actual condition leads to some disenchantment, moving many patients to discontinue association with the institution once they leave it. Yet the length of stay in hospitals is not determined by the desire of the patient but rather by the source of his financial support. One study on the cost of hospitalization in a chronic-disease institution found that the source of funding appeared to influence the average duration of hospitalization and attempted rehabilitation.[35] A comparison of patients with private and public funding revealed marked differences, and the patients with total or partial public funding had a considerably longer total hospitalization (and an even more markedly longer rehabilitation hospitalization) than patients with private funding (see Table VIII–5).

To understand this difference, a few factors need to be controlled. Disability (such as impairment in activities of daily living and/or mobility existing for six months prior to hospitalization) might prolong treatment and rehabilitation, but such prior disability was more prevalent in the group with private funding than in the group with public funding (29 percent versus 19 percent). An examination of the diagnostic categories did not produce significant differences between the two groups of patients. In view of such background data it may be of interest that, when the improved independence in mobility and ADL status during hospitalization and in the five-year follow-up period was examined, patients with public funding (total or partial) performed somewhat better than patients with private support. Patients with public funding showed slightly more gains in mobility and ADL during hospitalization and the follow-up period (66 percent versus 61 percent) and suffered slightly less failures in attempted rehabilitation (33 percent versus 40 percent).

Table VIII–5. Length of hospital stay for patients discharged from a rehabilitation hospital, by source of funding.

Source of funding	Number of patients	Average stay in days		
		In prior hospital	In rehabilitation hospital	Total
Private	107	66.9	70.3	115.3
Public	44	48.3	142.7	187.0
Private and public	26	67.1	191.3	240.1

Source: Morris W. Stroud, III, *et al.,* "Rehabilitation Patients' Needs: A Five-Year Follow-Up Study," unpublished manuscript.

It is evident that poor patients are kept, on the whole, almost twice as long in the hospital system than the better-off patients. Such an arrangement may, in part, help to meet some of the teaching and research needs of the institution involved; it may help in a major way to pay for the overhead and related costs of the hospital. At the same time, the data suggest two possible conclusions: either the lower-class patients come to the hospital sicker and more disabled than the higher-class patients, or they are less successful in obtaining release from the hospital. On the basis of available evidence, we are prone to discard the former and accept the latter explanation. The higher rate of previous disability among the privately supported patients as well as the finding of insignificant differences among the hospitalized poor and non-poor for hemiplegia, para- and quadriplegia, hip fracture, amputation, arthritis, and neurological disorders gives little support indeed for the former conclusion. As for the second one, it appears that the poor meet the needs of the institutions to have a stable population for income, teaching, and research purposes. Also, the poor are less likely to have family settings to which they can be discharged and have available sufficient nursing homes and financial support for nursing-home care; thus, they stay in hospital for a longer time. At the same time, the poor person can least afford to be absent from his family, neighborhood, and job, whereas the person of a higher social class, who has a much shorter period of recovery from a serious chronic illness, has more resources for handling the interruption and increased possibilities of being habitated into normal work and social roles.

Post-hospital Performance

Some data support the hypothesis of a direct relationship between the performance levels of patients after discharge from a hospital and the class status of their families. Insofar as mental illness is concerned, there appears to be a higher rate of rehospitalization among middle-class than lower-class patients, largely based upon the fact that families in the lower class have a higher tolerance toward deviant behavior than those in the middle class.[36] The family establishes the norm of tolerance, and although by professional criteria the patient may be sick enough to require rehospitalization, the family does not relinquish him to the institution. If the norm of tolerance persists and the sick person is no economic burden to the family, then a large number of individuals are unhospitalized and are widely scattered in the communities. The community in this sense becomes the therapeutic milieu for many mentally ill patients. One should treat with caution hospital readmission rates as criteria in determining the efficacy of a hospital treatment program.

The meaning and significance that illness has for the maintenance and interaction pattern of the family are determining factors affecting the patient's post-hospital performance. A long-term illness and disability is likely to be associated with a rallying among family members at the onset of the illness.[37] Once the illness passes the acute stage, the professional caretakers make an assessment of whether the patient can be returned to his family. Careful consideration is given to the financial capabilities of the family and the potential stresses, frustrations, and other reductions in achieving family and individual goals. These considerations enter into the decisions whether the patient should be kept in the home and influence the attention, empathy, and acceptance that family members can give to a disabled person. This does not mean that family members are devoid of sympathy, and many families function under great deprivation in order to give comfort and economic support to the ill person. Rather, the family as a system has its own needs for maintenance over time, and with the increased development of specialized institutional systems, it can be relieved of major burdens.

An examination of the work status of discharged mental patients points out that those who are gainfully employed have bargaining power, and they can develop new roles or revitalize old roles of high prestige within the family. Those in a dependent (non-working) situation have only short-term security and are subject to unilateral decisions on matters such as rehospitalization.[38] These findings support the theoretical notion of the family as a unit possessing exchange systems involving bargaining and reciprocities. To a large degree the success of a post-patienthood program depends upon the potential benefits to be received by the family as well as the patient.

The post-hospitalization care of the poor can be generally characterized as a state of medical deprivation. Considering our knowledge of poverty, one can agree with Edward Suchman that medical deprivation is a special case of over-all social and cultural deprivation.[39] An understanding of the problems of the poor in relation to medical care in the post-patienthood period can only be obtained by accepting the fact that a large number of social-psychological, economic, and cultural factors produce the conditions of poverty. Medical deprivation, whether it is induced by the institutional system or by the individual himself, is part of an over-all condition of deprivation.

IX · The Future of Poverty

by Arthur B. Shostak

Considerable progress has been made in the nation's antipoverty effort since the enactment late in 1964 of the Economic Opportunity Act and the establishment of the Office of Economic Opportunity (OEO). In the first three years of its operation, as the OEO estimates, perhaps 10 million of the nation's 32 million poor have been helped to begin to move out of poverty, and perhaps four million actually escaped from poverty between 1964 and 1968. Over 1,200 communities, including every major American city, formed antipoverty boards that attempted to bridge the wide gap between the community's poor and non-poor citizens. Some 90,000 poor people earned newly created paraprofessional jobs in local antipoverty programs or secured decision-shaping posts on antipoverty boards. Old-line agencies in education, welfare, and related fields were encouraged to sponsor their own antipoverty innovations, often in response to such stimulating government developments as Get Set, Upward Bound, Foster Grandparents Program, Neighborhood Health Centers, and Legal Services. Over a million youngsters participated in the summer pre-school program known as Project Head Start, and nearly a million adolescents were enrolled at one time or another in the Neighborhood Youth Corps. Other gross statistics readily available from OEO further augment this story of vastly expanded effort and coverage.

Nevertheless, the over-all record of the antipoverty program remains uneven. Its objective evaluation is a difficult, and perhaps almost impossible, task in view of the national controversy that has developed around the domestic and foreign policies of the Johnson administration. The issue of the Vietnam war versus the domestic program will not be discussed in the present context although one may question whether it is proper to assess the war on poverty without considering the national scene in its total complexity. We simply assume that the five years of the Johnson administration represent a meaningful and closed period of government-sponsored social action programs which as a unit can be evaluated in sociological terms and will yield general conclusions for predicting the success or failure of action programs dealing with poverty.

If viewed under such assumptions, the successes of the five years do not inspire unqualified confidence in the program's future. For one thing, the congressional friends of action programs have been unable to secure congressional enactment of critical large-scale programs to develop new jobs, low-cost housing units, or other tangible economic opportunities and community improvements. For another, the Office of Economic Opportunity itself has been stymied in its effort to coordinate often competitive, redundant, and thereby wasteful and under-effective local and federal, private and public antipoverty efforts. Of greatest significance, perhaps, OEO has failed to keep its political and public-relations losses at a minimum. Disequilibrium and disturbance have marred the national antipoverty effort from its inception. As it will be argued at length, some of this could have been expected in view of the nature of social intervention and of the basic American ambivalence concerning poverty. Other parts of the uneven record, however, are especially the responsibility of the Office of Economic Opportunity.

This situation raises the questions: What can be done about poverty? Can it be reduced or at least mitigated in some of its negative consequences, such as underdeveloped human resources and generational transference of cultural handicaps?

The answer is unequivocal. Regardless of whether poverty is defined as possession of material resources equal to the community's lowest acceptable standard of living, or as a lack of command over political influence sufficient to compel a meaningful change in public policy, or as the absence of confidence that one's own material resources and political influence will soon improve, poverty can be contained, alleviated, and even eliminated. Any of this can be done gradually or with dizzying speed. What is unclear is not how to do it, but at what cost are we willing to undertake effective actions; not what to do, but how much to do; not when, but, under what motivation, or under what compulsion should we act?

In order to gain some answers to these questions an exploratory attempt will be made to divide the many antipoverty projects that have gained public attention and political scrutiny since 1964 into those which have achieved comparative success and those which appear to have floundered. To this end, two representative programs are described: family planning and participatory democracy. By confining the discussion largely to these two, we may avoid being overwhelmed by complexity and detail and yet still draw certain lessons useful in evaluating the possibilities for programmatic antipoverty action.

CONTROL OF FAMILY SIZE AND POVERTY: A CASE STUDY OF RELATIVE PROGRAMMATIC SUCCESS

Birth-control or family-planning projects include both preconception methods (prophylactic measures and sterilization) and a single postconception method (abortion). Together the two types of methods offer the option of not conceiving at all or not conceiving out-of-wedlock. They make possible control of the number and spacing of children, and thereby, control of the allocation of scarce family resources among a planned number of dependents.

The large family is perhaps "the most disturbing constituent of poverty in the United States." [1] The incidence of poverty among families with a male head and with one or two children is 8 percent, but it reaches 36 percent among families with five or more children and a staggering 92 percent among families headed by a woman. Moreover, the large female-led families have only 41 percent of the income they need, i.e., what is thought necessary for a family to be "decently" poor. While the number of poor families has decreased slightly over the past five years, the number of families with five or more children has risen; these families now account for 46 percent of the nation's poverty-stricken children. [2] It is hardly surprising, therefore, that, as the annual reports on the national examinations of the Selective Service Test reveal, rejectees come disproportionately from large families of poor parents. Add to this the fact that 43 percent of the poor are presently under eighteen years of age, and a strong case is made for new aid to impoverished family life.

In 1966 the Office of Economic Opportunity asserted that family planning was the "single most cost-effective antipoverty measure." [3] Programs aimed at reducing the very considerable excess fertility or undesired childbirths among the poor have caught on dramatically in the past five years, and advances here overshadow much that has otherwise occurred in the current antipoverty effort. Related gains here include the following:

1. The Supreme Court has held that a state law prohibiting the use of contraceptives is unconstitutional.

2. Between 1963 and 1966 six states removed restrictive statutes, six other states authorized birth-control services in their public health programs, and four additional states adopted welfare policies making services available to all mothers on public assistance, regardless of marital status.

3. Satellite clinics, community aides, and mobile clinics are being employed for the first time on a large-scale, nationwide basis to disseminate the birth-control information and devices. Innovative here is the use of store-front operations, local people as aides, and vans equipped as traveling health centers.

4. The Office of Education has indicated its willingness to pay for family-life education and sex-education courses as an integral part of the curriculum from preschool to college and adult levels.

5. The state of Connecticut which in 1965 was one of two to ban the use of contraceptives, now provides welfare recipients with birth-control advice.

6. The Department of the Interior is promoting family-planning services on Indian reservations.

7. The OEO went from support of no birth-control clinics in 1964 to support in 1966 of 54 clinics in 24 states. As many as 300,000 women may have been aided.

8. The budget of the federal government for family planning has gone up from $2.3 million in fiscal 1965 to $14.7 in fiscal 1966, $25.3 in fiscal 1967, and $35 million in fiscal 1968. The President has requested $56 million for fiscal 1969.

Underlying all these advances is the finding of a Gallup Poll that six persons in every ten now think birth-control pills should be supplied free to all women of child-bearing age on relief.[4] Never before has public support been so considerable.

Related progress has been swift. As recently as three years ago, public and private agency workers were discouraged from discussing contraceptives with clients; poor women were thought to be neither interested nor responsible enough to participate in birth control; the opposition of the Catholic Church appeared firm; and the federal government was conspicuous in its fearful absence from the entire issue. At the time of this writing, the schools of New York, Chicago, and other large cities are introducing sex-education courses, and staff members in the welfare agencies do not hesitate to advocate family planning. Like seven million other users of oral contraceptives, the poor show an eagerness to sustain family-planning regimens. This is particularly so where the regimen is inexpensive, sensitively presented, and placed in the context of a total family health program. While there remains concern over the resistance of the Vatican, much of the previous opposition of American Catholics seems to be lessening.

For a realistic appraisal of the situation, it is also necessary to consider those matters where considerable resistance can still be observed, and a case in point is the sensitive and unpopular method of sterilization. In popular opinion, sterilization is erroneously thought to involve castration or depression of the sex drive. About 50,000 men and the same number of women annually elect this permanent method of birth control. What is even more, the nation's only concerned organization, the Association of Voluntary Sterilization, has made but small gains in its efforts to attract volunteers from among the poor. In 1966, only 26 of the 300 patients assisted by the association were supported entirely by welfare. While important government agencies (Health, Education, and Welfare, Defense, Medicaid Administration) have recently endorsed voluntary sterilization, the Office of Economic Opportunity remains firm in its refusal to finance this service for the clients of its family-planning clinics. Similarly, while a total of two million Americans have chosen this method of birth control, and 64 percent of a national Gallup Poll (1966) approved of the method, both the opposition of the Catholic community and the general unfamiliarity of physicians with the medical procedures involved greatly limit the possibilities for wide acceptance.[5]

Poorer still are the possibilities for positive action where abortion is concerned. In 45 of the 50 states, only a woman struggling for her very life can secure an abortion. No consideration is given to the general hardships an unwanted child brings on himself and his family, or to circumstances "such as more children than she could already hope to care for properly, with little money to feed them and clothe them and keep them from endless succession of diseases." [6] Indeed, while 71 percent of a national sample believe a woman should be able to obtain a legal abortion if her health is seriously endangered by the pregnancy, only 21 percent support legal abortions where the family has a very low income and cannot afford any more children. Abortion as a last-resort means of birth-control is firmly rejected.[7]

Ten thousand legal abortions and an estimated one million illegal abortions (or one abortion for every four births) are performed annually, with 80 percent involving married women. The poor are underrepresented in the first, and are overrepresented in the second category. In New York City, for example, the death rate from criminal abortions is 10 times higher among Negroes and Puerto Ricans than among whites. Indeed, criminal abortions may cause 20 percent of all known maternal deaths.

The possibilities for reform action are complicated by the well-known opposition of the Catholic Church. Less well known but equally significant is the lack of a public consensus on the questions: Does the state have the right to require the woman to bear a child against her will? Does the state have the right to punish the doctor for obliging such a woman? Also important is the public punitiveness inherent in the widespread opposition to legalizing abortions-on-request.[8]

Abortion as a social problem will become more complicated in the next few years when an effective and safe abortifacient pill becomes available. Such a development will challenge the present opposition to "abortions on request" recently voiced by

85 percent of a national sample of doctors.[9] Moreover, it could make this particular option of birth control evenly available across social classes. While twenty-nine states gave consideration during the 1967 legislative term to bills for liberalizing their laws on abortion, reform of any real magnitude waits finally on pharmaceutical, rather than legal advances—and on back alley, hallway, and under-the-counter sales, if enlightened and subsidized clinic dispersal practices do not stay abreast of the ensuing public demand for abortion pills. Abortion may yet become a matter of personal decision.

Of the major efforts at family limitation, the birth-control program of the Planned Parenthood Federation and its various public and private allies has clearly enjoyed the greatest success. A look, however, at its difficulties may prove uniquely instructive:

1. Less than one fifth of the hospitals with large maternity services recently surveyed by the American Hospital Association offer family-planning services.

2. Less than one third of all local public health departments offer any birth-control services.

3. Less than one fourth of the 54 OEO-aided clinics have been spared cutbacks, and 16 of the clinics are likely to close down entirely.

4. Less than one third of the counties and municipalities in the United States are supporting family-planning activities.

5. Less than half the $4,000,000 in grants expected in 1967 from OEO for support of birth-control clinics was actually distributed.

6. Less than half of the state health departments have official policies on family planning.

It is hardly surprising therefore that only 700,000 poor patients are thought to be receiving services from all public and private agencies combined, and 87 percent of the estimated target population of 5.3 million is left without access to subsidized services.[10]

Much of this bleak record finds its explanation in certain unstudied impediments to progress. For example, family-planning projects are often opposed by black nationalists who charge the enterprise with seeking to curtail the growth of the black community. More significant is the opposition of certain prospective mothers who believe men are owed proof of their virility, and feel poor women should be left alone to create the one form of riches available to all. Linked here is the ambivalence of many who think only more sweeping reforms have relevance to the elimination of poverty and thus would rather spend their money and energy to redo society so that all women can do justice to the children they choose to bear.[11]

The possibilities for vast new gains in the area hinge largely on five interrelated developments:

1. Public endorsement of birth-control programs for the poor must remain high. Such support and related programs must be broadened to include the large-scale provision of services to unmarried or deserted females.

2. Local antipoverty personnel must become more ingenious in surmounting present-day difficulties in communicating with, and affecting the attitudes of potential users.

3. The federal government may have to make birth-control services available as a matter of right, rather than as a local option. Good use could be made in this case of the 3,000 existing Public Health Centers.

4. The nation's leading private agency, the Planned Parenthood Federation, must secure vast new philanthropic support and increase its missionary campaign to engage more public and voluntary hospitals in educational and service clinics.

5. Above all, the federal government must invest more money in family-planning programs. Private efforts are inadequate. Even with its 12,000 volunteers in 400 clinics in 138 cities, the

privately financed Planned Parenthood Federation in 1967 was vastly unequal to the challenge.

The Office of Economic Opportunity estimates that it may cost $126 million over a five-year period to reach 4.5 million impoverished women, enroll half of them in a birth-control campaign and deliver services to the 40 percent of the volunteers who will practice birth control effectively. The Planned Parenthood Federation, more optimistic than OEO about the response and retention rates, estimates the cost at $100 million annually, or four times as much as OEO for the same five-year period. Partisans of government-aided family-planning programs point out that it costs the taxpayers $7,000 to raise one child through the age of 17 under AFDC, while it will cost only about $20 a year to supply a woman with a birth-control method for the same period. They also claim that $2 billion annually would be saved in welfare costs alone if all who needed birth control were given help.[12] Whatever the cost or savings, the response of the federal government remains critical.

The poor are ready, able, and willing to help themselves in this matter. Compared to the disaster of other antipoverty efforts, this one has momentum and promise.[13] It only remains for the affluent to determine how really willing they are to subsidize the necessary programs of self-help through family-size control.

CONTROL OF PARTICIPATION AND POVERTY: A CASE STUDY OF RELATIVE FAILURE

In the context of the antipoverty effort, participatory democracy may be understood to mean the fullest possible engagement of representative groups of the poor members of a community in the formation, execution, and evaluation of relevant public policy decisions.[14] The concept differs in several ways from conventional definitions of democracy. First, the adjective "participatory" is to underline the fundamental assumption that, historically, the poor have hardly participated in the community decision-making process, and have profited little from conventional forms of participation (such as a once-a-year exercise of the franchise). Second, the concept signifies the unfettering of democratic forms such as town meetings, open-house meetings with the mayor, and representation of the poor on the boards of social agencies. Finally, and above all, the name is meant to call into question the reality of decision-making in contemporary America. Participatory democracy compels attention to that most difficult of questions: How should men govern themselves?

In the antipoverty effort, participatory democracy has generally come to involve two options. First, OEO insures the poor seats on the board of directors of an OEO-funded community action program. This ranges in actual practice from domination by the poor of a Neighborhood Service Center to their token participation on the board of programs established by school authorities or welfare agencies. In the second option, the poor remain outside the formal community structures but seek to negotiate with such structures from an independent base of power (for example, a militant neighborhood association may seek to force concessions from a group of landlords by threatening a rent strike or office sit-in). Indeed, the OEO's *Community Action Workbook* suggests that a "promising method" of implementing maximum feasible participation is to "assist the poor in developing autonomous and self-managed organizations which are competent to exert political influence on behalf of their own self-interest." [15]

In the case of both options the poor are involved for the first time with issues of control, self-determination, and independence. Blacks and whites, in ghettoes and in rural areas, work to formulate and articulate issues and programs: What voice should they have in the allocation of local antipoverty funds? How can urban renewal be shaped by the people whose neighborhood is involved? In what ways can the community hold the police accountable? Who should be able to hear appeals from welfare rulings? And, how should power be divided in the ghetto? [16]

The campaign on behalf of participatory democracy has known some few successes:

1. The Office of Economic Opportunity has held that the nation's 1,050 community action agencies must reserve one third of their board seats for the poor.

2. National groups, including the Citizens Crusade Against Poverty and the Welfare Rights Council, have begun to promote participatory efforts of the poor. The Citizens Crusade, aided by a $375,000 grant from the Ford Foundation, is conducting a three-year, $4 million program to train 1,000 leaders from the ranks of the poor.

3. Elements of the major religious factions have begun to back up their endorsement of participatory democracy by making manpower and funds available to the poor.

4. College students, especially but not exclusively those of the New Left persuasion, have moved into northern ghettoes and southern towns to aid participatory democracy, many through the programs of VISTA.

5. Related movements of the poor to expand their influence in education, health, and urban renewal have been complemented by national legislation oriented toward participatory democracy (the 1964 Education Act, the 1965 Community Mental Health Act, and the 1966 Model Cities Act).

6. The entire effort has called attention to political voicelessness and lack of organization as root causes of poverty.[17]

Underlying all these advances is the considered judgment reached by many both in and outside of the welfare effort:

nothing short of the active involvement of the poor themselves will make possible far-reaching success in the antipoverty campaign.

Setbacks, however, have far outnumbered apparent successes. The public image of the poor has changed and, nowadays, the adjectives "aggressive," "greedy," and "dangerous" are all too often mentioned in popular discussions. The property riots in the cities during the summers of 1965, 1966, 1967, and 1968 are vindictively recalled all too often. Also cited are the HARYOU Act-LeRoi Jones alliance, the episode of the Mobilization for Youth red scare, the struggles in Syracuse and Newark over CAP control, the CCAP shouting down Sargent Shriver, and so forth. Some agency workers, city politicians, and representatives of vested interests speak of the "ungrateful insolence" of their formerly dependent clients, which they find hard to tolerate. Still others fear that the many race and poverty conflicts now brought to the surface may provoke a reactionary response, perhaps even in the majority of the white better-off citizens.

The provision of the Anti-Poverty Act permitted, at least theoretically, three alternative versions of participatory democracy: (1) containment, or confinement of the poor to essentially meaningless decision-making on petty issues: (2) co-optation, which would have meant luring the poor into voting as their elitist mentors would have had them vote; and, finally, (3) co-determination, or the independent and self-interested action of the poor in public affairs.[18] The history of participatory democracy in the War on Poverty to date has been the history of the rise to dominance of co-optation, the slow decline of the less-useful containment policy, and the near-devastation of hopes for anything approaching co-determination.

Co-determination, with its apparent antecedent condition, interclass hostility, was apparently doomed from the very start. As 30 percent of the poor are nonwhite, the new militancy of this group threatened the nation's elaborate caste system and deeply aggravated the classic *American Dilemma* of American race relations. The ascendancy of black power ideologies promoted a general confusion of participatory democracy with black power and prompted large elements of the dominant white community to reject both. The Negro poor were divided on the merits of co-determination, some preferring continued dependency on the whites, others, more separatism and retaliation, and still others, personal advantage of any kind.

The white poor, too, remained disinterested in co-determination because of ignorance, isolation, political apathy, and, often, because of their antagonism to any effort that they perceive as an aid to the Negro. For the white poor, the old-fashioned ethnic, religious and regional politics of ward heelers and machine bosses continue to substitute for participatory democracy. Hence, communities of the poor, as a rule, lack the important prerequisites of operating participatory democracy— command of substantial economic and social resources, extensive interactions among members, presence of experienced leaders, and commitment to a clear set of objectives.[19]

Containment also fell into disrepute, and partly because of the adverse reaction it received from the Negro community and the mass media as well. Above all, containment affronted two strong preferences of the dominant middle-class majority. It violated the principles that government programs should appear to promote the democratic way, and it violated a popular preference that previously disadvantaged groups should appear to be making progress. In short, containment proved anachronistic and embarrassing with few mourning its passage. Instead, many city politicians, welfare professionals, and OEO officials came to prefer co-optation as a viable alternative in participatory democracy. As a public policy, co-optation quickly gained advocates because it satisfied the city-hall authorities, gave positions of seeming stature and decision-making power to some of the poor, and preserved the appearance of progress and democracy.[20]

The hope that remains now for participatory democracy is confined largely to the difficult areas of education and welfare. Parents in certain ghetto areas are demanding a voice in hiring school staff and deciding administrative matters. The Welfare Rights Councils now emerging in many American cities bring together reform-minded welfare workers and mothers on welfare to right the procedures of local welfare administration.[21] The general failure of the participatory democracy efforts has deprived the OEO of a critical opportunity to secure strong political support among the poor and their liberal allies. The Economic Opportunity Act of 1964 has never had an organized, well-directed movement behind it. Accordingly, the bill has been weakened from year to year whenever it has come up for budgetary approval before the Congress and, in the summer of 1967, actually reached a stage where it was almost impossible to gather support for its mere renewal, least of all improvement.

A Paradigm for the Success and Failure of Programmatic Intervention

Analyzing the programmatic interventions of our two case studies as well as other anti-poverty projects, we can now postulate five conditions which we feel enhance the possibility for success. First, the program should center around a visible need. For example, the need for housing repairs in the slum ghettos is not especially visible because it is frequently hidden by the physical isolation of the ghetto from the rest of the community. Second, there should be a new and ready answer to the need. This, for example, has not been the case in the ill-fated effort to relieve school teachers in the ghettos with the untried members of the small-scale National Teacher Corps. Third, the necessary funds should be realistically available. Their absence, in the case of the Model Cities effort, has been disastrous. Fourth, there should be public support for the solution. Lack of such support is obvious in the case of the guaranteed annual income for the poor. Finally, any opposition to the solution should be limited and divided; this has been anything but the case where resistance to participatory democracy was concerned.

As summarized in Table IX–1, five noteworthy antipoverty programs have especially met the above conditions for successful action. In addition to the Family Planning Program, the successful five include programs that focus on closing the gap in educational attainment and career prospects that exist between the poor and the non-poor. They involve young people, permit the clients to make critical choices, operate at a modest cost, and quickly reach the experience of personal success. As might be expected, success is further ensured and enhanced when the projects can be interwoven with one another.

Keeping this paradigm in mind, we can now turn to a detailed analysis of the relative failure of certain antipoverty programs, and in particular, the failure of the program of participatory democracy. The latter never really found a hospitable setting in the antipoverty effort, failing as it did to complement any of the five critical conditions for program success.

To begin with, the relevant needs in the matter have not been apparent. Advocates of participatory democracy argue that the poor need new political power. But the number of poor people for whom political power was clearly salient has always been small. Nearly half of the nation's poor are under eighteen years of age, and another 20 percent are over sixty-five. The remaining 35 percent are sharply divided among themselves, and many of them live with chronic personal crises; comparatively few have been left who could rise to the challenge of getting engaged in community political affairs.[22] It is small wonder that only two percent of the poor have joined the organizations formed by Saul Alinsky in various cities, and that the turnout of the poor in OEO-sponsored elections has been so strikingly low.

Second, recommendations for participatory democracy were neither especially tenable nor imaginable. The concept of poverty neighborhood elections in poverty areas, for example, excited some interest at the beginning, but this was fleeting. Political and social reformers had long sought to dismantle the ethnic political-social organization of the big-city slums. As soon as it was apparent that community elections in community antipoverty programs operated to re-create the old target, the non-poor political and social reformers either lost interest or quietly opposed the entire effort.[23] Similarly, the cause was further set back by the failure of its advocates to maintain model organizations of their own, by the public suspicion of the New Left and similar groups, and by the disillusionment of certain intellectuals.[24] Handicapped from the start by baseless romantic notions about the inherent and superior wisdom of the poor, these intellectual commentators have been dismayed to find the poor much like Americans everywhere.

Third, the necessary funds were not available. The Office of Economic Opportunity was willing to support militant participatory democracy groups early in 1965, but soon had to comply with congressional statutes and pressures, and was forced to channel its financial grants through the official umbrella agencies of the cities. The latter, as well-publicized events in Chicago, New York, Philadelphia, and Syracuse soon proved, operated in a way rather similar to the usual dispensing of patronage by tradition-bound city halls. The situation was not improved by the 1967 congressional requirement that local community action programs raise 20 percent of their budgets in matching funds before making a grant request, since no program originated by the poor alone could readily meet this requirement.

Fourth, the public as a whole has never accepted, let alone

Table IX–1. Antipoverty programs of promise.

Clues to success	Birth-control projects	Compensation education [a]	Job training OIC [b]	NCY: Youth Work [c]	"New Careers" [d]
Had a visible need	Large families; crowded ghettos; expressed desire for help	Poor test scores; dropouts	Poor job record; high unemployment	Aid to continue school	Under-staffed welfare efforts
Had new and ready answers	The pill; Planned Parenthood Federation clinics; welfare workers	Special programs; federal aid	Esteem-enhancing training; race pride	Work in social agencies	Work in Office of Economic Opportunity related efforts
Had increased funds	1966 Community Health Act; 1964 Economic Opportunity Act	1964 Education Act; 1964 Economic Opportunity Act	1965 Manpower Development Training Act; 1964 Economic Opportunity Act	1964 Economic Opportunity Act	1964 Economic Opportunity Act
Had public support	6 in 10 favor free pills to relief mothers	Trade-off against integration; aid to "innocents"	Popularity earns replication in two dozen cases	Earmarked for increase by admiring Congress	Appeals as a bootstrap operation

Table IX-1. (Continued)

Clues to success	Birth-control projects	Compensation education[a]	Job training OIC[b]	NCY: Youth Work[c]	"New Careers"[d]
Had limited opposition	Catholic Church; antiwelfare forces	Antitax forces	Personal feuding; suspicion of race bias	Anti-make-work forces	Skeptical reception by anxious professions

[a] Getset, Headstart, Title I Programs.

[b] Philadelphia's Opportunities Industrialization Center is unusual in being Negro-formed, led, and oriented.

[c] Neighborhood Youth Corps has enrolled 800,000 youths.

[d] Programs to bring non-degreed neighborhood people into paraprofessional posts for On-the-Job-Training and advancement; focused on needs in social services.

actively supported, the idea of participatory democracy. A vocal opposition has arisen in the core-cities and the suburbs as well, in the former voiced mainly by the marginally poor whites who feel threatened by any advance made by Negroes, and in the latter, by those middle-aged suburbanites who seem to furnish a strong cadre of conservatism in the country as a whole. Indeed, opposition to participatory democracy has been considerable and cohesive. In due course, opposition has grown to include vocal segments of the poor and of the social work practice as well. In March 1967 a national meeting of community action agencies was told that the poor did not want a person to represent them who was no better off than they: "The thinking goes something like this: 'How can you get anything better for me, if you can't get anything better for yourself.'" The director of New York's Mobilization for Youth project suggested that bringing the poor into antipoverty programs as officials and board members had been a "mistake," and endorsed, instead, the direct funding of social action groups of the poor.[25]

In addition to the campaign for participatory democracy, at least four other antipoverty programs have been lacking in the prerequisites for success. These include programs to aid farm migrants, low-income renters, mentally ill indigents, and the seven million recipients of federally aided public assistance programs. The paradigm summing up their common characteristics is presented in Table IX–2.

In general terms, the possibilities for positive action are smallest when the strategy of intervention confronts issues of low visibility (as with the plight of farm migrants), of potentially great expenses (as in rehabilitating the mentally ill or raising AFDC allowances), and of minimal short-run results (relief from high rent has far to go before it aids transition out of poverty). In the case of all the comparatively ill-fated projects, adults are involved (poor adults are likely to be disliked, feared, or scorned, while poor children are general subjects of concern and pity). Decision-making by others is still another common characteristic. In family planning, the client acts on her need, but participatory democracy and similar ventures involve tightly interrelated decision-making networks with a high probability of effective resistance developing somewhere along the line.

To the extent that new efforts succeed in closing the gap between the five requisites of project success and the actual conditions of such floundering, antipoverty efforts as urban rehabilitation, Teacher Corps, Model Cities, guaranteed income, and participatory democracy, the prospects for the poor and for the war on poverty may finally shift in the right direction.

Agenda for Action

At the beginning of this analysis we assumed that government-sponsored intervention programs are of essentially political nature and that the Johnson administration, representing a specific constellation of political power, followed a specific policy on the issues of poverty. However, the analysis of the success or failure of the various action programs has sufficiently demonstrated that the policy of the federal government, paramount as it may appear, is only one of the many factors involved because the political forces that affect the problem area are inseparably interwoven with social forces. The two kinds of forces interact so closely that no assessment of the antipoverty program can be accomplished in purely political terms, with a disregard for the social understructure. Thus, the ultimate outcome of the war on poverty must await the resolution of the general ambivalence of America toward the grave social issues involved. Poverty is a reflection of all the ills of society, and the elimination of poverty must imply simultaneous advances against class hostility, racial

Table IX–2. Antipoverty programs with limited promise.

Clues to standstill	Participatory democracy	Aid to migrants	Aid to renters	Aid to mentally ill	Aid to AFDC families
Less-than-visible need	Illusion of power in machine politics and civil rights	Drifters need little; small numbers	"If they don't like it, let them move"	"Backwards" hide problems; unknown numbers	Local mores dominate
No new answers	Propose board seats; militant private groups	Propose shelter and health aid; ed. for children	Propose rent subsidies	Propose care subsidies	Propose aid subsidies
No available funds	Community Action funds cut by Congress	Minimal OEO funds	Expansion bill defeated, May 1967	No bill pending	Local option
No public support	Middle-class anxieties; professional suspicions	"Drifters deserve little"	"Everyone has housing problems"	"Remains a private, personal matter"	"Should not make poverty comfortable"

Table IX–2. (Continued)

Clues to standstill	Participatory democracy	Aid to migrants	Aid to renters	Aid to mentally ill	Aid to AFDC families
Strong opposition	Mayors, consensus theoreticians	Farmers; packers; county politicians	Landlords; real estate developers; low tax forces	AMA, antiwelfare forces	Ultra-moralists, low tax forces

segregation, and the powerlessness of the poor as well as middle-class, alienation, bureaucratic proliferation, and political elitism, in short, the condition of man in the modern world.

One has only to examine the nation's record in the support of compensatory educational programs to detect the ambivalence about America's determination to end poverty. Education is clearly the key to ending the poverty of those who are in the still educable age group. Nevertheless, very limited progress has been made to improve the quality of the grossly inferior schooling of the poor. Rather, economy-minded school administrators, anti-bussing neighborhood-school advocates, and prerogative-protecting local school officials have joined forces to contain efforts for narrowing the educational differences between the slum and the suburb. The Negro poor remain segregated; the white poor remain undersupported; the average poor child remains several years behind his grade level and is likely to drop out of school early.

Ambivalence gains further support from the fact that poverty may actually offer various social benefits to respectable America. For example, the poor provide a vast pool of manpower for the unskilled and undesirable jobs that society requires. The poor provide a negative reference model against which the working class can measure its own achievement and the middle class can affirm its own superiority. The poor provide eager enlistees for the Armed Services and eager recruits for membership in certain religious faiths. Above all, in their rejection of revolutionary dogma and in their focus on achievement within the nation's system of welfare capitalism, the poor provide a valuable confirmation of the American Dream and help it to retain its hold over all segments of our society. In an ironic way, poverty offers a proving ground for prevailing American ideology. The apparent eagerness of many poor people to help their children achieve the suburban life—and nothing more than that—flatters and comforts suburbanites, however reluctant they may remain to share that life.

Sociologist Harry C. Bredemeier offers a useful overview in this matter. "Poverty remains," he writes, ". . . profitable to those not in it. It is profitable because the comparatively rich consider the costs of remedies too great; because they receive several kinds of reward from having the poor on hand; because not many of them find rewards in carrying out the remedies; and because the costs of poverty are neither very great nor sharply perceived." [26] The nation appears to have settled for poorly interrelated, poorly funded, and poorly staffed demonstration projects which demonstrate not so much what might be accomplished against poverty as how good Americans are in providing funds for any purpose whatsoever. We do very little in the way of formal antipoverty programs of note and hope privately instead that our steady rate of economic growth will take care of the problem.

Yet proposals and suggestions abound, and it is worth listening to them. We could operate in the spirit of the multimillion dollar, ten-year Freedom Budget proposed by A. Philip Randolph as a sort of Marshall Plan for America's poor. Such a campaign could involve school, home, hospital, park and road construction, along with family allowance, guaranteed income, or negative income tax, to underwrite a poverty-eliminating standard of living. The program, however, seems unlikely, the war on poverty having gone long enough to undercut the case for sweeping radical action.[27]

The war has also probably gone long enough to dim the chance of the near adoption of the plans of Senators Javits, Kennedy, or Percy to draw the vast, untouched resources of private industry into the antipoverty effort. The nation's major businesses are already involved as Job Corps camp contractors and as cooperating parties in the job-training ventures of the ghetto.

But Senate critics are calling for much more, and their detailed, imaginative proposals warrant serious attention.

Other reform programs focus on the societal dimension of poverty and view the problem in terms of social change rather than individual rehabilitation. These programs seek to transform the social order by stirring all to examine the widespread anomia they believe is associated with a materialistic and mechanical society.[28] They accent blockages to group mobility and political power as the major causes of poverty, and they stress the intransigence of the Establishment in political and welfare matters. At their worst, programs of this sort indulge in an American propensity for assigning the failure of individual or group efforts to some vague aristocratic, monolithic, and revisionist conspiracy; at their best, they compel attention to the demand for large-scale sweeping social change.

In any case, future intervention programs are needed, but it would be irrealistic to expect that the future of poverty will be its smooth elimination through action programs. The future course of the antipoverty effort hinges, first of all, on the resolution of the American ambivalence toward social problems. Furthermore it is imperative that community militants, inspired by the civil rights movement, should prove to the whole nation that it does not pay to tolerate poverty. It is imperative that social planners and governmental change-agents work to reduce the costs of eliminating poverty. It is imperative that the practical utopians in pulpit, press, and seats of power raise the public's perception of the many benefits of poverty's elimination. And it is imperative that we all remember there is an organic relationship between the form of a campaign and its content: The chief "result" of an antipoverty program will be the means chosen to achieve the end.

Optimism is hardly encouraged by the present conservative mood of the nation. Signs abound that the majority of the nation judges the price too high, and the effort too taxing, to maintain even the inadequate antipoverty program of the last few years. As for the future, however, it is useful to warm one's hands and heart with the counsel of a man who may have known. In March of 1968 the late Dr. Martin Luther King advised: "I haven't lost faith even though the days ahead are still difficult. The problems are very real. Some of them are very frustrating. I still have faith in the future, and I will not yield to the politics of despair." The challenge is directly to us—the non-poor, socially alert, conscience-directed agents of change— who must activate, as well as analyze; act, as well as read; and endlessly press on.

X · The Future of Health Care

by John D. Stoeckle, M.D.

The care and treatment of the poor have always required special solutions.* The history of medical services for the poor is a history of special financing, special treatment-institutions and clinical organization, and even special therapeutic, health-education and human-relations methods.[1] Within this special system, the poor have had medical bills paid by taxes and charity rather than by their own funds, wards rather than private rooms, clinical teams rather than private doctors, school health examinations in place of office checkups, bureaucratic outpatient and public health clinics rather than private offices, and a greater reliance on authoritarian methods of inducing cooperation and education. Each of these familiar special solutions and accommodations within the health-care system has been the subject of both study and criticism.[2] The question is not how good or bad each of these solutions is. The important questions are whether special solutions are needed and, if so, how special and separate they should be. Should the organization of health services for the poor be something apart from the organization of health services for everyone?

A look backward might suggest reasons for such special ar-

* The author wishes to thank Dr. Stanley Reiser, History of Science Department, Harvard University, for the benefit of innumerable discussions and suggestions, Dr. Arnold Kish, University of California Medical School at Los Angeles for suggested references, and many other persons connected with Boston Health Centers.

rangements. Historically, these solutions have been attributed to limited economic resources, less money spent on the poor, cheaper and more separate care. More important than economic reasons, however, may have been our philosophy of reform. Implicitly at least the poor were to remain unchanged—poor but free of tuberculosis, dental caries, rheumatic fever, mental illness, and other diseases.[3] The major historical direction of reform was to make medical care more accessible. The poor needed the services brought to them, needed medical relief, if only to make life at the bottom less bleak. Health care was perceived as a sufficient goal. Once they had services, the poor could improve themselves through a do-it-yourself job. To bring the poor services and let them work out their own destiny has been the major orientation of public and private action in medical care.

Today, the ideas of reform are different; to be poor but healthy is no longer acceptable. Thus, the poor receive medical services and, in addition, opportunities to change their conditions and achieve full participation in modern technological society. At the same time, the federal government has introduced more money into health services, largely in recognition of the fact that the benefits of medicine are unevenly distributed. As a result, new beginnings and directions are being set. Health services, no longer medical relief, except for the aged, are to be instrumental in changing the poor, removing their handicaps to social, educational, and economic achievements. Criteria for the success of health services will be measured not in individual self-satisfaction but in group advancement. Action and innovation in health services today contain two ideas: (1) to bring services to the poor, and (2) to rehabilitate and save the poor with the help of health services.[4] The notion of health services for the poor has acquired a value connotation very similar to what health had for middle-class Americans.[5] As the poor—or more of them—become more like everybody else, treatments requiring special solutions may become less and less necessary or even politically viable.

Paying for Care

To get treatment, the poor have to be able to pay for it. Recent legislation, the Title 18, Medicare, and Title 19, Medicaid, Public Law 89-97, July 30, 1965, help them toward this aim. Title 18, a worker-employer contributory government insurance scheme, pays for the hospital care of the elderly, of a small segment of low-income persons, and of many older people with better incomes. For ambulatory care, Title 18 also offers insurance, although, for this coverage, the subscriber has to spend some of his own money. Since the services it covers are not comprehensive, this insurance, while paying for office diagnosis and treatment, does not pay for drugs and appliances, nor for the first fifty dollars of outpatient services.

Title 19 provides a comprehensive program for both hospital and out-of-hospital care. However, it is not an insurance but a welfare program and requires means test. It standardizes the medical care benefits of traditional relief programs (Aid to Dependent Children, Old Age Assistance, Disability Assistance, General Relief) and provides similar medical assistance for children of low-income families who would not qualify for these relief programs and for people who are disabled and compensated under the Social Security Act. As a welfare rather than an insurance scheme, it requires the negotiation of a personal contract with a municipal welfare office before payment of medical bills is authorized. Although broad in its coverage, including dental care among the medical services, Title 19 is not a new departure nor a general solution like Medicare. It makes children from low-income families eligible but not their parents. But it does promise a new orientation in welfare by encouraging people to seek financial medical assistance under the act and reverses the usual client management, as well as the traditional welfare procedures of limiting costs, services, and clients. For extensive public use of this medical assistance, resistance to the idea of welfare and to seeking help of the municipal welfare offices will have to be overcome. To facilitate its use but not remove its limitations, part of the administration of Title 19 might be handed over to hospitals or private groups, as has been done with other governmental help such as loans to college students.

Title 19 has other built-in limitations at a time when medical care aims to be more continuous and family-oriented. People go off and on welfare as their incomes rise and fall, and an analysis of the dynamics of welfare usage in New York has documented the transient welfare status of families.[6] At the end of three years, only 19 percent of the original welfare clients, enrolled in a hospital-based medical care program, remained on welfare. The implications are clear. Medical care can hardly be rationally organized for continuity of family services if financing is not similarly arranged. Medicare quite effectively deals with hospital and out-of-hospital care for the population over sixty-five. In the younger age group, voluntary private insurance still leaves some eighteen million persons uncovered for hospital care and has few plans to cover outpatient care for any sizable segment of the population.[7] A general solution, the long-advocated extension of insurance schemes for both hospital and ambulatory care, would be more effective than welfare and would furnish the necessary financing of community and hospital health services.[8] Hopefully, additional legislation for such comprehensive insurance will evolve under public pressures, but until a national health insurance—private, public, or a combination of both—evolves, economic barriers to the use of health services will continue and the development of the full scope of community practice outside the hospital will remain limited.

The passage of Titles 18 and 19 has brought expectations that the quality and organization of care available to the poor will change. The legislation, however, is primarily concerned with making care financially accessible by improving the paying status of the patient. The organization of health services may well remain fixed. The pressures for change will not come from the legislation, but, as such financing programs create more paying patients, the federal administration may stimulate popular demands to which the treatment institutions are likely to respond by organizational innovation.

Except for the Neighborhood Health Centers of the Office of Economic Opportunity, the Migrant Health Act, and part of the Children's Bureau program for maternal-infant-child care, the remaining federal programs are not specifically for the poor. Yet many of them may have implications for their treatment. Although no longer categorical, the program of heart disease, cancer, and stroke can create new referral centers or referral channels for some poor patients. Likewise, the Hill-Burton Act, the Community Health and Mental Health Service Acts, the Children's Bureau, Vocational Rehabilitation, the Health Professions Assistance Program, the Manpower Development and Training Program—all deal with particular problems of organization and with services equally available to everyone. By dealing separately with problems of facilities, equipment, education, health-manpower training, and organization and planning, these programs introduce tax moneys into a large number of treatment institutions. This approach is somewhat different from the classic pattern of tax-supported care for special diseases such as tuberculosis, venereal disease and mental illness hospitalization. In effect, the tax moneys properly subsidize some of the treatment institutions that could not be realistically covered by insurance alone. In teaching hospitals, some of these costs have, until recently, been inadequately and inappropriately derived from federal funds for medical research. These several programs may seem to be a temporary transfusion of tax moneys for ailing medical institutions, but, in all likelihood, they will be needed in future years as a form of indirect financing of health services for the poor and for everybody.

Yet even if the present subsidies continue and a general comprehensive insurance scheme does evolve out of public and private plans, some special problems of treating the poor will still remain and require different handling.

OUT-OF-HOSPITAL CARE

The health conditions and health care of low-income groups present four general problems. The poor have (1) many untreated dental caries, (2) much psychosocial distress and clinical psychiatric disorders, often compounded by congenital or acquired chronic medical disease, (3) high infant-perinatal mortality rates, and (4) many chronic diseases. Moreover, for the same illness, they generally have longer periods of disability than patients with high incomes.

Most of the care and treatment for these conditions and the rehabilitation of chronic-illness disability are given outside the hospital. In turn, nearly all the deficiencies in treatment resources for the poor are in those practices that are traditionally out-of-hospital and located in a variety of community settings—private doctors' offices, outpatient departments, clinics of local city health departments, public schools, factories, the Veterans Administration, mental health centers, and family agencies.

For the most part, out-of-hospital care in the United States is given by individual private practitioners; outpatient clinics at hospitals and other settings account for a small percentage of such care. Visits to outpatient departments make up but 14 percent of the 851.6 million visits each year to physicians; public health clinics account for a trifling 1 percent of them.[9] While these two sources of care are used proportionately more by low-income individuals, many poor receive at least some of their care from private practitioners, and many use more than one source of medical aid. These facts can easily be learned from clinical encounters with patients and from published studies documenting the expenditures of public funds for ambulatory care to private doctors. A Chicago study revealed that private practitioners received 29 percent of vendor payments for care, while the remainder went to institutions.[10] In the Charlestown district of Boston, near the Massachusetts General Hospital, two thirds of a sample of welfare recipients received some private care.[11] A survey of the sources of medical care used by the outpatient clientele of a voluntary hospital revealed that 57 percent of the clientele also used private physicians.[12] In a survey of New York municipal hospital outpatients, the private doctor use was 32 percent.[13] The National Health Survey reported that patients with annual incomes under $4,000 had 66.4 percent of their visits in private offices and 19.7 percent in a hospital clinic.[14] The percentages were similar for those with incomes under $2,000. In Massachusetts, 75 percent of the welfare vendor payments for medical out-of-hospital services, outpatient clinics, and physicians went to community practitioners; the pattern was reversed in the city of Boston.[15] The private-practice care of the poor, although sizeable, is less visible than their care in bureaucratic municipal and private hospital clinics; hence, the latter, and not private practice, is the usual target of critics. Although the private doctor is assumed to be good or better, we actually know less about his care. Certainly, if the care of the poor requires reforms, these will have to include private practices as well.

Regardless of the type of medical practice—public or private, group or solo—many ambulatory practices available to the poor are thought to have built-in barriers to their use.[16] Because of these barriers, the poor do not use office care with the same frequency as the affluent. The reason for this may not be that care is inconvenient and fragmented but, rather, that it may simply be less available. In areas where the poor live, there are, indeed, fewer doctors. A Chicago survey found that the ratio of physicians to residents was 0.62/1000 in poverty areas, compared to 1.26/1000 in a nonpoverty area.[17] In Boston the poverty areas have seen a steady decline in the number of doctors practicing there: the number of doctors having offices registered in two of the largest poverty districts of the city has declined by 50 percent and 30 percent within the last twenty years.[18] The South End Medical Club, an organization of general practitioners with offices in that area of Boston, had, in the 1920's, a large active membership engaged in community practice; with the exodus and death of physicians, membership gradually declined so that the organization disbanded in the 1950's.[19] Such findings suggest that the office care available to the poor within their residential areas is limited in quantity.* Some practitioners have left without replacement, some have changed from general to special, and some others have become centralized in other areas of the city. A solution to the problem presented by this trend is the establishment, or more accurately the re-establishment, of neighborhood health centers.

The Organization of Care in the Community

The neighborhood health center, one of the most popular current ideas for out-of-hospital care of the poor, is now established in Boston, Denver, and several other cities and rural areas.[20] The centers are miniature solutions to the major problem, examples of special medical institutions for the poor, and new bureaucratic efforts to organize the loose networks of community

* A different view is presented by Julius A. Roth in Chapter VIII of this book. The two views can be reconciled if we consider the fact that in many areas of the country, including Boston, the ratio of primary-care physicians per population decreased between 1940 and 1960.—Ed.

practice and involve the poor in the working of a health agency. The aspirations of the health centers, their locations, organization, staff, and treatment strategies reflect concern with the major problems of distribution, use, quality, and orientation of the whole system of health care. These general problems are germane to the care of the poor, for it is they, as critics commonly observe, who are often shortchanged in quantity, quality, and content within the system.

The idea of the health center as an institution for out-of-hospital care is not new, and, in the course of its historical development, it has come to denote a combination of five essential characteristics: (1) a common facility in the community for doctors, nurses, social workers, health educators and others concerned with out-of-hospital care and social welfare of patients; (2) the organization of the practitioners as the center's staff, which may range from informal contacts of independent practitioners to a tightly knit staff with specific tasks, roles, and duties assigned and interprofessional boundaries maintained; (3) a population or clientele usually restricted to residents of a district or those enrolled for services; (4) services rationally linked to other institutions by formal referral channels and agreement on specific tasks rendered by the center and other institutions; and (5) a program of preventive medicine and health promotion through work with individuals and the community. The total scope of the program may often be more extensive and include the curative treatment work. In any case, the forms of the various centers have been shaped by public needs for health services and professional concerns with efficiency, coordination, quality, and effectiveness of health care in the community.

Indeed, professional concern with efficiency was important in one of the first attempts of regional planning for health centers. In 1920 the British Ministry of Health Interim Report on the Future Provision of Medical and Allied Services proposed a "primary health centre" for "domiciliary services." [21] This was to be a facility located away from large hospitals, a place for the individual work of the general practitioner, the midwife, and the nurse. It intended to insure coordination in the work of independent practitioners and efficiency in the use of hospital consultants. Like military medicine, with its formal procedure for the movement of injured from the battalion aid station back to larger units, the regional referral promised a highly rational clinical efficiency in allocating patients to the right treatment institution—a perennial concern of planners.

In spite of ambitious planning for community care, no national system of health centers emerged in Great Britain, although this was again recommended in the National Health Act of 1946.[22] A few that were organized after World War II did not have notable success, and local councils planned the establishment of only sixty-eight such institutions by 1974.[23] The traditional separation between general-practice care and preventive care by public-authority clinics has continued and been maintained even when they were housed in the same center. In some other countries, however, national systems of health centers did emerge. The Soviet Union, Yugoslavia, as well as Chile, have health centers on a national scale.[24]

The idea of health centers took shape in the United States about 1910. It was stimulated by the dissatisfaction felt by the leaders of public health because of the serious limitations imposed upon their work. Indeed, the public health services were, at this time, restricted to the preventive and curative treatment of venereal disease and tuberculosis and the improvement of baby-infant welfare, the latter implying the vaccination and feeding of undernourished slum children. The public health leaders wanted a greater coordination among the separate clinics scattered about the city, and an expansion of the clinic services to the urban poor.[25] Beginning in 1910, several cities began to unite their public health clinics in one building and establish such centers in the various districts. Their intention was a decentralization of the health services by locating them closer to the users, but, in fact, only the preventive services were placed into district centers, while the curative care continued to remain in the scattered offices of community medical practitioners and outpatient departments of urban hospitals.

The first such centers were established in Pittsburgh and Milwaukee under W. C. White and W. C. Phillips.* In 1916 C. F. Wilinsky initiated the first district center for Boston, the Blossom Street Health Center of the West End, located within a block of the Massachusetts General Hospital, with the aim of correlating "all the health and social agencies under one roof with the beneficient result derived from contact of the workers." [26] He included in the center private social agencies as well as health services such as the Consumptive Hospital Department, Instructive District Nursing Association, Milk and Baby Hygiene Association, Visiting Physician of the Boston Dispensary, and the Hebrew Federated Charities. Periodic health examinations were given by the general practitioners of the community, but they were little used because of the other demands made on the practitioner's time during his brief attendance at the center.[27] Later, dental and "habit" clinics for mental health counseling were also added.[28] While there was no tie to the hospital's treatment departments, medical students

* The model for White's initial organization of health services for a district population was the system of public schools and districts for pupil assignment. As he reasoned: "In the educational field there has gradually developed a knowledge of the equipment necessary for a given population, and this equipment has been apportioned so as to be readily accessible to those whom it is to serve. The management of these units is centered in a legally constituted governing body, which also controls the expenditure of funds collected by taxation. The same form of control is applicable throughout to tuberculosis and other health problems." See William C. White, "The Official Responsibility of the State in the Tuberculosis Problem," *Journal of the American Medical Association,* 65 (August 1915), 512–514.

did use the well-child-care clinic to practice the examination of healthy babies. The centers were meant to decentralize services in order to maximize their use by the population, but reports of the quantity and nature of their use did not reveal their impact.[29] It was estimated that in some districts over 50 percent of all children were seen; in addition, nearly all babies were seen once by home visits following every registered birth.

In other major cities there was a similar development. Boston eventually had eight centers, one for each 50,000 people, while Philadelphia had nine with the district sizes ranging from 200,000 to 20,000, the latter a common number in the planning of centers. Not all centers throughout the country were under public auspices; some were sponsored by the Red Cross and other private agencies.[30] A survey carried out by Wilinsky in 1926 found some 600 centers operating. This number included the cooperatively housed public clinics and private welfare agencies, as well as "minor centers" which only contained clinics for well infants and children. From a 1926 survey, a White House conference on child health reported 1,511 such health centers.[31]

In Los Angeles County, J. L. Pomeroy had the most ambitious program.[32] By organizing the voluntary work of community medical practitioners, he included in each health center outpatient clinics which were to deliver ordinary medical aid. This contrasted with the similar practices of other places, where the centers operated under strong constraints against practicing medicine in order to assure the participation and approval of private practitioners. By adding medical practitioners, nurses, and social workers, but carefully restricting the clientele by means tests, Pomeroy had a combination of preventive and curative services quite close to the content of modern neighborhood health centers. His program was viewed as a decentralization of the outpatient system of the large hospitals as well as better distribution of medical services.

In Cincinnati, still another modern feature was added.* The organization of the district center included in its management public representatives of the district. This was the first attempt to get away from exclusively middle-class professional management, a tradition inherited from earlier social reformers. The intent of this participation was to arouse the interest of the public in health affairs.[33]

These district health centers for the urban poor, at least in most cities, have not flourished since the 1940's. Their impact on the health status of the poor cannot be assessed on the basis of the few studies of their use. One can hardly give them all the credit, as Sand does, for reducing infant and tuberculosis mortality during the period of their existence.[34] They faced several obstacles to lasting success. Over the years their clientele dwindled as many patients became able to use private doctors. Private care had also absorbed the preventive practices of the child health programs, and, with the advent of penicillin treatment, the curative program for venereal disease. The centers developed no systematic integration with other therapeutic institutions, and few of them were so enterprising as Pomeroy's to undertake comprehensive medical services. The present Gouver-

* Earlier commentators observed that the Cincinnati "social unit" organization of health and welfare services was resisted by conservative political forces in municipal government, welfare agencies, and the professions who saw "socialistic and bolshevistic tendencies in the venture." (Charles Bolduan and E. H. Lewinski Corwin, "Economic and Sociologic Aspects of Public Health," in *Nelson Loose Leaf System of Preventive Medicine Public Health*, vol. II [New York: T. Nelson, 1928]). Some of the voluntary spirit of World War I which swept the health center movement along may also have spent itself, no longer vital enough to keep the movement going (Lucy Candib, *A Social Study of the Health Center Movement*, unpub. undergraduate thesis, Harvard University, 1968). W. C. Phillips in his autobiographical account *Adventuring For Democracy* (New York: Social Unit Press, 1941), also attributes the failure of participatory democracy in health not to the local district residents but to city officials.

neur Clinic in New York, by linking with a nearby hospital, is a modern version of Pomeroy's plan.[35] If integration and links to hospitals did develop, it was not from the health center. The venereal disease clinics often left the centers to locate at hospital outpatient departments. More recently, a similar development has occurred with the treatment of tuberculosis. Ambulatory clinics for tuberculosis chemotherapy have also been established in outpatient departments of general hospitals.

The benefits arising from contacts among health and social agencies located in the same building are difficult to judge. If there was improved communication the leadership of private social agencies did not view this benefit as very large. Except for the Visiting Nurse Association, social agencies withdrew to more centralized offices, where they could engage in treatment rather than in services. The agencies originally preferred to have a district location in order to be available for direct relief and cash payments to the immigrant poor. As welfare took over this financial function and handed out relief by mailed check, the direct contact with the district did not seem necessary.

Other problems also contributed to the failure of health centers. In spite of special efforts, it was impossible to recruit public health physicians in sufficient numbers to manage the centers. Even the opportunity offered to the district health officer in Boston to get, while on the job, university training at the Harvard School of Public Health was not sufficient to attract staff. Many health centers attempted to involve actively the neighborhood residents in their programs, but "attempts to organize people of the district themselves into a local council . . . has generally yielded little result in proportion to the effort expended. The reasons for the difficulty lie deep in the characteristics of American neighborhood life whether among native or foreign born." [36] By 1958 Herbert Gans's neighborhood contacts in the West End community of Boston failed to mention the

Blossom Street Health Center often enough to be noted, although they reported their views of the hospital doctors and private practitioners.[37]

In spite of the obvious decline, public health planners continued to be hopeful about the future usefulness of the centers.[38] Their decline could be attributed to several factors, and, first of all, to their restricted program of health care in the face of increasingly complex health needs. Their program was limited to preventive action and remained unrelated to treatment; it was further hampered by the resistance of medical practitioners who did not want clinical functions dominated by public agencies and found the bureaucratic structure of the centers alien to the ideals of the medical profession. Others, however, might argue that the real cause of the decline was not the structure and function of the center but the insufficiency of public funds to combine curative and preventive care, hire salaried doctors, and pay for the treatment and prevention of all illnesses.

RURAL CENTERS

Another powerful public stimulus to the formation of health centers came from the efforts for rural rehabilitation. Poverty and deficient medical care in rural areas was a main social concern of the 1920's, which resulted in plans for providing medical facilities and equipment in the neglected areas. It was hoped that buildings and equipment would attract doctors to work in undoctored rural poverty areas and alleviate the maldistribution of physicians. The Milbank Fund sponsored comprehensive health demonstration programs, including public health centers. Herman Biggs, the health commissioner of New York State, also proposed a series of rural health centers "to insure cooperation and coordination between various branches of public health work through increasing efficiency, reducing overhead expenses of each, and making more money available for the actual conduct of work." He also proposed the addition of medical services for treatment. Much later, Caldwell Esselstyn's private group practice in rural upstate New York came probably nearest to Biggs' idea.[39]

After a series of studies on the distribution of doctors between rural and urban areas, Joseph W. Mountin of the U.S. Public Health Service recommended that health centers be built adjacent to hospitals. His view of the centers as workshops for ambulatory care was incorporated into the Hill-Burton Act for the construction of health facilities.[40] Yet, no such centers for the full scope medical group practices were built, and the money was used instead for the rehabilitation of outpatient departments and the construction of traditional public health clinics, mostly in the rural south.[41] The private and public efforts to finance facilities have continued. The impact of the new federal program under the Model Cities Act to guarantee loans for group practice facilities and equipment is yet to emerge, but private efforts have been most energetic. Over 10 percent of the nation's 6,000 hospitals have office buildings for private practice on their grounds. In addition, the Sears-Roebuck and the Kellogg Foundations have helped local communities to build centers to facilitate the recruitment of physicians.

Other parts of the world have also shown a wide interest in the health center as an institution for rural rehabilitation. Outside the United States the emphasis has not been on facilities and technical equipment, but on organized medical work and increased auxiliary help that would increase the output of the professional practitioners. John Grant, working with the support of the Rockefeller Foundation, established health centers in rural China in the 1930's and, later, with federal funds, in Puerto Rico.[42] Centers were also part of national health planning in India and other countries.[43]

Perhaps the most famous among all such attempts has been S. L. Kark's Phoela center in South Africa, begun in the 1940's and eventually incorporated in the national health scheme of centers for native districts. It emphasized environmental sanitation, preventive care, and some curative treatment—a program dictated by the community's medical problems of infectious diseases and malnutrition.[44] The center worked with a health team, combining physician, nurse, and health educator. Participation of councils made up of the natives was anticipated in the management. Yet the center ran into difficulties in attracting staff and creating comprehensive care in alliance with hospitals. Because the center was a governmental agency, it proved to be difficult to establish links to private-voluntary hospitals for coordinated treatment of patients and staff exchange.[45]

Besides the usual health centers for the rural and urban poor, there are isolated examples of health centers established by physicians interested in the ideology of health as an optimal way of life and in the practice of family care as a means to achieve that life. The best-known example, Pioneer Health Center (Peckham, England), included resources for recreation, education, and preventive care, chiefly periodic examinations.[46] This communal grouping of living activities and medical aid has not been repeated, with the possible exception of health centers of the *kibbutzim* in Israel. In the tradition of the Peckham experiment, George Silver, in the 1950's, established a family care practice at Montefiore Hospital, New York, and introduced the combined clinical work of the doctor as internist and pediatrician along with the nurse and social worker for the care of private patients.[47] This health team was responsible for the comprehensive care of the family, a job which no longer seemed to be within the scope of a general practitioner working alone. Similar innovations were tried with the urban poor within established hospital outpatient departments. Comprehensive clinics offering a broad range of therapies and preventive family care orientation were initiated in a number of outpatient departments. Most often, these clinics were demonstration projects for teaching medical students and dealt with that small fraction of clinic users who opted to enroll in them when offered. In spite of its utopian appeal, comprehensive family care may not be the most marketable project even for the new family with young children.[48] In any case, these clinics have, so far, stimulated no basic change in the organization of ambulatory hospital practices. Nonetheless, they are efforts of reform to alter the orientation, if not the structure, of the bureaucratic traditions in patient care.

The history of health centers presents a series of attempted reforms in providing medical care outside the hospital. It has a fascinating aspect: it attempted to rehabilitate rural and urban communities, help the poor in their health problems, and, at the same time, reform medical practice itself. Yet the history is a partial one because the group practice of medicine in its various forms has represented another effort to establish health centers, although on a private rather than public basis, and directed toward the middle-class rather than the poor.[49] This private movement has been a response to medical specialization and technology rather than to needs of special groups of patients; at any rate, it has never focused around the idea of helping the poor. Those who criticized group practice, or such examples of it as the now defunct United Mine Worker's hospital and clinic services or the Kaiser-Permanente plan, took issue with their orientation. In their efforts to be as good as or better than the private doctor, group practices have efficiently marketed a conventional brand of medical specialists with little of the ideology of family care, preventive medicine, social-psychological treatment, the view of health as an optimal way of life, or any other part of the utopian ideals of the health center movement.

THE NEW NEIGHBORHOOD HEALTH CENTER

At present, urban reform is again a major social concern, and the neighborhood health center is part of our concern. The new interest in this old institution is noteworthy because it originates not only in the historical past but also in the recent findings of social science studies on the culture of poverty, interprofessional work, bureaucratic organization, and community structure.

As the present-day advocates of the plan visualize it, the poor will receive services closer to home and, moreover, receive instant medical aid; their care will be prepaid involving no further negotiations. Local health aides—neighborhood therapists without degrees—will help them recognize treatable conditions, overcome indifference to treatment, use the center, and follow advice. More appropriately designed for lower-class culture, the neighborhood health services will be used more often by more poor people, and the later will, thus, approach the middle-class pattern of use.[50] The poor will also participate in other ways than as patients and acquire the social and political experience to initiate social change and have a sense of community cohesion.

There will be new groupings of therapists or new arrangements of interprofessional work at such centers. The doctor, nurse, and social worker of Silver's program will be supplemented by health aides and psychiatric consultants to the team. These additions are planned to recognize that treatment tasks in the community are complex and require specialized therapy, different from that of the hospitals; they also represent an effort to extend the clinical-care output of specialists. The practitioners do not work in the traditional part-time pattern, dividing their hours between public clinic and private practice. Their full-time commitment is a modern necessity to evolve team work as a new style of interprofessional work. The orientation of the care will be family centered and comprehensive, with a general strategy of "out-reach" to nonattending patients.

Do these features insure the center's long-range success as an organization and provide the best care of the urban poor? One of the most promising features for success is that the management of the centers is private. They are not operated by public health departments, with the exception of the Denver center, but by private or university hospitals and their practicing staff. This arrangement should guarantee more flexibility in recruitment and management than the traditional public health departments could offer. Moreover, the new centers have another advantage in linking their staff activities to hospitals, and this arrangement, if it occurs, gives us a hope that every physician will have some connection to an institution where the quality of practice is of continuous concern.[51]

A second feature in the success of the centers will be their size. One might argue that there is an optimal number of staff members for any medical institution, optimal not only in the potential for delivering a broad range of therapies but also for creating conditions most attractive for professional work. The currently popular community planning, based on epidemiologic analysis of health needs and the many demonstration projects, envisions small centers with small staffs. However, small centers (for example, one that would not support diagnostic radiological equipment) have the disadvantage that they serve only as registration points: their physicians cannot function properly without the everyday use of common technical aids, and their patients have to be referred, for diagnosis or treatment, to other facilities. If there is an optimal size for professional staff, then planning based on small districts or on a few but not all neighborhood health needs, will need re-examination.

The size of the centers determines not only the degree of professional complexity but their location. Major importance has been attached to having the centers visibly located within poverty areas. In a day when there is the possibility of convenient intra-city transportation and distance is no longer the same barrier it was, this strategy does not seem necessary.[52] Centers could be located outside, or at the border, of poverty areas, where the poor as well as the working-class and middle-class patients can use them; this arrangement would insure a variety of patients, a feature beneficial in many respects.

There are still other limitations to the district idea, the limitations of the district itself. Such district centers may create segregated institutions and perpetuate the existing status quo for the district and its people. True enough, not everyone wants a change. Professionals often complain about the many poor who show little willingness to change in their health-care practices, and this is particularly frequent in reference to the elderly and those beyond rehabilitation, who are to be found in every district.

The centers offer curative as well as preventive services, with attention to the major health needs in dental, chronic medical, psychiatric and maternal-infant care. As the scope of the psychosocial work of the centers will be enlarged with health teams, mental health care will be decentralized. Whether the mental health clinics will be local centers for post-hospitalized mental patients or will be modeled like general practice, available for a mixture of specific medical therapies and general psychosocial help, is yet uncertain. If both services are going to be delivered as community practices, they could be delivered together for the benefit of the poor and other groups as well. However, the planning of medical and mental health services is generally divided. Currently, the mental health services in Massachusetts are organizing around districts much larger than most of those conceived in the health center movement, and with more central authority than medical practices have ever had.

The success of the centers will depend, too, on their ability to attract full-time staff and enroll poor clients. The former may be easier than in the past because of a new orientation within medical schools. While no schools have adopted a curriculum of educating doctors to work in groups or with auxiliaries in ambulatory care, they have implicitly favored group practice by their policy of not training general practitioners. Hospitals also have come to favor group practice over solo practice where use of hospital facilities is concerned. Yet, where private group practice is the only practice form at the hospital, significant numbers of the poor are usually left out.

The strategy of services at the centers will include "out-reach" programs of active case-finding by home visiting and the use of neighborhood health aides. These programs, however, raise two problems. What is the certainty of determining what can or cannot be effectively treated and prevented? Also, does everyone want the kind of package care that the centers propose? Clinical experience and studies suggest that everyone does not opt for continuous comprehensive care in spite of its professional endorsement. It may indeed be that discontinuity in using medical help is not disadvantageous.[53]

Finally, the health center may be viewed in the context of established institutions. It is, at once, a decentralization of services and a centralization of community medical practices—a response to the view that personal care cannot be given in large-scale institutions and that, in solo practice, the care given is not efficient enough nor qualitatively as good as it should be. Are there other alternatives?

Some reservations about centers, especially their location, strategy, size, complexity, and clientele, have been mentioned. Even within the existing large institutions, the issue of size and impersonality can be met.[54] Professional staffs can work with smaller numbers of colleagues and patients. In some mental hospitals, the idea of a district has been the basis for decentralization of treatment, with wards designated for patients from the same district. In established practices, such as the prepaid group practice used by industrial employees, the poor could just as well be enrolled and treated, even if they are not located in the poverty area. Convenient transportation could be arranged, and better access to urban outpatient clinics could be insured. At present, the largest outpatient clinic in Boston is two blocks away from the subway exit, a major walking distance for handicapped older persons.

The dimensions of the health needs of the poor are so large that fifty new health centers would be insufficient to service the poor across the country. Therefore, the use of group practice in and out of poverty areas has to be considered. The organization and management of successful group practices have been demonstrated (an achievement that, at the present writing, does not hold for the new health centers), and, for example, the Health Insurance Plan in New York has enrolled 20,000 persons under Medicaid.[55] In view of such facts, it is desirable that private group practices be encouraged, not only through financial guarantee for the construction of facilities but also through an extra payment for poor patients.

Many proponents argue that economy and efficiency in providing health services recommend the health centers and pay particular interest to the cost-effectiveness of health programs.[56] Part of the attraction of the community health movement and health centers is the expectation that care and treatment outside the hospital will be simpler and cheaper because treatment problems will be contained and managed in the community at less cost than at hospitals.[57] The need for auxiliaries and technical innovations are seen as cost-cutting production measures which increase clinical output at the same cost. A nurse, in effect, is cheaper than a doctor, an aide cheaper than a nurse, and a machine-taken history cheaper still.

Evidently, the centers are concerned with economy, making the existing care as cheap as possible. Yet the center's dual purposes must have an effect which cannot reduce costs. The addition of people to the treatment team and the agency, the provision of more centers and group practices, the organization of more comprehensive services will make the care more costly and, although, hopefully, more personalized, not necessarily more efficient. The unit cost of a health center can hardly be judged against the usual criterion of what it costs to be treated in the doctor's office. A social account sheet of the effects of the health center on people and their health will be difficult to determine.[58] In any case, no health program should be judged by its economy alone.

THE IMPACT OF TREATMENT AND CARE
ON HEALTH STATUS AND POVERTY

So far, the organization of health services in the community has been our major concern. Looking beyond this problem, two further questions arise. First, what care is most important for improving the health status of the poor? Second, what medical intervention might be important for reducing poverty? The first raises an issue of priorities, the second, an issue of strategy.

The improvement of health programs in dental, psychiatric, and maternal-infant care is most needed. In dental care, fluoridation and restorative work must have the highest priorities, but both of them have to face great obstacles. Fluoridation, although endorsed by health authorities, still has limited application because of political and social resistance. The restorative work is hampered by manpower shortage, although the profession and the dental schools are now willing to train and employ dental aides. Furthermore, public resistance to reasonable dental treatment must also be considered. In clinical practice, it was observed that regular dental care given to children in a free municipal program did not carry over into later years, when private sources were expected to be used.[59] While these findings indicate a need for continuing dental services, they also raise questions about the effectiveness of health centers.

If the centers, along with other institutions, are successful in remodeling people to fit the economy, they may become victims of their own success. Leaving a district to live in a better place may be a mark of successful change, but such people will no longer be around to use the center or, supported by their improved economic status, will seek the offices of private practitioners. In this respect, health centers may be institutions of transition leading to something else. In the past, health planning for the poor often worked in the expectations that any plan would only be temporary. For example, the hospital outpatient department was not always viewed as a "medical soup kitchen" for the poor, but, rather, as an institution teaching good standards of practice and correct utilization of services for those who later could afford to see private doctors. The center, however, may still be needed even after its patients are no longer poor, because, as previous studies have observed, the patients will not "go private" as soon as they have more money. Accordingly, one can expect that the instant medical help and crisis medicine of health centers and hospital emergency rooms, so often disparaged, might still be with us for quite some time to come.

It is even more difficult to evaluate the long-range effect of the health centers upon the treatment of psychiatric problems. The specific nature of clinical psychiatric disorders, including alcoholism, is so complicated that no simple prescriptions for preventive intervention can be written for them. Yet, appropriate and comprehensive services at general hospitals and in the community are certainly needed.[60] It is doubtful that they can be organized at the centers without employing a too large and complex staff. The neighborhood center's health side may be of some importance in this respect by recognizing treatable situations, surveying families at certain critical points, and generally making accommodations for the early symptoms of clinical disorders.

Probably the most important point of interaction of health services and poverty is the connection between educational methods and techniques of psychotherapy. If psychotherapy is viewed as a means of emotional re-education, conducted either in a one-to-one relationship, or in family and group therapy, then it may be important in dealing with some of the developmental problems of the dropouts, slow learners and overactive children. However, it is rarely considered whether therapeutic group work will be offered by the health center staff or be built into the educational bureaucracy of the school health programs, student counseling, or into education itself. The results of conventional school health programs are not impressive, and their historical bases are no longer tenable.[61] An important function of the health center could be for referral from local schools. The other important task of psychiatric intervention, consultation with teachers on classroom problems, has been done by psychiatry but, in the future, may be done by educators with special skills.

The much publicized social class difference in perinatal mortality rates requires renewed efforts in the field of maternal and infant care. The clinical team of pediatrician, nurse, and health aide may be able to make this care available, although one cannot expect that the provision of more care and treatment alone would reduce these rates.[62] Part of the increased perinatal mortality rate seems related to prematurity, which, in turn, is related to the early age of the mother's conception and antecedent periods of nutritional imbalance in her earlier life.[63] The basis for early conception is rooted in lower-class life, where early sexual intercourse is the norm. One may argue that the potentialities of birth control might be useful in this respect, but, at the same time, one must not forget that in the same lower-class culture the fact of having a baby has a very special psychological significance and, often, a desirable feature for many unwed mothers.

Some time ago, John B. Grant, like many others, viewed the local health centers as a means for the social rehabilitation of the community.[64] Indeed, to some extent they were, for through improved environmental sanitation and the control of infectious disease, more people had longer lives to live in the community; through improved nutrition they had greater physical vitality for living. While our expectations of health centers today may be the same, the modern problems and the means are not. The centers now have complex problems of chronic medical and psychological disorders as well as dental and maternal-infant health. The major means of the center are still comprehensive personal health services but its scope is changing. Much of this is because the boundary between health and illness is becoming blurred and thus what constitutes "medical treatment" is also undergoing change. Just as the halfway house, now a first step going out of treatment institutions, becomes a necessary variety of living and so a preventive first step for containing illness in the community, the health centers may do the same. They can offer relief and rehabilitation to many handicapped so that such persons can be their best even with their disorders, provided, of course, that the center's services are sufficiently complex to deal with complicated illness. An expectation that the medical care at the centers can offer more, that treatment will result in a cure, is true in but a few instances. Yet the limited outcomes are no less important. While medical therapies and the use of personal health services at the health center, the office, and the hospital do not promise cures, they do promise some control and relief. By making such services more available and accessible, we can achieve much in patient satisfaction and relief from health problems, and such an achievement will make life better in our communities for the poor and the not poor alike.

XI · Health and Poverty Reconsidered

by John Kosa, Irving K. Zola and
Aaron Antonovsky

The preceding chapters of this book have discussed the various aspects of health and poverty and presented much empirical material and many views on the topic. The contributors have attempted to assess what the medical and social sciences, two productive and research-oriented disciplines, have to offer for a better understanding of our problem. The faithful reader who has followed their discussion may end up with a feeling rather akin to the embarrassment of riches. Such a feeling is common and perhaps unavoidable in the present stage of academic productivity; fortunately enough, it can be resolved by summarizing the gist of the detailed analysis. By necessity the following summary will be brief and perhaps all too general, but it is intended to serve the convenience of the reader.

For this summary we assume that poverty (as discussed in Chapter I) represents a specific social environment which affects most, and perhaps all, aspects of life, including health, illness, and related behavior. Furthermore we assume that the social significance of health-related events can be most conveniently analyzed with the scheme of morbid episodes described in Chapter II. Following the two assumptions, the basic question is: What effects can be attributed to poverty in the health and illness of people?

Lerner and Fried, surveying the morbidity status in the fields of physical and mental health respectively, reach rather similar conclusions. "The poverty population is today considerably less healthy than the rest of the population of this country," states Lerner, and Fried sums up the evidence thus: "The lowest social classes have the highest rates of severe psychiatric disorder in our society." This similarity, however, is due to different dynamic forces that operate in the two fields. In physical health the social distribution of morbidity (dependent as it is on the different ways of life of the different classes) shows some diseases (coronary problems, lung cancer, etc.) to be more prevalent in the better-off classes, while others (contagious diseases, diseases resulting in infant mortality) are shown to be more prevalent in the poverty class; the net balance is more unfavorable to the poverty-stricken class. In mental health the cumulative effects of the diverse forms of deprivation, disruption, and difficulty, common scourges of the poor, tend to create an environment in which the serious psychiatric disorders become more common.

There is no discernible sign that the morbidity gap between the poor and the not-poor is narrowing in the field of mental health. The question of the morbidity gap in physical health, however, is more complex. There is no question whatsoever that differences among social class above the poverty line have narrowed considerably. The evidence is strong, too, that in those disease areas which are open to control by public health measures the poor are not as relatively disadvantaged as they once were. Whether these trends will continue or not, or whether the differential patterns on those diseases on which the poor seem advantaged at present will be maintained is, however, more a matter of blind faith in progress than a reasonable inference from the evidence.[1]

The Health Deficit Among the Poor

Is it reasonable to transfer these findings into the scheme of morbid episodes by saying that the poor class experiences more health disturbances and, accordingly, evaluates the disturbances in a different way than the more affluent classes? The social distribution of morbidity being as complex as it is, it would be unjust to make a purely quantitative statement on the frequency of disturbances without considering the seriousness of the event. In fact, the differentiation between less serious and more serious events is a very important analytical tool in understanding the health care of our times. As the contributors to this book repeatedly warn, there are more minor illnesses reported today than were reported in the past and there might be more minor illnesses reported among the well-to-do than among the poor.

Some observers claim that the poor perceive more episodes as nonserious, or in other words, that their perceptual threshold, beyond which an event is judged to be a symptom, is higher than that of other classes. This might be so in case of medically unsophisticated people; but speaking of present-day America, the poor, and particularly the urban poor, can hardly be characterized with such a lack of sophistication. Moreover, the observed differences in the morbidity of social classes show up in the serious illnesses where the likelihood that a symptom would not reach the perceptual threshold is greatly diminished by the nature of the illness. In view of all these it is perhaps more reasonable to suggest that the social-class differences exist along the line of rational versus irrational assessment of the morbid episode where rational is the assessment that conforms with the current medical practice and such a rational assessment is more common among the educated classes. This conformity with the expectations of medical practice also affects the next stage of the morbid episode, the management of anxiety.

The contributors to this book seem to disagree on the point whether or not the poor are less concerned about illnesses than the well-to-do.[2] The concern about illness evidently reflects the anxiety (either specific or floating) which naturally accompanies every morbid episode. Fried, speaking about the class differences in mental health, suggests that either the poor have a greater amount of floating anxiety than the well-to-do or there is a qualitative difference between the anxieties prevalent in the two classes, the poor having to face more oppressive stresses and strains. In any case it is warranted to assume that the extent or the form of the floating anxiety varies by social class, but it is not easy to make the same kind of statement about the specific anxiety. The latter, which is evoked by the health disturbance, is related to the perception of the disturbance. Since this perception varies along the rational-nonrational line, one is inclined to believe that specific anxiety shows a corresponding variation: in the well-to-do class it tends to conform, on the whole, with the expectations of the medical profession, while in the poor class it tends to deviate from such expectations. The situation implies certain negative consequences for the poor. It poses serious obstacles in the line of effective communication between the physician and the poor patient, and creates difficulties in the professional treatment of the anxiety component of the poor patient's illness.[4]

People assess their health disturbances and control their health-related anxieties with the aid of the knowledge that they have on matters relating to health. But knowledge is unequally distributed among the social classes; it is a part of those privileges which mark the differences between the poor and the non-poor. The results can be well observed when examining preventive behavior and health maintenance. As Rosenstock sums it up, "there is a marked association between income and possession of correct knowledge about a wide variety of health-related matters," and a similar association exists "between income and extent of belief in the efficacy of alternative procedures for preventing or controlling various health conditions." Accordingly, the poor are less likely to seek preventive services or seek diagnostic services in the absence of symptoms. The consistency in the health actions that Rosenstock discerns can be extended as far as the poor are concerned: they consistently fall short of meeting medical standards and expectations in assessment, anxiety, knowledge and preventive behavior as well. This situation, then, compounds the consequences of the initial threats of deprivation and environmental stress.

The full extent of the disadvantaged status of the poor becomes visible when we examine the manipulative actions that people take to remove illness and resolve morbid episodes. Manipulation as a rule implies that the patient uses the help of other people—lay as well as professional—and attempts to interact with them in an ordered way to regain health. But the possibilities of interaction, available to any person, depend on social power, mastery, and other privileges which vary in accordance with social class. Thus, the interaction pattern available to the poor is restricted when compared to that of the better-off classes; it is weaker, less efficient, and less conforming with the requirements of the professional standards. The studies assess this deficiency and its consequences.

Mechanic sums up clearly: "Low socio-economic status is associated with a lower level of utilization of medical services based on consumer decision," and he adds immediately, "income . . . does not explain this in full." The essential difference is that in its manipulative actions the low-income group tends to use the lay referral system rather than the medical referral system or, in other words, uses the network of the primary group (family, neighbors) rather than the network of the secondary group (medical system, social agencies) to obtain the help needed. The difference refers not simply to the greater competence that the medical system and its auxiliaries can insure but also to those social-psychological services that the two groups render.

Both types of networks serve to inhibit our instinctual actions and to furnish us with nurturance, but they do so in their own ways, which differ by social classes. In their system the patient of the poor class is shortchanged and is unable to receive the optimal services from any of the sources. From his primary group he can expect nurturance but not much in the line of inhibitory services to check his instinctual responses to illness-related anxiety. After all, his family and neighbors, with their insufficient medical knowledge and often disrupted routine of life, can inhibit rather inefficiently his gratificatory manipulations and move him just as inefficiently toward the therapeutic ones.

At the same time the patient of the poor class cannot expect much nurturance from the service pattern of the medical system and social agencies. Roth, in his compassionate description of the formal treatment of patients, points out how the principle of fee for service—the essential ordering principle in the health care system—divides the service pattern of medicine into two segments, those of private practice and public clinics. Medical competence (which by its nature restricts the gratificatory manipulations) is available in both segments, but nurturance is not equally available in the two. In the private segment the extent of nurturance received by any patient is regulated by the principle of fee for service, that is, by the financial status of the patient; but in the public sector the same is regulated by formal policy and institutional behavior. The public sector, as it is structured today, can never match the flexibility and personal orientation that physicians in private practice offer because any public clinic has to fit the treatment of any group of patients into the complex totality of institutional goals. In this fit the poverty patient with his reduced social power is likely to come off worse.

The same conditions accompany the patient on his road toward the desired cure. As Sussman's analysis makes it clear, in the area of readjustment and rehabilitation the effects of poverty are somewhat blurred by many specific factors, such as the relatively old age of the average patient, the chronicity and disabling nature of the illness, and so on. Nevertheless the availability and utility of rehabilitative treatments "show conspicuous variations by income classes" and "the post-hospitalization care of the poor can be generally characterized as a state of medical deprivation."

The line of analysis that follows the process of the morbid episode, clearly shows the effects of the poverty-health complex: the detrimental effects of poverty as a social environment lead to more (or more of the serious kind of) morbidity, hamper the poor in maintaining or regaining their health, and make any morbid episode more threatening and unpleasant for the poor than for the more fortunate people. This total difference can be best visualized as a health deficit existing among the poor and affecting every important aspect of their health and illness.

POVERTY AS A CAUSATIVE FACTOR

The picture is clear. Whatever aspect of health, whatever stage of the morbid episode is examined, the poor are at a disadvantage. In this case one has to ask the question: What part of this sad situation can be attributed to poverty and what part of it to other factors, including chance, which are always present in human life and inflict inequities on so many people?

In any answer to this question we shall overlook the possible role of genetic factors in the causation of pathology. It seems safe to assume that hereditary traits are unable to explain to any significant extent the observed relationship between health and poverty. Moreover, we think that poverty is a social environment, created by man or by his negligence, and can be interpreted in terms of social factors. But if we look at social life, we find there all too many phenomena which are interrelated. In this lattice of phenomena it is extremely difficult to single out for any social fact one or several distinct causes, that is, antecedent variables the occurrence of which is regularly connected with the occurrence of the social fact. Hence the theories explaining complex behavior (for example, health behavior) usually involve multiple causation, as is the case with Rosenstock's motivation theory, Mechanic's theory of ten sets of response patterns, or Zola's theory of five triggers of patient's decisions.[3]

The previous pages have specified a great many social causes related to health and poverty. They have pointed out that a poverty-producing factor is not necessarily pathogenic and, vice versa, a pathogenic factor is not necessarily a cause of poverty; but there exist some factors that can be described as both poverty-producing and pathogenic. In order to clarify this point, it might be useful to consider such causes in a systematic order and reach a better understanding of the role that poverty plays in the health of a society.

Age and sex are two conspicuous causative factors related to both health and poverty. Their functioning illustrates rather well the general complexity of causation. Advancing age generally increases the likelihood of both ill health and poverty, while the sex division outlines a more difficult pattern. Females have lower mortality rates and lower morbidity rates in the major illnesses than males but females face a higher risk of poverty. Thus, a given age group of women may fare better in health characteristics than a younger age group of men but may be more impoverished than an older age group of men.

Race and ethnicity represent a different set of causes. Although certain ethnic groups have higher mortality rates in certain disease categories, there is no reason to believe that any of the races or ethnic groups would be biologically weaker or generally more morbid than others.[4] Rather, the racial and ethnic groups should be viewed as subcultures in our country which maintain specific cultural traits different from those of the middle-class majority. The cultural differences refer not only to such traits as diet, housing, and sanitation (which, although strongly affecting the health status, are changeable) but also to such more fundamental traits as the approved ways of handling anxiety, acquiring medical knowledge, and carrying out preventive and manipulative measures.[5] In this context one may often hear the statement that the risk of poor health status and material poverty in any subculture is in direct relationship to the extent to which the subculture deviates from the standards of the middle-class majority.[6] While there is more than a grain of truth in this statement, it should be remembered that cultural deviation is a multidimensional phenomenon that is likely to include both negative and positive traits. For example, the Jewish immigrants living in the American cities of the 1910's represented a poverty group with cultural traits greatly different from those of the middle-class majority, yet, they had a surprisingly good health status and, for example, the lowest infant mortality rate among all the groups studied.[7]

Another group of causes, implicated in both health and poverty, refers to the individual's place in the social interaction pattern and includes such items as marital status, social isolation, anomie, social mobility, migration, loss of status and personal inadequacy. It is evident that any condition that weakens a person's place in the generally established pattern of social interaction, tends to increase for him the risk of poor health and poverty.

A different set of causes can be best summed up under the name of habits—drinking, eating habits, smoking, and sedentary life. In daily language we often refer to them as "bad" habits and just as often we launch popular, moralistic, and highly emotional campaigns against them. For example, the old prohibitionist campaign consistently indicted drinking as a cause of poverty, but at present no unemotional student of the problem would attribute such a pauperizing impact to any of the habits. The bionegative effect of any habit depends on its intensity. Altogether, such habits cannot be entirely neglected in the studies of morbidity, but, the claims of the moralists notwithstanding, they do not affect the specific poverty-health complex.

If, finally, we come to regard poverty itself as a cause of morbidity, it should be remembered that poverty is a social environment of many facets. It can be equally well measured in terms referring to the means of subsistence (income, education, social class, occupation, residence) and in terms referring to the lack of privileges of life (unemployment, powerlessness, loss of status, inadequacy, social disruption.) Altogether poverty is a collective noun which covers a wide variety of the undesirable features of social life. It is therefore an extremely difficult task to parcel out the morbid causation among the various facets of poverty. When speaking of health in general as one compact entity, it might well be impossible to determine whether income, education, or social disruption is the most potent causative factor; in all probability the importance of each facet varies according to the specific health phenomenon under investigation. Thus when the question was examined what kind of families are likely to have a private physician for their children, income was found to be a more important contributing factor than the social class of the family or the education or occupation of any of the parents.[8] On the other hand, when the effect of socioeconomic status upon perinatal mortality was investigated, the education of the mother turned out to be the most important factor.[9]

This might be the proper place to point out some practical consequences of this situation. Each of our antipoverty programs is designed to attack one concrete facet of poverty; thus, one program is aimed to enlarge the income, while another focuses on the education of the poor. From the first we can expect health-related improvements only to the extent to which a health problem is related to the lack of income; from the second, to the extent to which a health problem is related to the lack of education; but none of them can promise to improve the whole spectrum of health problems. The same limitations refer to the medical programs also. A neighborhood clinic can promise to improve those health problems which are related to the un-availability of medical services in the given neighborhood; it cannot promise anything more nor anything outside of its neighborhood. In other words, there is no single prescription, no magic formula (short of ending poverty itself) which would solve the entire poverty-health complex.

Both poverty and ill health have multiple causes which are interrelated among themselves and affect in varying degrees the various facets of poverty and health. Thus, the question must be raised: What kind of causation exists between poverty and health?

When attempting to explain any phenomenon we usually distinguish among sufficient, necessary, and contributory causes. For example, myocardial infarction is a sufficient cause to explain one man's death, but it is not a necessary cause because many other diseases also cause death; when speaking of deaths in a given population, myocardial infarction is a contributory cause which contributes its share to the total deaths experienced in the population without sufficiently or necessarily explaining all of them. It is evident that poverty is neither a necessary nor a sufficient cause of poor health; the rich people, too, suffer from ill health. But can it be a necessary or sufficient cause of that health deficit that characterizes our poverty population? The example of dental caries, mentioned earlier in this book, will help to formulate the answer. Dental caries is noticeably related to lower socio-economic status in communities which do not have fluoridated water but in communities which use fluoridation, the social-class differences in caries tend to disappear.

Poverty is a specific social environment, but the elements of this environment change and vary; through man's work (such as fluoridation) they may improve. Hence, poverty must be considered as a contributory cause in the health deficit of the poor. A contributory relationship might be, and in this case is, grave enough to appeal to our emotions and prompt intervention. At the same time it permits us to believe that, through proper actions, the poverty-health complex can be alleviated and greatly improved.

There remains, however, one more question to be answered. Our conclusions on the relationship of the health deficit of the poor are based on the many detailed measurements and observations that are relevant to our topic. But if both poverty and health have so many facets, how can we be sure that our measurements, observations, and conclusions are correct, that we are not laboring under illusions and self-deceptions? The history of medicine, and the historical treatment given to poverty as well, give innumerable examples of misconceptions and self-deceptions, of slogans and stereotypes taking hold of the minds of the best-educated people. What is the guarantee that in the present case we are not entertaining similar, albeit moralistic, misconceptions?

In any issue of social medicine, the problem of methodology is crucial; to this problem Haberman addresses himself in the Appendix of this book. His careful analysis of the method is reassuring. In spite of the serious inherent obstacles that the field of health presents to any research worker, in spite of the difficulties that encumber communication between the middle-class research worker and the lower-class patient, it is possible to obtain information on the health of poor which is just as reliable and valid as the information that can be obtained on the health of the middle class. At the same time Haberman voices a warning that is very appropriate for a timely and popular topic which has ignited its own publication explosion. Only research which carefully complies with the requirements of methodology can yield acceptable data, and the more exciting a topic is, the more it touches upon action programs, the more rigorous must be the method.

THE POSSIBILITIES FOR ACTION

There are few sights in life that would strike us with a stronger force than the sight of poverty and ill health: they appeal to our conscience and prompt us to take actions. The works of conscience make up a natural part of human psychology, their examples show up in the history of medicine and poverty of all ages. But ours is a particularly action-oriented age, due perhaps to our advances in technology and human organization which render it so much easier for us to translate our dreams, desires, and the suggestions of our conscience into meaningful actions. Aided by such circumstances, modern medicine shows an activity unparalleled by previous epochs in research, teaching, and, especially, in efforts toward making competent care available to the broad masses. Due to the same circumstances, our present-day preoccupation with poverty is far advanced beyond traditional charity and philanthropy, advanced to the stage where communities and entire nations are launching planned, large-scale action programs.

Yet, our activity does not follow directly and impulsively our dreams, desires, or the suggestions of our conscience. Between the actions and the dreams there stands an inhibitory system which in its own way scrutinizes and weighs the possibilities and consequences, the motives and difficulties, the taboos and rewards that surround the action. With the aid of the inhibitory system man makes a decision, often in the form of a reasoned judgment, before acting. In case of community actions (such as the poverty programs) we like to resort to a special and sophisticated instrument of the inhibitory system—research.

The aim of research is to collect and consider systematic knowledge which can then be used in rational action. Through its protracted work with data, research takes on a second function that often becomes more important than the first one; it inhibits impulsive actions and delays decisions. Thus it becomes a piece of safety equipment that those who embark upon a major activity like to carry with them. It helps to find the best plan for any action, saves us from missteps and mistakes and removes the errors from our trials. It is an eminently useful activity in our action-oriented society, which supports a great deal of research in the hope of making its actions safe and efficient. In fact we come to rely too much on research and expect from it not only safety and success in actions but also the services of a cookbook giving us the recipes that, if followed step by step, make a good cake. Thus a spokesman of the field of public health asked the sociologists to furnish the "human values and goals" for health-related actions and promised that public health as a nationwide organization would implement those values and goals.[10]

But far from being a recipe in the cookbook, research is (in the words of Wordsworth) "something between a hindrance and a help." Research and action are separated by a chasm much wider than the one separating personal desire and action. A research, if completed, yields bases for inferences about what should be done, but the best reasoning abilities are needed to reach the proper inferences. After that, other logical steps must follow—planning, decision-making, responsibility-taking, administration—each of them requiring the optimal psychological input before safe and good actions can be taken. Research is helpful in making plans and decisions, but does not relieve us of the necessity of reasoning and working; neither does it furnish us with a sure-fire solution of any vexing problem.

An often-heard criticism of community actions and antipoverty measures claimed that those programs acted first and reasoned, if ever, only after the action. Yet it would be unrealistic to expect that knowledge and research should always be rationally linked to planning and action; after all, irrational elements usually intrude upon the psychological process leading to action. When it comes to community action, one irrational element that perhaps unavoidably intrudes is politics. To be sure, the basic role of politics is not entirely negative. It is a useful process that permits the different segments of the community to voice their opinions and partcipate in making decisions; it permits the legitimate use of political power and the advocation of any just cause; it facilitates a satisfactory compromise among the different segments of the community. It makes the issues public and initiates debates about them; in the course of public discussion it moves the interested parties to introduce slogans and stereotypes.

In the public discussion of emotionally loaded issues a great many slogans and stereotypes are bound to emerge which in their total impact obstruct the clear view of the issue and hamper the formulation of reasoned judgments. For example, the relatively high infant mortality rate of the United States, which is causing quite some concern, has produced a set of stereotyped answers such as demands for more doctors (especially obstetricians), more maternity wards, more medical attention and, generally, more money. A careful study, however, compared infant mortality in the United States and in fifteen other countries with more favorable mortality rates. It found that the obstetrical care given in the United States surpassed in quality and quantity that given in the other countries. In the United States, over 97 percent of births were delivered in hospitals and institutions and virtually all of these were attended by physicians. In England and Wales only 66 percent of all births occurred in hospitals and only 14 percent of them were delivered by physicians; in the Netherlands only 27 percent of live births were delivered in hospitals and 65 percent of the deliveries were attended by physicians.[11] The countries with better infant mortality rates lagged behind the United States in medically attended and hospitalized deliveries; in most cases the midwives worked well enough.

One may infer from such data that more obstetricians, more maternity wards, and more money spent would not suffice to make any perceptible change in the infant mortality rate of the country. As it appears, the stereotypes give the easy but wrong answer. When looking for better answers, one may speculate how much two well-known factors—illegitimacy and young age of the mother—contribute to the infant mortality rates in the United States and the other countries. Assuming that these two high-risk factors explain the difference, one may again speculate about what kind of action programs could lead to an improvement of the existing situation. Illegitimacy has been a social problem since time immemorial and the numberless efforts made to eradicate it have been futile.

The role of politics and slogans should be kept in mind when we consider any community action or social policy in the field of poverty. In his chapter on the future of poverty, Shostak builds this role into a general theory of intervention programs and sums up in two paradigms the probability of the failure or success of any program. But the forces contained in any program cannot explain the ultimate outcome without regarding the forces operating outside of it; thus, Shostak concludes with some remarks on a general American ambivalence toward poverty programs. One is tempted to enlarge this ambivalence into broader perspectives and use it to discern a natural feature of American reform movements. Let us think back to the decade of the muckrakers and big trusts, the decade of the depression and social unrest, and, finally, our own decade of poverty amidst affluence. In each case one can witness a slow, diffident and often-bungling series of reforms which, in spite of its conspicuous shortcomings, somehow managed to restrict the rule of monopolies, prevent an economic collapse and a seizure of power by the extremists, and at present promises to remove hopelessness from the lives of millions of poor. They seem to represent the American way of reforming conditions which finally manages to solve a problem without force and revolution, and establish a workable balance among the desires and the realities.

Perhaps one should not overlook what may be called the utopian streak in American mentality, which usually shows up in our general but enthusiastic determination to wipe out the social problems in their totality. Yet at every point this utopian mentality has to be reconciled with the realities of power, politics, and interest groups, with a scheme of counterpressures. Utopias generate enthusiasm, commitment, and determination, much needed to reach great goals; but the realities of power and politics determine the boundaries within which reform work is feasible. It would be unwise to abandon the dream of ending poverty and wiping out class differences in health, but it would be even more foolish to forget about the smaller goals which lie within the politically feasible boundaries. Then the only serious way to deal with poverty and illness is to follow the American way of reforming and search for a workable compromise.

Just how much optimism can this American way of reforming instill into us? In the case of poverty programs the danger lies not only in politics and stereotypes interfering with rational planning but also in the steam running out of the social movement that supports the endeavors for reform. What will happen a few years from now when our national concern and interest will be diverted into other directions and the management of the poverty programs will represent nothing more than the bureaucratic routine of a governmental agency in charge of welfare administration? Can anything be done for the survival of the present popular concern beyond the short life span of social movements?

The cycles of popularity greatly interfere with health-related community actions also. Stoeckle, in his analysis of the health-related interventions, gives a striking illustration: the idea of neighborhood and community centers has passed through several peaks of popularity and just as many valleys of decline although stable development is the first requirement of success for any efficient medical institution. What are the safeguards against the whimsical effects of popularity? As Stoeckle points out, our presently emerging health policy (which has evolved rather late after the emergence of a national social policy in the 1930's) moves along two lines: nationwide and local actions. The first nationwide action of our health policy was the Medicare-Medicaid legislation which was called a first timid step toward a national health insurance system and was designed to extend its benefits to all citizens of the country. The local actions were exemplified in the health centers established in crucial areas of a few large cities for improving the health services of a neighborhood. The experiences show that the local actions are much more subject to the whimsical effect of popularity and that any action that aims to be effective in the field of health, must be nationwide.

At the same time it should not be overlooked that every intervention program operates with a built-in social bias. We never try to intervene into the affairs of the middle class and we seldom see any good reason for doing so; but we are ready to launch an intervention program whenever we contact the lower class with a behavior pattern different from ours. Hence, the intervention is directed toward a different class of people and, no matter how "good" its' aims are, it implies the danger of discrimination among classes. If we establish neighborhood clinics for the poor, this policy in itself perpetuates and expands the existing double standards of medical care which offers private practice for the middle class and public clinic for the poor. It would be a great naiveté to expect that the two will ever render the same kind of services.[12]

The principle of a single standard of medical care must govern our health policy. "The need is imperative," the Medical Care Section of the American Public Health Association stated, "to eliminate the two classes of medical care, to abolish the means test as the implement of segregated service, and to replace the whole concept of charity medicine with a single high standard." [13] Yet, how realistic is this aim? As long as there is social and economic inequality, there will also be a class of people with some health deficit. As long as the complete elimination of poverty cannot be accomplished, a reasonable plan has to be worked out for the nationwide application of the principle of a single high standard. It would be unrealistic to demand that private-practice medical care should be made available to all citizens of the country, but it would be even more foolish to strike out for abolishing private practice or denying it to those who wish to use it and can pay for it. The realistic compromise requires that private-practice medical care should be made available to more people than at present and that the existing system of public clinics should be maintained and improved in its quality of care: in this way we may make a few steps toward approaching the ideal aim of a single standard of medical care.

With this aim in mind we submit three propositions in the hope that they may influence future actions.

First, a nationwide, federally administered health insurance scheme is needed for all citizens, without a means test which offers uniform services but a selective content of coverage. The opponents of health insurance (a large and powerful group on the national scene) are wont to voice two momentous arguments.

They assert that a general insurance scheme would be financially prohibitive and perhaps outright ruinous for the national economy and that it would favor the hypochondriac in a nation which has more than its fair share of hypochondriacs. Hence, the insurance scheme must be selective and cover only those major diseases (cancer, tuberculosis, congenital diseases and deformities) which are anyhow beyond the financial possibilities of the average famly. Within this limitation of coverage the patient's right to select his physician, and select a physician in private practice must be maintained. The insurance should be for the whole medical cost of the disease and for loss of income due to the disease. Its administration cannot show the same state-by-state inequities as the administration of welfare and medicaid shows.

This proposal should make sense to almost all Americans in the poor and in the middle classes as well, although it may run up against the vested interests of a few. However, it will not solve all the medical care problems of the poverty population, and particularly not the problems arising out of acute or other "usual" illnesses. Therefore, as a second point, the general medical care of the poverty population should be assigned to the state and local public health authorities. In the majority of the states these authorities are now entrusted with the care of the indigent patients, but carry out those duties by their own standards determined by the local governments. In order to make such services nationwide, uniform, and efficient, federal standards and federal subsidy must be established for the state and local public health administration. Federal standards will insure the quality and range of the services (such as mobile clinics in areas without a doctor), while the subsidy will free public health from the political and budgetary pressures of the local governments.

Third, effective measures have to be taken to assure the necessary number of physicians and perhaps even of auxiliary medical personnel. In 1966 the medical schools of the country furnished exactly one half of the physicians who started out on a professional career, while the other half of the physicians taking up practice in the country were furnished by the immigration of foreign-trained doctors who were most willing to take up the less attractive and less remunerative positions in America.[14] The reluctance of the medical schools to face the doctor shortage can be overcome through the systematic financing of medical education by the federal government, but the future system must contrast the present haphazard financial support given in the form of many small, short-term grants and contracts. At the same time, the federal financing must maintain the competition for quality and distinction that presently exists among medical schools.

Such reforms will undoubtedly increase the role of the federal and state governments in medical care but, as a great many Americans feel, the enhanced power of government and bureaucracy is dangerous unless the proper control and balance are applied. One of the usual regulatory agencies of the federal government would not be able to exert the desired control, but one may think of the solution developed in our system of public education: elected health boards could be entrusted with the control on national and state levels and such boards (much the same way as the school boards represent the voters on the local level) would represent the public as a balancing power.

The three propositions, if carried out, will essentially contribute to reducing the health deficit of the poor. But let us remember the biblical warning about the poor always being with us. Indeed, whatever achievement our decade will accomplish in the field of poverty and illness, it will still leave a task unfinished. Poverty and illness are timeless problems. We can do much for their solution and, hopefully, we shall do more than a little; but, at the end of our labors, we still have to bequeath upon future generations the warning that much needs to be done.

Appendix

Appendix · The Reliability and Validity of the Data

by Paul W. Haberman

How accurate and consistent are the existing sources of morbidity and mortality data? * When distortions do appear in existing data, is there any systematic bias by socio-economic class? These are the questions upon which our attention will be focused. Relevant methodological studies will be examined to indicate the nature and extent of distortions in present morbidity and mortality data and differences in such distortions by socio-economic class.

The first section of this appendix will deal with the different sources of morbidity and mortality data. Then, the terms reliability and validity will be discussed with some emphasis placed upon their applicability to morbidity and mortality. Methodological studies will be presented separately under the broad categories of mortality and morbidity. The studies on morbidity will be further subdivided by the type of methodological procedure used in evaluating the validity or reliability of existing data. The concluding section will take up some general considerations as well as the implications of the methodological findings for the relationship between poverty and illness.

* Acknowledgements to Jane Cadwallader for her able assistance in abstracting the relevant literature, and to Dr. Jack Elinson and Cyrille Gell for many constructive suggestions. The work on this chapter was supported by the Health Research Council of the City of New York, Contract U-1053.

SOURCES OF MORTALITY AND MORBIDITY DATA [1]

The Death Certificate. The basic record for mortality data in the United States is the death certificate, on which the funeral director enters the personal details of the deceased supplied by an informant and the certifying physician enters the particulars regarding the cause of death. The funeral director files the death certificate with the local registrar having jurisdiction over the civil government unit, after which the certification goes to the state Vital Statistics Office for data tabulation. A copy is then sent by the state to the National Center for Health Statistics in Washington, D.C., for tabulations on national and state basis.

The personal data recorded on the standard certificate of death include city or other location of death, length of stay therein, usual residence, age, sex, race, marital status, usual occupation, and birthplace. The medical certification includes the immediate cause of death, conditions giving rise to this cause, stating specifically the underlying cause, and other significant conditions contributing to death but not related to the terminal disease condition considered the immediate cause. The underlying cause of death has been defined as "(A) the disease or injury which initiated the train of morbid events leading directly to death, or (B) the circumstances of the accident or violence which produced the fatal injury." [2] Information is also obtained about the interval between onset and death for the immediate and related causes of death and about any autopsy performed. Detailed description of the data recorded on death certificates is available in a U.S. Public Health Service Report.[3]

The reporting of deaths in the United States is virtually complete. The standard certificate, although not binding on registration areas (the fifty states, District of Columbia, and three cities—Baltimore, New Orleans, and New York), has been used as a model in every area. Up to now, the National Center for Health Statistics tabulations have been based on the single diagnostic entity selected as the underlying cause of death. Very little use has been made of past tabulations of multiple causes of death published by the Bureau of the Census, except for the cross-classification of the underlying and contributory cause without reference to personal characteristics.[4]

The International List of Causes of Death has undergone periodic revision so that some adjustments may be necessary for analyses of mortality trends, according to these changes in classifying mortality as well as morbidity data.

Reporting morbidity. No comprehensive system of morbidity reporting comparable to that of mortality reporting has yet been developed. Physicians are required by state laws to report certain communicable or occupational diseases to local or state health officers. Summaries of these reports by the states are published by the U.S. Public Health Service. However, only a limited number of conditions are reported, the conditions required to be reported vary by states, and the reporting may be incomplete.

Under Congressional legislation enacted in 1956, the Public Health Service introduced a continuing Health Interview Survey, with a sample of the civilian population, as part of the National Health Survey program. There have also been state and community health and screening surveys as well as studies of health in special populations. The National Health Survey studies include measures of illness by characteristics such as family income, family size, age, and color, as in the report on *Selected Family Characteristics and Health Measures*.[5]

The principal sources of morbidity data are the various publications of the Public Health Service, e.g., the annual *Vital Statistics of the United States;* the monthly *Public Health Reports;* the *Morbidity and Mortality Weekly Report;* and the *Vital and Health Statistics,* which are irregularly released reports of the National Center for Health Statistics. Other sources are vital statistics reports of the states and cities, and data on state mental hospital patients. In addition, data have been obtained from various nongovernmental sources, the most important of which are records of hospitals, clinics, health insurance plans, life insurance companies (particularly Metropolitan Life), health agencies, and practitioners.

RELIABILITY AND VALIDITY

Defined in simple terms, reliability is the consistency or precision with which something measures that which it actually does measure.

Two aspects of consistency are stability and equivalence.[6] Stability is determined by the extent to which consistent results are obtained using the same measure on the same subjects at different times. Equivalence is determined by the extent to which consistent results are obtained by using different measures or different observers with the same subjects during the same time period. Validity, in similar terms, is the accuracy with which something measures that which it is intended to measure, or the degree with which it approaches perfection in measuring what it purports to measure. Validity can also be expressed in terms of relevance or degree of agreement between one measure and some acceptable or standard yardstick. However, as Elinson has observed, reliability and validity "no longer serve as useful terms in an unqualified sense." There are instead "several operationally definable reliabilities and validities." [7]

Types of reliability. Observer reliability is the measure of correspondence between two or more observers (inter-observer) or correspondence between two or more observations by the same observer at different times (intra-observer). Instrument reliability is the measure of correspondence between two or more instruments or between different versions of the same instrument. Inter-observer and instrument reliability involve estimates of equivalence, whereas intra-observer reliability involves estimates of stability. With regard to stability, it is important to distinguish inconsistency due to a genuine variability in the observed phenomenon, e.g., blood pressure and moods or feelings, from inconsistency due to unreliability.

Observer reliability also has been differentiated on a case-by-case (individual) and a sample frequency (group) basis.[8] The former deals with the correspondence of specific cases and the latter deals with the correspondence of sample proportions (or for comparable samples). A study of 1,348 psychoanalytic clinic records presents an excellent example of individual and group observer reliability among clinical coders evaluating the records.[9]

Types of validity. There are at least four operationally definable types of validity, with two subtypes. The definitions of validity presented here are related to those described by Cronbach and Meehl and the other sources cited.[10]

Content validity involves the demonstration that the measure used is generally accepted as defining that which is to be measured. Construct validity involves the demonstration that the measure used does measure what it claims to measure. When there is no content generally accepted as defining what is to be measured or no standard criteria for the measure used, construct validity becomes important. Consensual validity is assessed by the degree of group agreement, the group consisting of experts, colleagues, and/or staff members at various levels. General acceptance of the accuracy of a diagnostic procedure as a test of the condition in question involves content validity. If there is no fully accepted diagnostic test for the condition, the investigator's demonstration of the accuracy of his procedure involves construct validity, and such demonstration of its accuracy by group agreement involves consensual agreement.

Criterion validity is the association between the measure used and some other "more valid" or criterion measure. Criterion validity can be concurrent or predictive. If concurrent, it involves two measurements of the same phenomenon in the same time period by different measures. If predictive, it involves assessment of the measure used against some future criteria, e.g., functioning, condition, or outcome, which can only be supplied by a prospective study. Criterion validity has been described as pragmatic; it is judged in terms of the association between the measure used and a criterion measure of present or future status.[11]

The only type of validity which is evaluated to any extent in morbidity and mortality studies is concurrent criterion-oriented. However, it has been noted that criterion validity implies either consensual validity, with ad hoc criteria established by group consensus, or construct validity, with the investigator establishing his own criteria.[12]

Validity of morbidity measures. Validity involves the concepts of sensitivity and specificity. A highly specific measure of morbidity will correctly identify a large percent of the population which is not ill, i.e., the true negatives. A highly sensitive measure of morbidity will correctly identify a large percent of the ill cases present in the population, i.e., the true positives. A perfectly valid measure of morbidity will correctly identify the population as either ill or well; there will be no false positives or false negatives. In practice, however, a high degree of specificity and sensitivity can seldom be attained, since an increase in one usually results in a decrease in the other.

Two major groups of morbidity measures have been distinguished: (1) those derived from the findings of physicians or clinicians on the bases of autopsies, exploratory operations, diagnostic tests, clinical examinations, or routine medical observations; and (2) those derived from the reports on diseases and symptoms by survey respondents or by patients during the course of medical care.[13] The morbidity reports of respondents or patients are based either on previous medical diagnoses or lay impressions. In general, only the findings of physicians and clinicians have been considered as more or less valid criterion sources against which other medical sources and respondent or patient-reported morbidity can be verified.

METHODOLOGICAL STUDIES ON MORTALITY

Although mortality statistics have been used extensively and have provided much information for epidemiological studies of disease, their value has been questioned because of inaccuracies in cause-of-death statements. All of the methodological studies dealing with mortality have measured the extent of diagnostic agreement between matched medical sources (criterion-oriented validity). The degree of agreement between matched medical sources varies as expected by the quality (type and amount) of diagnostic information and the number of diagnostic categories used. There is also considerable variance by the stated cause of death on the more valid criterion source, and by personal data, e.g., occupation.

Most studies on the accuracy of mortality statistics have compared either clinical and pathological reports with death certificate information or death certificates with autopsy findings. It is difficult to generalize to over-all mortality statistics from the results of these studies since they have been limited by necessity to deaths in hospitals or deaths with autopsy reports. These deaths are weighted with surgery cases, acute illnesses, and the more difficult diagnoses. Moreover, less than half of all deaths occur in hospitals, and autopsies are performed in only about 15 percent of the hospital cases.[14]

Clinical evaluation of reported cause of death. In an alternative approach, Moriyama *et al.* have worked back from the death certificate and have queried the physician.[15] This study, using a sample of 1,837 deaths occurring in Pennsylvania in 1956, classified the quality of supporting diagnostic information by cause of death (excluding accidents, suicides and homocides) as very good, good, or sketchy. In general an autopsy or clinical finding with some supporting evidence was considered very good, and strongly suggestive clinical and/or laboratory findings were considered good. Using this classification, 39 percent of the death certificates had sketchy supporting diagnostic information. For the two major causes of death, 47 percent of cardiovascular-renal diseases (CVR) and 15 percent of malignant neoplasms had sketchy supporting diagnostic information.

The same study classified the consistency of medical certification with diagnostic evidence as "most probable diagnosis," "another diagnosis equally probable," or "another diagnosis preferred." Of all the certificates, 13 percent were classified as "another diagnosis equally probable" and 5 percent as "another diagnosis preferred." A reviewing internist evaluated the diagnostic information as "in doubt" for 10 percent of these deaths certified by physicians and as "probably wrong" for 8 percent. It was suggested that the certifier was more certain of the accuracy of diagnosis than the reviewer because the certifier may have used unreported information or his impressions might have been misconveyed.

The quality of diagnoses was better among urban medical practitioners than among their rural counterparts. The quality of diagnoses was poorer for deaths in the older ages, a finding attributed to medical problems presented by these patients and to less frequent attempts to reach definite diagnoses.

Another paper from the same study deals exclusively with deaths from CVR diseases, accounting for more than one half of the annual deaths in the United States.[16] The consistency of medical certification and the reviewing internist's evaluation of diagnostic information for CVR diseases were similar to those reported for all diseases. The medical certification of CVR diseases was grossly incomplete or incorrect in 4 percent of the cases. In these CVR cases, 6 percent had an incorrect sequence of events reported, and 8 percent had poor terminology used by the certifying physician.

Matching reported cause of death with autopsy findings. Two large-scale studies matched clinical diagnoses of hospital patients with autopsy findings for 25,066 deaths in New York and New Jersey hospitals in the decade from 1930 to 1939, and for 1,106 deaths in Veteran's Administration Hospital, Washington, D.C., in the period from 1947 to 1953.[17] In the earlier study, 30 percent of the clinical statements on cause of death were not in accordance with autopsy findings. There was a large variation in the accuracy of clinical statements by anatomical site and type of disease. Infectious diseases, primarily tuberculosis of the respiratory system, were more often correctly stated than organic heart diseases, while for malignant tumors, cancer of the stomach was more accurately stated than cancer of the liver or biliary passages. In general, the accuracy of clinical statements was similar with regard to both the anatomical site and the underlying cause of the disease.

In the later study, 6 percent of the clinical diagnoses were incorrect. Slightly more than half (53 percent) of the patients who were misdiagnosed had been hospitalized less than one week, including about one quarter who were hospitalized less than twenty-four hours; and only about one fifth (19 percent) had been in the hospital more than one month. Almost half (47 percent) of the misdiagnosed patients were unable to give any history whatsoever because of acute alcoholism, confusion or toxicity, shock, coma, or aphasia. Incorrect diagnoses were more frequent in atypical cases which did not present the usual systemic manifestations. Correctable diagnostic errors seemed to be due to deficiencies of medical judgment, alertness, and thoroughness rather than a lack of medical knowledge. These correctable errors included failure to obtain routine screening tests, investigate pathology that did not fit the diagnostic impression, pursue indicated procedures, recognize new illness where some other disease had been previously diagnosed, anticipate that laboratory reports, particularly X-rays, occasionally fail to disclose pathologic changes, and review the record and repeat the physical examination in prolonged illnesses.

A study of 1,889 consecutive deaths in twelve upstate New York hospitals in the years 1951 and 1952 matched cause-of-death statements on the death certificate with the "true" findings at autopsy.[18] The percentage disagreement was 29 percent, suggesting serious doubts about the validity of cause of death data as bases for epidemiological studies. The inaccuracies were attributed to the physician not listing available data on the death certificate, insufficient clinical or laboratory data, or difficulty in selecting one underlying cause out of multiple causes of death. Because of compensating errors, the variance in the underlying cause from death certificate to autopsy report was minimized. For example, although pneumonia, except of the newborn, was the stated cause on the same number of death certificates and autopsy reports, there was only 44 percent agreement between the two cause-of-death statements. Similarly, the over-all frequencies of cancer and heart disease as causes of death did not vary appreciably from death certificate to autopsy report due to the offsetting shifts in underlying cause listed on the two medical sources. These examples of compensating errors refer to over-all frequencies of diagnoses, and an equivalent compensating effect for diagnoses by basic personal characteristics, e.g., age, sex, and race, would seem to be most unlikely.

Some important causes of death were decidedly underrepresented among the autopsies, arteriosclerotic heart disease, vascular diseases of the central nervous system, and diabetes. These three diseases had percentage agreement between the death and autopsy certificates of 73, 60 and 31 percent respectively. The fact that a large number of such deaths do not occur in hospitals suggests that there are even greater errors in present mortality data for these conditions.

Comparability among mortality studies. Although all the studies cited found inaccurate causes of death on death certificates or hospital records, their results are not comparable. Some of the differences between these studies in the amount of error was undoubtedly due to improvement in diagnostic techniques over time and variations by locale or hospital. However, the extent of differences due to time period or site cannot be measured because of the influence of periodic classification revisions in the International List of Causes of Death, the different medical sources analyzed, and the varying number of diagnostic categories used. The lack of comparability among studies due to differences in diagnostic grouping is frequently overlooked although it is evident that agreement between medical sources varies inversely with the number of diagnostic categories used. To illustrate this, for hospitals in San Jose, California, during 1951 and 1952, the percentage of agreement between the final diagnosis on hospital records and death certificates increased from 77 percent using 800 diagnostic categories to 91 percent and 95 percent using 100 and 15 categories respectively.[19]

There is very little mention of socio-economic factors in the methodological studies on mortality statistics. Some aspects of the effect of class on mortality have been reported in two studies dealing with cirrhosis mortality and alcoholism prevalence rates. The effect of arbitrary assignment of city boundaries on cirrhosis mortality rates has been evaluated by comparing San Francisco and Los Angeles, which in 1950 had crude cirrhosis mortality rates of 42.2 and 19.6 per 100,000 respectively. In San Francisco, with limited room for internal growth, many middle-class families reside in adjoining suburbs outside the city limits. In contrast, Los Angeles is much more decentralized and has a much greater capacity for internal growth. By expanding San Francisco to Los Angeles dimensions, with the inclusion of adjoining suburbs, or by constricting Los Angeles to a central city area, the two cities were more comparable socio-economically, and the difference between the observed cirrhosis mortality rates in the two cities was greatly reduced.[20]

In the same study it was suggested that "the apparent economic influence upon cirrhosis mortality could be partly a function of protective forces manipulating death certification in higher economic areas." A recent study dealing with the reluctance to certify alcoholism as the cause of death, pointed to "the social stigma involved" which "may be a significant factor in the recorded differential between whites and nonwhites in death rates from alcoholism." [21] Thus, a considerably larger proportion of deaths ascribed to cirrhosis of the liver is likely to be associated with alcoholism than the one third so reported. Moreover, deaths in accidents involving alcohol or resulting from a combination of drugs and alcohol are usually not attributed to alcohol. Such manipulation of causes of death might also affect the death certification of other "socially unacceptable" diseases, e.g., syphilis. Known diagnoses may also be misstated in order to aid surviving relatives in securing certain death benefits. Cirrhosis of the liver was more likely to be certified as the underlying rather than the contributory cause of death in areas which were more populated, where autopsies were more often performed, and for younger decedents.[22] Therefore, the validity of regional comparisons of alcoholism prevalence estimates based only on the certification of cirrhosis when it is the underlying cause of death, and not when it is a contributory cause, has been questioned.

In order to make the tabulation of mortality trends and the assessment of disease complexes more complete, the multiple coding of diagnoses has been proposed, as it has been suggested by the close clinical association between alcoholism and cirrhosis mortality.[23] Such multiple cause tabulations for mortality statistics would permit counting of all reported diseases and conditions as well as an unduplicated count of deaths.

A result of the underlying cause concept is that deaths due to therapeutic misadventure are grossly underreported. At present, a death is classified according to the disease or condition for which the therapy is given, rather than according to the consequences of the therapeutic intervention even if reported. In 1955, in the United States, 617 deaths had some therapeutic misadventure listed as the underlying cause, although 2,644 other deaths specified therapeutic misadventure in transfusions or infusions and in the administration of anesthesia, drugs, and biologicals. In addition, some surgical procedure was reported in about 140,000 deaths. Similarly, postoperative death rates for hospitals are distorted when such rates are obtained by dividing deaths within ten days after the operation by the total number of operations including minor ones, e.g., dental extractions.[24] It is more meaningful to calculate death rates for specific diseases or operations; and since life can be prolonged for long periods due to medical advances, to include all deaths rather than only those within ten days of the operation.

To summarize, the distortion in mortality statistics varies inversely with the quality of the diagnostic information on the medical sources. Some of this distortion is due to medical deficiencies and could be corrected by obtaining more complete clinical or laboratory data or by reporting the available, pertinent data on the death certificate. Some unavoidable misdiagnoses occur because medical history cannot be obtained, the usual systemic manifestations do not occur, multiple causes are present, or because the patient's condition or sudden death did not permit taking adequate medical history. Multiple cause tabulations would remedy the problem of selecting a single underlying cause when death was due to the combined action of two or more diseases or conditions including therapeutic misadventure.

It was observed earlier that the quality of diagnosis was poorer among rural practitioners and for older decedents. Since older patients and those attended by rural practitioners are more apt to have lower incomes, inaccuracies in mortality statistics generally would seem to vary inversely with socio-economic status. The manipulation of death certification as a "protective function" was believed to be a phenomenon in the higher income areas.

Although mortality data are not precise measures, they do seem to be more than adequate in suggesting leads to be elaborated by other approaches. Their reporting in the United States is almost complete; the patient is not important as a source of distortion; no range of possible outcomes or severity exists; and the total population is exposed to the risk, minimizing inaccuracy of the denominator in the computation of rates.

METHODOLOGICAL STUDIES ON MORBIDITY

In contrast to the methodological studies on mortality, all of which involve a diagnostic agreement between two matched criterion sources, there have been several types of studies on the reliability and validity of morbidity data. These morbidity studies fall into four main groups: (1) survey responses compared with the results of clinical evaluations, physical examinations, or multiple screening tests; (2) survey responses compared with records of hospitalization or other medical care; (3) comparisons between survey responses obtained at different times or by using different respondents, interviewers, or instruments; and (4) multiple measurements of medical diagnoses and of clinical or laboratory procedures. The studies dealing with medical verification of survey responses involve criterion-oriented validity, and those dealing with intrafamily responses or multiple diagnoses primarily involve inter-observer or intra-observer reliability. Although morbidity can be classified in terms of chronic or acute and physical or mental illness, the studies on the accuracy or consistency of morbidity data will be discussed in appropriate subsections categorized by methodological typology.

The essential factor in deciding whether to classify morbidity studies under validity or reliability is the presence or absence of a criterion medical source. A study on hospitalization-reporting in three household survey procedures verified by hospital data is useful as an illustration.[25] Admission and discharge data on hospital records are criterion medical sources, so that a comparison of the three procedures matching each with hospital records is a validity study. On the other hand, a comparison of the three procedures without reference to hospital records would be a reliability study—a measure of the correspondence between different instruments.

Generally speaking, reliability is a prerequisite of validity. If an instrument is valid, i.e., measuring what it is supposed to measure, it has a minimum of constant or transitory distortion. Thus, there would be little reason to investigate its reliability, since this is the extent to which it is inconsistent and thereby a source of distortion. However, a measure may be highly reliable and yet have low validity because the high reliability was achieved with a loss of clinical relevance—a failure to ask the important questions.[26]

Validation of survey-reported disease by diagnostic procedures. The underlying assumption in this subsection is that clinical evaluations, physical examinations, or multiple screening tests are generally speaking more valid measures of disease than one-time household interview surveys. It has been observed that clinical examinations, while only the preferred—but not absolute—standard, do yield morbidity data closer to reality than household interviews.[27] However, clinical examinations of a general population sample have had poorer response rates than interview surveys, resulting in a greater problem of nonresponse bias.

By far the most important methodological problem in household morbidity surveys has been the extent of unreported disease, the large number of false negatives. Although some of these false negatives have represented asymptomatic and/or undiagnosed conditions, most unreported conditions could have been reported by family respondents. With regard to the opposite situation—interview-reported disease unsubstantiated by diagnostic procedures—Dorn has contended that a person believing himself to be ill should be so considered even if a physical cause cannot be identified and the person's statement about the cause may be erroneous.[28] This viewpoint emphasizes one facet of morbidity for which survey techniques are particularly well adapted.

A most important source of information about morbidity validation has been the single-visit household surveys such as the Hunterdon County and the Baltimore studies sponsored by the Commission on Chronic Illness.[29]

In the Hunterdon County study, 78 percent of the conditions clinically evaluated in diagnostic examinations as present during the year preceding the interview were not matched to any degree by conditions reported in the family interview, with each responsible adult found at home at the time of the call interviewed separately. Similarly, 53 percent of the conditions reported in the family interviews were not matched by clinically evaluated conditions. A physician determined the degree of match between the interview-reported and clinically evaluated conditions as perfect, close, general, or remote, with perfect and close matches making up the category in which epidemiologic confidence could be placed. About one fifth (19 percent) of the matches were either general or remote. However, all matches were considered in the comparisons between family interviews and clinical evaluations.

The proportion-of-match for interview-reported conditions was directly related to their recency and seriousness. Seventy-four percent of the interview-reported conditions not present "yesterday" did not match to any degree with some clinically evaluated condition, compared with 44 percent of those conditions which were present "yesterday." The median interval between the family interview and the diagnostic examination was 20 months, with a range of 13 to 25 months. However, the proportion-of-match did not decrease by time interval between the family interview and the diagnostic examination except when the interval was as long as 22 months.

Taking the type of reported treatment as an index of seriousness, 23 percent of the conditions involving hospitalization, 54 percent of conditions otherwise medically attended, and 67 percent of unattended conditions did not match with any clinically evaluated condition. All persons covered by interviews had been divided into six strata according to the reported seriousness of the condition. About one third of the conditions reported for persons in the institutionalized and disability strata were not validated, compared with two thirds of the conditions reported in the "well" stratum. Other measures of severity which had the expected relationship to the over-all proportion-of-match were conditions which left a defect or curtailed ordinary activities.

In the proportion-of-match for clinically evaluated conditions by personal characteristics, there was little sex difference and no meaningful age trend. However, the proportion-of-match varied inversely with family income and was less for persons who had graduated from high school. Two possible explanations for this unexpected class relationship were suggested: (1) the diagnostic examinations were more thoroughly conducted for persons in the upper socioeconomic groups, resulting in relatively more conditions definitely established on diagnostic examination; and (2) persons in the upper socio-economic group were better able to recall symptoms existing at the time of the family interview which assumed more importance in the diagnostic examination.[30] Since the proportion-of-match for interview-reported conditions was directly related to their seriousness, a third possibility may be that lower-class persons had relatively more serious conditions clinically evaluated.

Some characteristics which are relevant to the comparison of clinical evaluation and interview are medical disability, chronicity, need for medical supervision, and preventability. The over-all proportion for unmatched, clinically evaluated conditions considered to be disabling was not much smaller than for nondisabling conditions —76 percent compared with 82 percent. For disabling conditions the unmatched proportion was the same for chronic and nonchronic cases and varied directly with preventability and the need for medical supervision. Because of the amount of unreported conditions involving medical disability as well as chronicity, need for medical supervision, or preventability, a severe limitation is placed on the usefulness of the family interview in eliciting information about disease prevalence.

In the Baltimore study mentioned earlier, a case-by-case comparison similar to the one in the Hunterdon County study showed the same over-all proportion of conditions diagnosed in clinical evaluations not matched by conditions reported in the household interviews (78 percent).[31] Three quarters of the conditions were considered to have been reportable, i.e., known to the respondent. Limiting the match to reportable conditions, 70 percent of those which were clinically diagnosed did not match interview-reported conditions. Less than one quarter of all matched conditions and of those matched conditions which could have been reported did not match to a high degree, and this finding is similar to the proportion of general and remote matches in the Hunterdon County study. On the other hand, 30 percent of the interview-reported conditions did not match the evaluation diagnoses, with a median interval between interview and clinical evaluation of four months. For reportable conditions, those considered severe were reported slightly more often than those considered moderate, with mild conditions reported least often. However, there was less direct relationship between seriousness of condition and validity in Baltimore than in Hunterdon County, perhaps due to different methods of rating seriousness.

By personal characteristics, reporting in household interviews of reportable evaluation diagnoses in Baltimore was a little more complete for white persons and for women; part of the sex difference in reporting was due to women being self-respondents much more frequently. The completeness of reporting was not substantially affected by age or income group.

In both the Baltimore and Hunterdon County studies, the variance in morbidity from household interview to clinical evaluation was primarily due to unreported diseases rather than to differences in disease classification. In Baltimore, for example, more than twice (2.3 times) as many conditions were diagnosed in clinical evaluations as were reported in interviews. Moreover, in both studies, the ratio of clinically evaluated to interview-reported conditions varied tremendously among diagnostic groups.

In the Baltimore study, some reasons were suggested for the failure of respondents to report conditions in interviews and for the large differences in the proportions reported among the various diseases. Some of these reasons probably apply equally to all diagnostic groups, while others apply to different diagnostic groups in varying degrees. Without attempting to differentiate by diagnostic groups, these reasons were: deliberate withholding of information, loss of memory, lack of medical attention, information not given to patient, respondent's ignorance of other family members' conditions, different concepts of what constitutes a disease or a symptom of disease, the presence of diseases considered socially stigmatic, e.g., syphilis, mental disorders, and tuberculosis, and reasons attributable to the interview procedure, e.g., number of conditions covered, types of questions or probes, and interviewer variability. In basic agreement with the Hunterdon County study, the Baltimore study staff concluded "that the one-time household interview . . . is when used alone, of little value in measuring the prevalence of all or even of diagnosable chronic disease known by the respondent to exist." [32]

An alternative to the one-contact household health survey is the longitudinal study involving periodic observations over a relatively long span of time. The so-called health calendar or diary can be utilized as an aid to recall or to reduce underreporting morbidity, with an advance mailing or perhaps one repeat visit. Research tools and techniques such as these, which have been used infrequently, will be discussed subsequently.

Two studies conducted in Pittsburgh for two specific classifications of chronic disease, arthritis and heart disease, had similar results to the Hunterdon County and Baltimore studies.[33] In all three areas, the proportion of clinically evaluated arthritis and heart disease previously unreported in family interviews (false negatives) was greater than the proportion of interview-reported arthritis and heart disease not clinically evaluated (false positives). Interview-reported heart disease was unsubstantiated by subsequent clinical evaluation less often than arthritis, only two or three times out of ten in each of the three areas. The conclusion regarding arthritis and heart disease, that "household interview data on the prevalence of clinically diagnosable disease are more likely to be inadequate or incomplete . . . than to be inaccurate or false," confirms previous observations.

In the Pittsburgh arthritis study, the prevalence rate for clinically diagnosed "classical" or "definite" arthritis was 218 per 1,000 including false negatives at the rates per 1,000 of 173 in response to the household survey, and 94 each in responses to individual interviews or physician inquiries. The rates of false positives in response to the household survey, individual interview, and physician inquiry were 30, 85, and 86 per 1,000, respectively. It was observed that "much of the difficulty here stems from the fact that the terms 'arthritis' and 'rheumatism' are not sufficiently clearly defined, even in the minds of the rheumatologists. It should, therefore, not be surprising that survey respondents are imprecise in their use of these terms." [34]

In a comparison between diagnoses of hypertension and heart disease made by the Health Examination Survey during 1960-1962 and those reported on a self-administered medical history and by a personal physician, the survey examination yielded the most definite and borderline or suspect cases, from 61 to 88 percent more cases for each condition than medical history or physician's diagnosis.[35] Diagnoses reported in the self-administered medical history were likely to be corroborated by the survey examination only when the physician's diagnosis, rather than self-diagnosis, was indicated. Self-reported hypertension symptoms were found not to be associated with hypertension diagnosis on examination. Reports of heart disease and hypertension by a personal physician, although less frequent than survey examination diagnoses, were likely to be corroborated by the examination.

To summarize the findings on the verification of survey-reported disease by clinical evaluation, the extent to which respondents did not report the reportable conditions and diseases indicates a low degree of sensitivity for the household interview survey. Thus other procedures are necessary for an accurate measure of morbidity prevalence. There was no conclusive relationship between the accuracy of interview-reported conditions and socio-economic factors. However, in the Hunterdon County study, agreement between survey reports and clinical evaluations unexpectedly was inversely related to family income.

Multiple screening tests and periodic health examinations. Screening tests and health examinations not linked to previous household interviews for the purpose of validating survey responses do provide some relevant information about unreported disease in morbidity studies. Descriptive data on multiple screening surveys and periodic health examinations have indicated on the basis of confirmed diagnosis that many seemingly healthy individuals had diseases or conditions unknown to themselves or to their doctors, even if they had been under medical care.[36] However, abstracts of these screening surveys and health examinations rarely reported socio-economic class differences.

In a study of periodic health examinations of 1,513 business executives, two fifths were found to have previously unrecognized diseases.[37] Almost three fifths (57 percent) of the newly diagnosed diseases were regarded as serious, i.e., resulting in death or major disability if unchecked. Moreover, therapeutic measures were deemed available for more than nine out of ten conditions (93 percent), but with only a small proportion requiring immediate care. Persons in professional occupations are likely to have more frequent health examinations than persons of comparable ages in lower occupational classifications. Thus it may be inferred that health examinations and screening tests would reveal an even larger proportion of previously undiagnosed diseases for persons in lower socio-economic groups and in sparsely populated areas with fewer medical facilities and personnel.

An analysis of the literature on patient delay in the diagnosis and treatment of cancer has some relevant findings.[38] Although the results were not conclusive, the majority of the studies that examined socio-economic characteristics of cancer patients reported delay inversely related to lower income, education, and/or occupation, and directly to age. Moreover, several studies found that delay or resistance in seeking medical advice was likely to be the usual behavior of the patient in case of any symptom, not only cancer.

Willingness to participate in health examination surveys was observed to be directly correlated with middle income, younger age, fewer chronic conditions, and recency of last physician visit.[39] Stated willingness to cooperate was greater for nonwhites and rural residents. In the Pittsburgh arthritis study, which included a clinical examination, some factors directly associated with participation were interview-reported arthritis or manifestations thereof, more utilization of medical services, younger age, and for persons under forty-five years of age, higher family income.[40] Among low-income families, those who refused to take part in a pediatric care program were characterized by relatively better health status and fewer health needs than the participants.[41]

The amount of unknown conditions diagnosed in multiple screening tests and periodic health examinations attests to that part of the unreported disease which could not have been reported in morbidity studies. Although survey reports of verified disease were not found to be conclusively related to socio-economic class, an inverse relationship between undiagnosed and, thus, unreported disease and class was inferred by the less frequent health examinations among lower-class persons. The data on patient delay and cooperation in health examination surveys seem to confirm this suggested survey morbidity-class relationship.

Validation of survey-reported disease by medical records. Hospital data about inpatient or outpatient care and the reports of physicians in prepaid group or private practice have been used as criterion medical sources to verify interview-reported conditions and medical utilization. One obvious limitation of validation by medical records is that unattended or undiagnosed conditions cannot be verified in this manner. On the other hand medically attended conditions are more likely to be symptomatic and, for the most part, diagnosed. Thus, the attended condition or symptom would be reportable by respondents. Although medical records can be used to validate survey reports of medical care and illness, the prime concern in this subsection is verification of events of illness for which medical care has been given, and secondarily, diagnostic accuracy, rather than medical care per se.

From subscribers and their dependents who were enrolled in the Health Insurance Plan of Greater New York (HIP) in 1957, a representative sample of 1,400 families, continuously insured for the preceding twelve months were interviewed in the National Health Survey. The reports on chronic illness made by these respondents in household interviews were compared with the reports from HIP physicians on their patients who sought care during this one-year period.[42] The medical record used was the "Med 10" form, the basic reporting document of HIP physicians on which each entry represents a single patient-physician, face-to-face contact.

Since the Med 10 reports furnish no information on date of onset, it was not possible to define chronicity in terms of the duration of symptoms or diagnoses. Therefore, chronicity was defined solely on the basis of Med 10 terminology, with a maximum number of conditions included as "possibly chronic." The possible chronic conditions were grouped into three classes according to comparability with National Health Survey classifications: Class 1, conditions covered by NHS terminology; Class 2, conditions suggested by checklist terminology; and Class 3, conditions not obviously suggested by checklist terminology. The correspondence between survey-reported conditions and those inferred from the Med 10's was then determined, with a condition reported in the interview allowed to be matched to any number of Med 10 conditions. In addition, hospitalizations inferred from the Med 10's or reported on interview were followed back to hospital records to provide exact dates of admission and discharge.

About two fifths of the possibly chronic conditions on the Med 10's were in Class 1, slightly more than one quarter were in Class 2, and one third were in Class 3. The proportions of Med 10 conditions unreported in interviews for Classes 1, 2, and 3 were 56, 72, and 80 percent, respectively, making the magnitude of medically recorded conditions unreported by respondents the most striking finding. The probability of a condition being reported by a respondent was strongly related to the frequency and recency of physician contacts for that specified condition within the study year. Only one fifth of the chronic conditions with ten or more physician contacts was not reported on interview. About two fifths of the conditions last attended by a physician within two weeks preceding the interview compared with three quarters of those with no service in four months preceding the interview were unreported. There was great variation in the percent of survey-reported conditions by specific diagnostic categories, with only eight such categories for which more than half of the Med 10 conditions were reported on interview. However, there was very little difference between unmatched respondent reports of nonchronic and chronic conditions for the two weeks preceding the interview.

Self-reporting of chronic conditions was slightly more complete than proxy reporting, with poorer reporting of conditions in children largely responsible for this small differential. By personal characteristics, there was no consistent pattern except for more complete reporting of conditions in older adults and in the lowest income class (under $4,000). The better reporting in the lowest income class in part reflected the larger proportion of self-respondents and older adults among the families with incomes under $4,000.

Survey-reported conditions unmatched to those inferred from the Med 10's differed in several important respects from the matched conditions. Larger proportions of the overreported conditions were stated either to have been never medically attended, last attended before the study year, or last attended by a non-HIP physician, and not to be disabling.

In contrast with the level of correspondence in reporting medically attended conditions, only 13 percent of the HIP patient hospitalizations which had been inferred from the Med 10's and confirmed by the hospital were not reported on household interview. Similarly, there was a difference in average duration of stay of only 2 percent between the record source and survey report, and disagreement on duration of stay of more than one hospital day in about 15 percent of the episodes reported. Interview-reported hospitalizations were not confirmed by the record sources in 4 percent of the cases, including one percent which were overreports telescoped into the study year from the preceding year. Hospitalizations in families in the lowest income class, were reported least completely, and the time interval between hospitalization and household interview was inversely related to completeness of reporting.

In the 1951–1952 San Jose study, survey reports of hospital conditions and other medically attended illness were checked against the records of hospitals and against other medical records. Only 11 percent of the survey-reported hospital admissions did not match hospital records, and these almost balanced the 14 percent which were underreported.[43] Almost half of the underreports were for persons with multiple admissions, who reported at least one other hospitalization.[44] The average length of hospital stays and the percent of admissions with surgery were calculated accurately from the interview data. For most of the sources of other medically attended illness, checks were limited to the degree of underreporting in the survey. The degree of agreement for other medically attended illness depended on the type of medical records used as the criterion and the number of diagnostic categories used. Underreporting was largest for records containing the widest range of diagnoses, e.g., disability insurance claims, ranging from about 60 percent with 800 diagnostic categories to 30 percent with 15 diagnostic categories.[45]

In the Hunterdon County study, the physicians named by the respondents were asked to furnish diagnoses for the specified visit of the patient.[46] A random half of the physicians were informed of the conditions reported by the family, and the other half were not informed. Identical proportions (85 percent) responded to the request for verifying information. Over-all, 17 percent of the conditions reported in the families as medically attended were not verified by the physician's reports. Only 8 percent of the physicians informed of the conditions did not verify the interview diagnoses in some degree compared with one quarter of the physicians not so informed. Of all physician-reported conditions, 30 percent were not mentioned in the family interview, 20 percent for the informed physicians and 40 percent for the uninformed physicians.

Validation of survey-reported hospitalization. Several studies have dealt with the verification of survey-reported hospitalization through hospital data. For eighteen Detroit hospitals, in the comparison of three survey procedures, the proportions of known episodes not reported were 17, 16, and 9 percent, with apparent overreports of 2 or 3 percent.[47] Underreporting was lowest for the most inclusive procedure, which involved an experimental interview similar to the 1961 Health Interview Survey, but included additional probe questions and explanatory statements, in addition to a follow-up, self-administered questionnaire. Thus, more complete reporting of actual hospitalization was related to more comprehensive questioning.

In a study designed to evaluate the amount of underreporting of hospital episodes, the total underreport was 10 percent (12 percent excluding deliveries).[48] In a typical county of the Great Plains area (Kit Carson, Colorado) a comparison of household schedule data with the records of four hospitals in the state indicated underreporting and overreporting of 8 and 6 percent respectively.[49]

Underreporting of known hospitalizations in surveys was found to be directly related to the time interval between hospital discharge and household interview, and inversely related to income. Underreporting of hospitalization tended to be greater among persons who were nonwhite, older, less educated, proxy respondents, and reported to have fewer ailments. In addition, respondents more often failed to report episodes involving shorter stays, nonsurgical treatment, and socially threatening or embarrassing diagnoses.

Length of stay reported in household interviews, although similar to that reported in hospital records, was overstated more often than understated. Excluding overreports, the exact length of stay was reported by respondents for roughly half of the hospital episodes, with about 30 percent of the respondents overstating and 20 percent understating the actual length of stay.

In a validity check of interview information regarding the use of outpatient clinics, slightly more than one quarter of the sample patients (27 percent) either failed to name the clinics used during the preceding 12 months or erroneously reported clinics never used.[50] This 27 percent included 7 percent simultaneously underreporting and overreporting the specific clinics used, 16 percent exclusively underreporting, and 4 percent exclusively overreporting clinic use.

However, in a check on the actual number of visits to outpatient clinics, almost one half of the mothers reporting for their families overreported, and almost one third underreported utilization.[51] The tendency for erroneous reporting was associated with the number of actual visits during a one-year period. Those mothers reporting correctly had the least number of actual visits (4.1); overreporters had a somewhat higher mean number of visits (5.1), whereas underreporters had a much higher number of actual visits (10.4).

The conclusion based on the San Jose study that reports of hospitalization obtained in household sample surveys are sufficiently accurate to be used for many purposes in lieu of hospital data, seems to be applicable for the most part to the other studies dealing with verification of inpatient and outpatient hospital care.[52] Other medical record sources do not provide the same opportunity for a comprehensive check on both over- and under-reporting of illness. However, the findings for medically attended conditions without hospital care, particularly from the HIP survey, indicated a much less adequate reporting of chronic and nonchronic conditions. The magnitude of possibly chronic conditions recorded by HIP physicians but unreported by respondents compared roughly with the findings on clinically evaluated conditions unmatched by interview reports.

The accuracy of survey-reported disease was directly related to socio-economic class in all of the studies involving validation by hospital records. The only case in which underreporting was inversely correlated with income was in the main part of the HIP study on correspondence between survey-reported conditions and those inferred from medical records (Med 10's). However, the HIP population differed from the other samples because HIP subscribers were essentially New York City residents in the labor force, a working population substantially younger and with somewhat higher family incomes than the total population in New York City. Moreover, as previously mentioned, HIP patient hospitalizations were reported least completely for families in the lowest income class.[53]

Reliability of survey-reported disease. The reliability of survey data can be tested in several ways. With regard to morbidity studies, the same respondents can be asked at different times about diseases or conditions present during a given time period. The same morbidity questions can be repeated using a different but comparable sample of respondents, or interviewer variability can be evaluated. Comparable instruments or different versions of the same instrument can be administered to the same or comparable samples.

Tests of the validity and reliability of morbidity data obviously involve the use of two or more procedures. Since the overriding type of distortion in household morbidity surveys is the inadequate reporting of clinically diagnosed conditions, additional survey procedures might be most advantageously employed to reduce the number of false negatives and increase survey validity. Even though reliability is subsumed to a great extent by validity, reliability studies can suggest ways to make morbidity surveys more valid. Since unreported disease is the major methodological problem, the positive response in negative-positive response patterns about the presence of disease is more likely to be valid. Thus, in situations involving the reliability of several morbidity survey techniques, the one which elicits more positive responses about the presence of disease is apt to be more accurate.

Respondents' reports on illess made one to two weeks apart have been found to be quite reliable.[54] For some symptoms, however, there was a relatively low degree of reliability. It was suggested that the reliability of reported symptoms can be increased by asking only for serious or frequent conditions. In general the relative reliability decreases as the interval prior to reinterview increases. In reliability studies involving different household respondents, there has been more illness reported by self-respondents than by proxy respondents. When household informants have been used, reporting of illness tended to be more complete for women.[55] Moreover, in some studies, more positive responses about personal illness have been elicited from household informants when reinterviewed for themselves only.[56]

In the California health survey, reinterviews with self-respondents, adults having proxy respondents at the original interview, and proxy respondents for children were conducted shortly thereafter, 70 percent being reinterviewed within two weeks.[57] On reinterview, there were many more reconciled underreports (conditions which the respondent should have been reported on the original interview) than reconciled overreports which should not have been reported on the original interview. Reconciled underreports and overreports were 35 and 3 percent respectively of the total conditions on original interview. Underreports and, to a slight extent, overreports were both higher for proxy respondents than for self-respondents.

Recall was found to be better in the California health survey when the relationship between the proxy respondent and the household member for whom he was reporting was closer. Thus, adults for whom a nonspouse was the original proxy respondent accounted for a disproportionate share of the differences between original interviews and reinterviews. The proportion of adults having proxy respondents, either spouses or nonspouses, increased with family income for all age-sex classes. Therefore, in the higher income classes, a disproportionate share of the interview-reinterview differences was attributable to more proxy respondents for adults in households with larger family incomes.

Retest for chronic disease. In two situations involving chronic diseases, re-examinations (or reinterviews) were used to increase the number of survey positives. Because of the remittant nature of rheumatoid arthritis, subjects with specific symptoms observed at either of the two examinations were considered to be affected with this disease.[58] A group of 274 male blue-collar workers were screened monthly by a nurse for manifestations of arthritis. Simultaneous observed swelling, pain on motion or tenderness, and reported morning stiffness, without trauma, formed the most common basis for a probable diagnosis of rheumatoid arthritis. The initial determination of an episode, coupled with one subsequent redetermination for men not initially in episode, was highly sensitive, as checked by further examinations. The study made "a major contribution to the epidemiology of rheumatoid disease, and chronic disease in general . . . by making it quite clear that . . . the disease process occurs as a continuum of disturbance, not as a have-it or don't-have-it phenomenon." [59] The same general scheme may be applicable to other chronic diseases in which periodicity and variable progressiveness are so important.

Probable alcoholics and matched comparison group persons, originally identified by a survey in the Washington Heights Health District of New York City in 1960, were reinterviewed three years after the original interviews.[60] Although lifetime prevalence was sought, 25 of 99 reinterviewed cases giving evidence of drinking problems in the first interview failed to confirm the problem on reinterview; and 29 of the 331 comparison persons, who had given no evidence of drinking problems in the first survey, indicated such problems in the second. In almost every case, the drinking problems of previously presumed nonalcoholics reported on reinterview antedated the original interview. As with arthritis, respondents giving clear evidence of drinking problems in either of the two interviews were classified as presumed alcoholics for subsequent analyses. Thus, for chronic diseases which are episodic and/or have a high degree of social stigma, underreporting can be reduced by supplementing the usual point prevalence surveys with additional examinations or interviews.

In order to minimize the underestimate of alcoholism prevalence, persons in the Washington Heights survey were identified by interviewers as probable alcoholics on the basis of evidence other than verbal admission of difficulties due to drinking. This other evidence was either acknowledgement of too much drinking while denying resulting problems or grossly pathological drinking behavior during the interview. One quarter of the 132 probable alcoholics in the first interview were interviewer-identified. The proportion of these interviewer-identified cases who verbally admitted difficulties due to drinking on reinterview was 70 percent, which was similar to the 75 percent for reinterviewed cases verbally acknowledging difficulties in both surveys.

Respondents in the highest and lowest income categories were more likely to deny an existing drinking problem in the family.[61] In families with better living standards, the social stigma attached to alcoholism is likely to be greater, increasing the chances of concealment. In families with low living standards, there is apt to be less social pressure against alcoholism, as indicated by more inappropriate drinking during the interview or by admission of excessive drinking while denying resulting problems. Moreover, the very low living standard for the poorest families may have made it more difficult for them to associate excessive drinking with specific economic and family problems. Morbidity surveys attempting to estimate the prevalence of other socially unacceptable conditions or diseases are likely to have similar problems.

Field studies of psychological disorder. Four sociocultural factors —age, sex, race, and socio-economic status—have been studied sufficiently in field studies of psychological disorder to show a pattern of relationship to rates of judged psychopathology. The studies yielded no trends for age, sex, and race, but fourteen of eighteen studies presenting data on the relationship with social class found the highest rate of psychopathology in the lowest economic stratum.[62] The results obtained in the readministration of a mental health scale to subsamples of the 1960 Washington Heights survey have implications related to this association of low socio-economic status with a high rate of judged psychopathology and to the validity of community mental health surveys.

The mental health scale, developed from the Midtown Manhattan Study, was a twenty-two-item series of questions about psychophysiological symptoms usually associated with mental disturbance.[63] It was repeatedly given to presumed alcoholics and matched comparison persons. The distribution of symptom scores for the two periods was quite similar, but there was considerable symptom score shift among respondents so that only moderate correlation between the two scores was observed.[64] The occurrence of environmental stress factors seemed to be significantly related to patterns of change in symptom scores, indicating relatively high sensitivity of the twenty-two items to such stress. This same relationship between intervening events and Midtown Study score changes was confirmed in reinterviews with a different subsample of Washington Heights respondents.[65] Several hypotheses have been suggested linking social class to this symptomatology-stress relationship which may be summarized as follows: (1) a large portion of symptomatology reported in field studies is induced by contemporary stressors, and a large portion of such stressor-induced symptomatology is transient; (2) the extent to which such symptomatology is defined as maladaptive as well as the incidence of contemporary stressors vary inversely with social class.[66]

The higher rates of psychopathology found in the lower social classes seem to represent, to an appreciable extent, more situational stress and transient reactions to this stress rather than more chronic psychological disorder in the lower-class environment. According to this interpretation of a class-symptomatology-stress relationship, such mental health scales administered in community surveys tend to overstate the morbidity of the poor.

Differential morbidity reporting among interviewers and by types of questions. In two studies, the use of nonmedical or medical interviewers did not have a consistent effect on the frequency of reported symptoms and disorders. About the same amount of symptomatology was reported to nonmedical interviewers and to physicians in the Pittsburgh arthritis study, although there was some inconsistent variance by specific arthritis symptoms.[67] Lay interviewers and nurses trained in interviewing obtained equivalent frequencies of reported symptoms and disorders in a study of different medical-history techniques.[68] However, there was a tendency for nonuniformed nurses to obtain higher frequencies of symptoms and illnesses than nurses in uniform.

In contrast to these findings, female medical students in the Pittsburgh Arsenal Health District studies had much more illness reported than other female or male enumerators.[69] In this case as well as in the Kit Carson County survey, there was a large amount of individual variation in reported illness among interviewers with equivalent training and experience, using the same questionnaire, and with random (systematic in the Kit Carson County survey) household assignments. In fact, the latter survey concluded "that most of the variance with respect to average number of prevalent conditions is contributed by the interviewer." [70]

In addition, there has been considerable variation in yield among the several questions utilized to elicit reports of disease. These questions have been classified in the Hunterdon County study along two dimensions (recall-recognition and direct-indirect) which permit questions to be classified into four types: [71]

1. Direct recall—questions about illness or effects of injury during various time periods

2. Direct recognition—a chronic disease list

3. Indirect recall—questions about any conditions not causing illness

4. Indirect recognition—a symptom list

Together, the symptom list and the chronic disease list accounted for over one third of the reported conditions, even though they were placed at the end of the questionnaire. Some explanations for the failure of the open-ended questions to elicit more reported conditions were suggested, including the possibility that respondents did not ordinarily feel that some very common and/or mild conditions were worth mentioning unless the interviewers specifically asked about them. It was also observed that the usefulness of the four types of questions in eliciting reports of disease differed considerably among broad diagnostic categories. In some confirming data from the Kit Carson County survey, a check list of chronic conditions plus one question about any recurrent ailments or conditions accounted for almost three quarters of all morbidity and chronic conditions reported.

In the previously mentioned study a self-administered questionnaire obtained about the same reported frequency of symptoms and illness as a closed-interview form.[72] An open-interview form elicited considerably lower frequencies for the symptoms specifically asked about in the closed-interview questionnaire. In the open questionnaire, the problems which bothered the respondent most were reported with the greatest frequency; and more information on the background of the problem was obtained.

Mooney has reported that health diaries maintained on a current basis for a month produced higher rates of minor acute illness than interviews with a month recall period. Similarly, a health calendar mailed in advance of a four-week recall period resulted in a substantial increase in illness reported on subsequent interviews, particularly of acute illness. The "repeated observations" in the form of reinterviews or repeat diaries "appear necessary for full reporting of chronic conditions, especially those not currently causing trouble." [73]

In a longitudinal study of low-income families with at least one child who had used the emergency clinic of Children's Hospital in Boston, a health calendar yielded about five times as many episodes both for families and for children as a questionnaire on utilization of health facilities.[74] A health index for children had the lowest yield, but it was constructed to give an over-all view of health rather than the frequency of episodes. Repeat applications of health calendars in both California and Boston elicited fewer positive responses on illness or symptoms, although in Boston seasonal variations in health and related behavior were observed to have affected the results.

The consistency of survey-reported morbidity has been found to be affected by the length of time between interview and reinterview, the relationship between household informants and other household members, the episodic nature or social undesirability of the conditions, interviewer variability, and differences among questions or instruments. However, class differences in the reliability of morbidity data obtained from surveys have been noted very infrequently. Generally speaking, the survey technique with the larger morbidity yield will be more accurate with respect to prevalence estimation of disease because of the magnitude of unreported disease in surveys. For the most part, the survey techniques involving more extensive questioning, e.g., additional interviews, probes, or aids to recall, have elicited more positive responses about illness.

Reliability of medical diagnosis. Since medical diagnoses based on clinical evaluations, physical examinations, and screening tests are the main criterion sources for verification of morbidity survey data, any conclusions based on the results of this method of validation must take into account the reliability of the diagnostic procedures used. Inconsistent medical diagnoses obviously limit the effectiveness with which the accuracy of survey-reported illness can be measured.

The reliability of medical diagnoses has been assessed in community surveys and in specially designed reliability studies. The several types of reliability (inter-observer, intra-observer, and instrument) have all been used to measure the consistency of diagnostic procedures and judgments.

In the Hunterdon County study, there was about a 50 percent variation in proportions-of-match for clinically evaluated conditions between the two internists who did the clinical evaluations. For one internist 29 percent of the conditions diagnosed had been previously reported in family interviews, while for the other only 19 percent, with little change in this pattern by sex, age, education, or income groups. Since the assignment of persons to the two internists for examination was essentially random, there seems to have been a real difference in their reports of diagnostic workups. This inference was supported by the difference between the internists in the mean number of conditions per person found on diagnostic examination —2.8 for the internist whose interview adequacy was higher, compared with 3.5 for the other one.

In the Baltimore study, two cardiologists who reviewed the medical records were in close agreement on the total number of persons with heart disease and on the results of the clinical evaluations. Each cardiologist decided that the medical record did not support the diagnosis of heart disease in 6 percent of the cases and that the record supported this diagnosis in 11 and 17 percent of cases not diagnosed as having heart disease. The results suggest that the cardiologists were more sensitive than the internists to the less obvious signs of disease, and thus classified a somewhat larger number of cases as heart disease.

The three different screening procedures for heart disease used in the Baltimore study resulted in a rate of 33 cases subsequently confirmed by personal physicians per 1,000 screenees. An electrocardiogram (EKG) was more sensitive than a chest X-ray or questionnaire, using the two items about symptoms of heart disease. The EKG was positive in 21 of the 33 cases per 1,000—the only positive test in eight of these cases—while the chest X-ray and questionnaire had positive findings of 16 and 9 per 1,000 respectively. It was observed that a questionnaire does not seem to increase the yield of cases significantly if an EKG and chest X-ray are being used. In the absence of both these tests, however, the questionnaire was considered sufficiently specific to be of value in detecting a small proportion of cases.

The proportion of doubtful and abnormal results was much greater among nonwhites than among whites for both EKG and chest X-ray tests. Since the average age of the nonwhite group was lower and positive results were directly related to age to a marked extent, the nonwhite-white differences in yields are even more significant. The proportion of persons giving positive answers to both symptom screening questions for heart disease tended to increase by age and was higher for women than for men in all age groups. Among women, nonwhites gave positive answers to both questions more often, although there was no such difference among men.

In the Midtown Manhattan Study the two psychiatrists who evaluated the mental health of the respondents on a six-point scale disagreed on more than half (53 percent) of the cases. Setting aside one-step differences between the ratings, disagreement decreased to 13 percent. A mental health rating derived from the symptomatic data alone had a Pearson correlation of .75 between the two psychiatrists. The addition of social functioning data to formulate a second mental health rating slightly decreased the correlation between the two raters to .68. As might have been expected, the psychiatrists had the greatest agreement at the extremes of the mental health continuum—serious disability or freedom from significant symptoms—and the least agreement upon mild or moderate symptom formation. The observed agreement for each mental health category, however, did occur more often than would have been predicted by chance.

The uniform single-visit examination used for population studies has been compared with the usual clinical examination since survey objectives and procedures are different from those involving the evaluation and management of individual patients. In one such investigation, the results of a single-visit cardiovascular examination were comparable to those obtained by a complete medical workup in good clinical practice.[75] There was diagnostic disagreement on the absence, suspicion, or presence of heart disease in 22 percent of the 296 cases, including 4 percent positive-negative disagreement. For an additional 8 percent, the disagreement was in regard to specific diagnosis. Replication of 80 single-visit examinations demonstrated that the procedure was reliable, with diagnostic agreement irrespective of specific type in 83 percent of the cases. However, there was a higher level of positive findings on the medical history and physical examination and a lower level of electrocardiographic abnormalities on the single-visit examination.

The extent of variability of blood pressure confirmed the necessity of incorporating some measure of such variability in the long-term study of hypertension.[76] However, no single reading or group of readings obtained on a single day was found to serve as an index of blood pressure variability over a three-week period. Thus, the reliability of variable phenomena, e.g., blood pressure readings, cannot be measured because of its variability.

Diagnostic errors in pediatrics have been sometimes made by imposing a replicated pattern of diseases of adults on childhood although illness in children tends to be much more acute and sometimes presents an entirely different clinical picture, e.g., in tuberculosis.[77] Misconceptions, masked clinical pictures, misinterpreted symptoms or signs, and overpopular diagnoses are all factors in pediatric misdiagnoses.

A study of 1,002 consecutive patients undergoing operations for primary appendicitis in five Baltimore hospitals indicated some class differences regarding necessary surgery, with implications for the poverty-illness relationship.[78] Categorizing appendectomies as necessary in cases with acute or ruptured appendices, unnecessary in cases with normal appendices, and doubtful in cases with chronic appendices, ward patients were found to have a much higher number of necessary appendectomies than private or semiprivate patients. Similarly, nonwhite, older, and male patients were found to have a significantly higher number of necessary appendectomies.

In a summary of findings on clinical and laboratory tests dealing with observer error, Garland reported a considerable amount of disagreement among professionals on a wide range of tests including diagnosis of emphysema by expert internists, nutritional status of children by pediatricians, interpretation of electrocardiograms by expert cardiologists, disease of the tonsil by groups of observers, laboratory procedures by hospital laboratories, and taking of medical histories by observers.[79] With regard to interpretations of chest roentgenograms, experienced radiologists in several studies missed about 30 percent of the films with positive evidence of disease (false negatives) and overread about 2 percent of those negative for disease (false positives). In one study evaluating pairs of serial films obtained three months apart for alteration in disease status, an experienced physician was apt to disagree with another in about one third of the cases and to contradict himself (on review) in about one fifth of them.[80] Garland concluded that "comparable degrees of error occur in many forms of clinical practice. Indeed, if all branches of medicine could be tested, the phenomenon would be found to be quite universal." [81] The recommendations that accuracy in diagnosis can be improved by independent, dual readings of films, interobserver or intra-observer, seems applicable to many other diagnostic procedures.[82]

In respect to the reliability of psychiatric diagnosis, a review of studies mainly using inter-observer techniques suggested that there was clearly a need for greater reliability in diagnosis, although the situation was not as uniformly bad as is often reported.[83] However, useful comparisons between studies cannot be made unless variables relating to the psychiatrist, psychiatric examination, nomenclature or reporting, patients, and manner of analysis are controlled. It also has been observed that inconsistency of diagnostic opinion varied according to diagnostic group, being smallest on organic disorders and largest on neuroses, and was smaller for more severely disturbed patients.[84]

Although clinical evaluations, physical examinations, and screening tests have been used as criterion medical sources to validate survey-reported illness, these medical diagnoses have been found to have varying degrees of inconsistency in a number of studies on diverse subjects, e.g., heart disease, psychiatric judgments, pediatrics, and X-ray films. Thus, the usefulness of validation by diagnostic procedures is not as great as might generally be supposed. Unfortunately, there has been virtually no analysis by socio-economic class in reliability studies on medical diagnoses, but it seems likely that consistent class differences in the reliability of most diagnostic procedures, except perhaps for psychiatric diagnoses, would occur rarely.

As previously suggested to reduce the extent of underreporting in morbidity surveys, dual observations obtained independently can be used to improve the accuracy of medical diagnoses and their effectiveness as criteria for validation. In addition, a range of normal clinical values, such as those compiled by Sunderman and Boerner, must be accepted as standards against which pathology in the various fields of clinical medicine can be measured.[85]

GENERAL CONSIDERATIONS

The three essential elements of a rate are the population exposed to the risk of some event, the denominator; the occurrence of the event in the risk population, the numerator; and the unit of time in which the rate is expressed. If the denominator excludes institutionalized persons or is limited to those who either had sought medical care, were covered by a specific type of health insurance or were members of a select group, e.g., labor union, the rates obviously cannot be generalized to the total population in the community. Moreover, some excluded groups, because of the reasons for exclusion, seem likely to differ substantially from the sample population with regard to the morbid events being studied.

In all studies involving the participation of the general public, the problem of the bias introduced by those who do not respond is present. If there is a high refusal rate, those interviewed may no longer be a representative sample of the population. In addition, the refusals and respondents may have real differences in rates of morbidity. It has been previously observed that poorer response rates have been obtained in clinical examinations than in interview surveys and that patient delay and nonparticipation in health examinations were directly related to lower socio-economic class, older age, and relatively good health status.

In an analysis of hardest-to-obtain interviews, initial refusals or noncontacts, the late cases did not differ from the early cases with regard to reported chronic conditions, impairments, limitations in ordinary activities due to illness, and medical care.[86] In addition, the early and late cases were similar with regard to family income, public assistance, and occupation of employed persons. Other class characteristics that had different distributions among early and late cases, e.g., lower level of educational attainment among the late cases, seemed to be related to the larger proportion of smaller families or older persons among the late cases. In some confirming data, the only bias related to cooperation in a sample survey was that the proportion of success was greater for children than adults so that noncooperators tended to have smaller families and to be older.[87] Thus, differences between respondents and refusals or noncontacts would tend to reflect differences between these groups according to survey status in age and family size.

The usual numerator unit is the case of illness or disease, although in some studies this unit of tabulation is the person or very rarely, but occasionally in recent years, the family.[88] Where the numerator is the morbid condition or even a single episode, a person can be counted more than once in computing a single rate or the rates for a number of different conditions. Focus on the patient as a whole person rather than as a series of discrete diseases has applicability to morbidity statistics. Moreover, in studying the consequences of ill health, the health status of the entire family may well be the most suitable tabulating unit since the health status and expenditures for medical care of any family member might affect the family income. Despite the gradual attrition of panel membership and the difficulties of follow-up with repeat interviews, longitudinal studies seem to be required in order to investigate many long-term aspects of illness, particularly chronic disease, and the interrelations between illness and other factors, e.g., family income.

Since morbidity surveys have varied so widely in their scope, pattern, locale, and timing, and since the National Health Survey is relatively new, there are no firm grounds for inferences regarding trends for the most important causes of illness.[89] Some inferences regarding morbidity trends may be drawn from mortality data, however, despite the periodic revisions in the International List of Causes of Death. Along with the sharp reduction in mortality from conditions for which immunizations or improved methods of treatment have been developed, there seems to have been a corresponding drop in the cases of illness from these conditions.

For mental illness, in particular, there is considerable difficulty in computing rates and discerning trends. Most studies usually cited in this connection cover too short a time span and many fail to provide age specific rates or even rates adequately adjusted for age changes in the population.[90] Fashions in diagnosis have been governed by the interpretations and preferences of individual clinicians and hospitals so that illustrative data presenting diagnoses taken twenty-five years apart from 1900 to 1950 are not conclusive regarding the type of patients admitted to three hospitals selected, the incidence of mental illness in the population served, or diagnostic inconsistencies among staff psychiatrists.[91] The bulk of untreated mental illness can only be estimated, and the rate of treated illness is strongly affected by the availability of treatment facilities and by community attitudes about mental illness and its treatment. The range of rates for eleven community surveys of mental illness from 1916 to 1958 was so great as to defy generalization because of differences in study design, definitions, and classification systems.

It has been stated that "hospitalization data overestimate the extent of totally disabling mental disorders," since many hospital patients are unable to care for themselves, but would not require inpatient treatment if there were persons or agencies available to assist them. On the other hand, "hospitalization data underestimate the actual extent of mental illness," since many equally disabled persons are not hospitalized and many others suffer from illnesses which either are treated outside a hospital or remain untreated.[92] It has been estimated that for every mental hospital patient, there are probably at least two other persons unable to care for themselves who are receiving assistance outside a hospital.

An increasing tendency for physicians to give psychiatric labels before excluding physical diseases has been observed.[93] In this respect, psychiatric diagnoses made by internists in the Baltimore study were not allowed to stand unless the medical records supported the diagnoses on review by a psychiatrist.[94] As a result, one third of the patients for whom the examining physician recorded a psychiatric diagnosis had this diagnosis deleted by the reviewing psychiatrist, although in some cases, all the information available to the internists may not have been recorded. In addition, the much lower prevalence of mental illness among Negro respondents in Baltimore seemingly reflected, at least for psychosis, mental illness of old age in a noninstitutionalized population. This is supported by lower life expectancies and higher first admission rates to mental hospitals for Negroes.

Hollingshead and Redlich found a direct relationship between class status and the extent of treated neuroses in the population, and an indirect relationship for class and psychotic disorders.[95] Class status was, however, also found to be a significant factor in the diagnoses of essentially similar symptoms. Responding to the same varieties of behavior, physicians tend to diagnose upper-class persons as neurotics, while lower-class persons are more often treated as psychotics. In a somewhat related situation, private practitioners dealing with middle-class patients may often avoid noting socially stigmatizing conditions which would be recorded for the poor being treated at public clinics. Such socially undesirable diagnoses in the case of business executives go beyond alcoholism and tuberculosis, and include less obvious conditions, e.g., heart disease or obesity.

Other factors related to interpreting class differences in the reliability and validity of morbidity data are sociocultural differences in utilization of medical care, class differentials in labeling disease, subjective perception of health versus actual medical status, limitations of and variation in evaluation of patient care, and the cause-effect or reciprocal relationship between socio-economic status and chronic disease. Moreover, distortions in reports of family income, personal earnings, education or occupation, which are used as indicators of socio-economic status, and the lack of comparability between the various class measures in different surveys present formidable obstacles.

IMPLICATIONS

While mortality data seem to be more than adequate, most sources of morbidity data except for reported hospitalizations do not seem to be satisfactory, primarily because of underreported diseases and undiagnosed illnesses. Furthermore, medical criteria used for verification of reported morbidity have been observed to be somewhat lacking in reliability. Completeness of reporting seems to be directly related to the degree of saliency of the illness in question; and the degree of saliency can be inferred from such factors as self-reports versus proxy reports, recall period, severity of condition, and length of time for which medical care is required.[96] Unfortunately, the evidence on class differences in the reliability and validity of morbidity statistics is inconclusive, partly because many researchers either fail to analyze their data by class factors or fail to report their findings related to class.

Despite the inadequacy of existing morbidity data for purposes of ascertaining class differentials in reliability and validity, the available evidence does suggest the existence of such class differences. On the one hand, actual medical care and accuracy in reporting such care as well as cooperation in household morbidity surveys and health examinations do seem to be directly related to reported socioeconomic status. Therefore, community health surveys and examinations tend to favor more observed attended conditions among the middle class.

On the other hand, the poor tend to go to public clinics where their diagnoses are recorded; and much of the reported morbidity data relies on the records of public facilities. Middle-class patients are more likely to see private doctors who do not always note the complete diagnosis and are prone to omit socially stigmatizing diagnoses. Moreover, few studies in the field of health care other than community surveys include data from private practitioners having middle-class patients. Thus, class differentials in the utilization of public facilities and the labeling of illnesses together with reliance of much of the reported morbidity mainly on public records would seem to increase the observed morbidity of the poor.

Notes

Index

Notes

CHAPTER I—THE NATURE OF POVERTY

1. William Graham Summer, *What Social Classes Owe to Each Other* (New York: Harper & Bros., 1883), pp. 19–20.

2. Suzanne Keller, *The American Lower Class Family* (Albany, N.Y.: State Division of Youth, 1966); and Arthur B. Shostak and William Gomberg, eds., *Blue-Collar World* (Englewood Cliffs, N.J.: Prentice-Hall, 1964).

3. Henry E. Sigerist, *Medicine and Human Welfare* (New Haven: Yale University Press, 1941).

4. W. Lloyd Warner and Paul S. Lunt, *The Social Life of a Modern Community* (New Haven: Yale University Press, 1941).

5. John Hope Franklin, *From Slavery to Freedom* (New York: Alfred A. Knopf, 1948), p. 70.

6. John Kosa, "Hungarian Society in the Time of the Regency, 1920–1944," *Journal of Central European Affairs,* 16 (October 1956), 253–265.

7. Marion D. de B. Kilson, "Towards Freedom: An Analysis of Slave Revolts in the United States," *Phylon,* 25 (Summer 1964), 175–187.

8. Walter B. Miller, "Lower Class Culture as a Generating Milieu of Gang Delinquency," *Journal of Social Issues,* 14 (1958), 5–19; Oscar Lewis, *La Vida* (New York: Random House, 1965), pp. L–LI.

9. R. H. Tawney, *Religion and the Rise of Capitalism* (New York: Harcourt, Brace & Co., 1926).

10. Charles Nordhoff, *The Communistic Societies of the United States* (New York: Hillary House, 1960).

11. Karl Polanyi, *The Great Transformation* (New York: Farrar and Rinehart, 1944).

12. Robert L. Heilbronner, *The Worldly Philosophers* (rev. ed.; New York: Simon and Schuster, 1961).

13. Michael Harrington, *The Other America* (New York: Macmillan Company, 1962).

14. Dwight MacDonald, "Our Invisible Poor," *The New Yorker*, January 19, 1963, p. 84.

15. Concerning the theory of the paradox see Hubert H. Humphrey, *War on Poverty* (New York: McGraw-Hill, 1964); Burton A. Weisbrod, *The Economics of Poverty: An American Paradox* (Englewood Cliffs, N.J.: Prentice-Hall, 1965); Robert E. Will and Harold G. Vatter, eds., *Poverty in Affluence* (New York: Harcourt, Brace & World, 1965).

16. Max Weber, *The Protestant Ethic and the Spirit of Capitalism* (New York: Charles Scribner's Sons, 1948).

17. Robert Staughton Lynd and Helen Merrel Lynd, *Middletown* (New York: Harcourt, Brace, 1929); David Riesman, *The Lonely Crowd* (New Haven: Yale University Press, 1950); William H. Whyte, Jr., *The Organization Man* (New York: Simon and Schuster, 1956); Mark Lefton, "The Blue Collar Worker and the Middle Class Ethic," *Sociology and Social Research,* 51 (January 1967), 158–170.

18. Robert H. Bremner, *From the Depths* (New York: New York University Press, 1965).

19. Jacob A. Riis, *How the Other Half Lives* (New York: Charles Scribner, 1890; W. I. Thomas and Florian Znaniecki, *The Polish Peasant in Europe and America* (5 vols.; Chicago: University of Chicago Press, 1918–1920).

20. John Kosa, *Land of Choice* (Toronto: University of Toronto Press, 1957); and Kosa, "Patterns of Social Mobility Among American Catholics," *Social Compass,* 9 (1962), 361–371.

21. Donald J. Bogue and Calvin L. Beale, *Economic Areas of the United States* (New York: Free Press of Glencoe, 1961).

22. Harry Caudill, *Night Comes to the Cumberland* (Boston: Atlantic-Little, Brown, 1963); Mary Jean Bownian and W. Warren Haynes, *Resources and People in East Kentucky* (Baltimore: Johns Hopkins Press, 1963).

23. Also see Oscar Ornati, *Poverty Amid Affluence* (New York: Twentieth Century Fund, 1966); Herman P. Miller, *Rich Man, Poor Man* (New York: Thomas Y. Crowell, 1964).

24. St. Clair Drake and Horace R. Cayton, *Black Metropolis* (New York: Harper & Row, 1962); Franklin E. Frazier, *The Negro Family in the United States* (Chicago: University of Chicago Press, 1930).

25. Albert K. Cohen and Harold M. Hodges, Jr., "Characteristics

of the Lower-Blue-Collar Class," *Social Problems,* 10 (Spring 1963), 303–334; and W. B. Miller, "Lower Class Culture."

26. Louis Schneider and Sverre Lysgaard, "Deferred Gratification Pattern," *American Sociological Review,* 18 (April 1953), 142–149.

27. W. Lloyd Warner, *American Life, Dream and Reality* (Chicago: University of Chicago Press, 1953), p. 87.

28. August B. Hollingshead, *Elmtown's Youth* (New York: John Wiley & Sons, 1949); and Seymour M. Lipset and Reinhard Bendix, *Social Mobility in Industrial Society* (Berkeley: University of California Press, 1962).

29. Alfred C. Kinsey, Wardell B. Pomeroy, and Clyde E. Martin, *Sexual Behavior in the Human Male* (Philadelphia: W. B. Saunders Company, 1948), chap. 10.

30. Alfred C. Kinsey *et al., Sexual Behavior in the Human Female* (Philadelphia: W. B. Saunders Company, 1953), pp. 239–241; August B. Hollingshead, "Age Relationships and Marriage," *American Sociological Review,* 16 (August 1951), 492–499; and Lee G. Burchinal and Loren E. Chancellor, "Social Status, Religious Affiliation, and Ages at Marriage," *Marriage and Family Living,* 25 (May 1963), 219–221.

31. James West, *Plainville, U.S.A.* (New York: Columbia University Press, 1945); and Lewis, *La Vida.*

32. Herman R. Lantz and J. S. McCrary, *People of Coal Town* (New York: Columbia University Press, 1958); John Kosa *et al.,* "Crisis and Stress in Family Life," *Wisconsin Sociologist,* 4 (Summer 1965), 11–17; Sheldon Glueck and Eleanor Glueck, *Unraveling Juvenile Delinquency* (Cambridge, Mass.: Harvard University Press, 1950); August Hollingshead and Frederick C. Redlich, *Social Class and Mental Illness* (New York: John Wiley & Sons, 1958); and Thomas S. Langner and Stanley T. Michael, *Life Stress and Mental Health* (New York: Free Press of Glencoe, 1963).

33. Erving Goffman, *Stigma: Notes on the Management of Spoiled Identity* (Englewood Cliffs, N.J.: Prentice-Hall, 1963).

34. Lawrence D. Haber, *The Disabled Worker Under OASDI* (Washington, D.C.: U.S. Department of Health, Education, and Welfare, Social Security Administration, Division of Research and Statistics, Research Report No. 6, October 1964); Wayne E. Thompson and Gordon F. Streib, "Health and Economic Deprivation in Retirement," *Journal of Social Issues,* 14 (1958), 18–34.

35. John L. Gillin, *Poverty and Dependency* (3rd ed.; New York: Appleton-Century, 1937), p. 22; Raymond W. Murray, *Introductory Sociology* (2nd ed.; New York: Appleton-Century-Crofts, 1946), pp. 859–860.

36. John Kenneth Galbraith, *The Affluent Society* (Boston: Houghton Mifflin Company, 1958).

37. See Harrington, *The Other America*; Humphrey, *War on Poverty*; and S. M. Miller, "The American Lower Class: A Typological Approach," *Social Research*, 31 (Spring 1964), 1–22.

38. Leon H. Keyserling, *Progress or Poverty* (Washington, D.C.: Conference on Economic Progress, December 1964); Milton Friedman, *Capitalism and Freedom* (Chicago: University of Chicago Press, 1962).

39. Saul D. Alinsky, "The War on Poverty: Political Pornography," *Journal of Social Issues* (January 1965), 41–47; Michael Harrington, *The Accidental Century* (New York: Macmillan, 1965), chap. 4.

40. Tom Levin, "The Child Development Group of Mississippi," *American Journal of Orthopsychiatry*, 37 (January 1967), 139–145; and George A. Brager and Francis P. Purcell, *Community Action Against Poverty* (New Haven: College and University Press, 1967).

41. Arthur B. Shostak, "Urban Politics and Poverty," a paper presented at the meeting of the American Sociological Association, 1966. See further Harry Gottesfeld and Gerterlyn Dozier, "Changes in Feelings of Powerlessness in a Communty Action Program," *Psychological Reports*, 19 (December 1966), 978.

42. See for example Irving Kristol, "Poverty and Pecksniff," *New Leader*, March 30, 1964; S. M. Miller and Martin Rein, "The War on Poverty," in Ben B. Seligman, ed., *Poverty as a Public Issue* (New York: Free Press of Glencoe, 1965), pp. 272–320.

43. Martin K. White, Joel J. Alpert, and John Kosa, "The Hard-to-Reach Families in a Comprehensive Care Program," *Journal of the American Medical Association*, 201 (September 11, 1967), 123–128.

CHAPTER II—THE SOCIAL ASPECTS OF HEALTH AND ILLNESS

1. Galen, *De sanitate tuenda*, 1.5.20, ed. K. Koch *et al.*, *Corpus Medicorum Graecorum* (Leipsig: Teubner, 1923).

2. World Health Organization, *Official Records,* no. 2 (June 1948), p. 100.

3. Robert P. Hudson, "The Concept of Disease," *Annals of Internal Medicine,* 65 (1966), p. 600.

4. Richard H. Shryock, *The Development of Modern Medicine* (Philadelphia: University of Pennsylvania Press, 1936).

5. Edward Zigler and Leslie Phillips, "Psychiatric Diagnosis and Symptomatology," *Journal of Abnormal and Social Psychology,* 63 (July 1961), 69–75.

6. Hudson, "The Concept of Disease," p. 599.

7. George L. Engel, "Is Grief a Disease?" *Psychosomatic Medicine,* 23 (January–February 1961), 18–22.

8. Owsei Temkin, "The Scientific Approach to Disease," in Alistair Crombie, ed., *Scientific Change* (New York: Basic Books, 1963); René J. Dubos, *The Mirage of Health* (New York: Harper & Row, 1959); and George L. Engel, *Psychological Development in Health and Disease* (Philadelphia: W. B. Saunders Company, 1962).

9. Saxon Graham, "Social Factors in Relation to the Chronic Illnesses," in Howard E. Freeman, Sol Levine and Leo G. Reader, eds., *Handbook of Medical Sociology* (Englewood Cliffs, N.J.: Prentice-Hall, 1963).

10. Stanley H. King, "Social Psychological Factors in Illness," in Freeman, Levine and Reader, eds., *Handbook of Medical Sociology.*

11. Hans Selye, *The Stress of Life* (New York: McGraw-Hill, 1956).

12. Harold E. Simmons, *The Psychogenic Theory of Disease* (Sacramento, Calif.: Citadel Press, 1966).

13. Hans J. Eysenck, *Smoking, Health and Personality* (New York: Basic Books, 1965).

14. Stanley H. King, "Psychosocial Factors Associated with Rheumatoid Arthritis," *Journal of Chronic Diseases,* 2 (September 1955), 287–302.

15. Roger J. Meyer and Robert J. Haggerty, "Streptococcal Infections in Families: Factors Altering Individual Susceptibility," *Pediatrics,* 29 (April 1962), 539–549.

16. Richard H. Rake *et al.,* "Social Stress and Illness Onset," *Journal of Psychosomatic Research,* 8 (July 1964), 35–44.

17. Daniel H. Funkenstein, Stanley H. King and Margaretta E. Drolette, *Mastery of Stress* (Cambridge: Harvard University Press, 1957).

18. Kurt W. Back and Morton D. Bogdonoff, "Plasma Lipid Responses to Leadership, Conformity and Deviation," in P. Herbert Leiderman and David Shapiro, eds., *Psychobiological Approaches to Social Behavior* (Stanford: Stanford University Press, 1964).

19. Roy Coleman, Milton Greenblatt, and Harry C. Solomon, "Physiological Evidence of Rapport During Psychotherapeutic Interviews," *Diseases of the Nervous System*, 17 (March 1956), 71–77; Alberto Di Mascio, Richard W. Boyd, and Milton Greenblatt, "Physiological Correlates of Tension and Antagonism During Psychotherapy," *Psychosomatic Medicine*, 19 (March–April 1957), 99–104.

20. Howard B. Kaplan, Neil R. Burch, and Samuel W. Bloom, "Physiological Covariation and Sociometric Relationships in Small Peer Groups," in Leiderman and Shapiro, eds., *Psychobiological Approaches to Social Behavior*.

21. Seymour S. Kety, "Biochemical Theories of Schizophrenia," *Science*, 129 (June 1959), 1528–1532, 1590–1596.

22. Stanley Schachter, *The Psychology of Affiliation* (Stanford: Stanford University Press, 1959).

23. Robert R. Sears, Eleanor E. Maccoby, and Harry Levin, *Patterns of Child Rearing* (Evanston, Ill.: Row, Peterson, 1957).

24. Barbara S. Dohrenwend and Bruce P. Dohrenwend, "Stress Situations, Birth Order, and Psychological Symptoms," *Journal of Abnormal Psychology*, 71 (June 1966), 215–223.

25. U.S. National Health Survey, *Family Income in Relation to Selected Health Characteristics*, Vital and Health Statistics, Public Health Service Publication, no. 1000, series 10-no. 2, Washington, D.C.: Public Health Service, 1963.

26. Warner Wilson, "Correlates of Avowed Happiness," *Psychological Bulletin*, 67 (April 1967), 294–306.

27. "The Special Position of the Sick," originally published in 1929, and reprinted in Henry E. Sigerist, *On the Sociology of Medicine*, ed. Milton I. Roemer (New York: M.D. Publications, 1960), pp. 9–22; see further Henry E. Sigerist, *Medicine and Human Welfare* (New Haven: Yale University Press, 1941).

28. Talcott Parsons and René Fox, "Illness, Therapy, and the Modern Urban American Family," *Journal of Social Issues*, 8 (1952), 31–44; Talcott Parsons, "Definitions of Health and Illness in the Light of American Values and Social Structure," in E.

Gartly Jaco, ed., *Patients, Physicians and Illness* (Glencoe, Ill.: Free Press, 1958), pp. 165–187.

29. John Kosa *et al.*, "The Place of Morbid Episodes in the Social Interaction Pattern," a paper presented at the Sixth Congress of the International Sociological Association, 1966.

30. Stanley H. King, *Perceptions of Illness and Medical Practice* (New York: Russell Sage Foundation, 1962).

31. David Mechanic, "The Concept of Illness Behavior," *Journal of Chronic Diseases*, 15 (February 1962), 189–194; and "Some Implications of Illness Behavior for Medical Sampling," *New England Journal of Medicine*, 269 (August 1963), 244–247.

32. Edward A. Suchman, "Stages of Illness and Medical Care," *Journal of Health and Human Behavior*, 6 (Fall 1965), 114–128.

33. Stanislav V. Kasl and Sidney Cobb, "Health Behavior, Illness Behavior and Sick Role Behavior," *Archives of Environmental Health*, 12 (February 1966), 246–266.

34. Monroe Lerner and Odin W. Anderson, *Health Progress in the United States* (Chicago: University of Chicago Press, 1963); James L. Halliday, *Psychosocial Medicine* (New York: W. W. Norton, 1948); John Fry, *Profiles of Disease* (Edinburgh: Livingstone, 1966).

35. Thomas S. Szasz, *The Myth of Mental Illness* (New York: Harper & Row, 1962).

36. John Kosa, Joel J. Alpert, and Robert J. Haggerty, "On the Reliability of Family Health Information," *Social Science and Medicine*, 1 (July 1967), 165–181; John Kosa *et al.*, "Crisis and Stress in Family Life," *Wisconsin Sociologist*, 4 (Summer 1965), 11–19; Joel J. Alpert, John Kosa, and Robert J. Haggerty, "A Month of Illness and Health Care Among Low-income Families," *Public Health Reports*, 82 (August 1967), 705–713.

37. Paul R. Robbins, "Some Explorations into the Nature of Anxieties Relating to Illness," *Genetic Psychology Monographs*, 66 (August 1962), 91–141; Gene N. Levine, "Anxiety About Illness," *Journal of Health and Human Behavior*, 3 (Spring 1962), 30–34.

38. Kosa *et al.*, "The Place of Morbid Episodes in the Social Interaction Pattern."

39. Rose K. Goldsen *et al.*, "Some Factors Related to Patient Delay in Seeking Diagnosis for Cancer Symptoms," *Cancer*, 10

(January 1957), 1–7; Leta McK. Adler, Marcia Goin, and Joe Yamamoto, "Failed Psychiatric Clinic Appointments," *California Medicine,* 99 (December 1963), 388–392.

40. John Cassel, "A Comprehensive Health Program Among South African Zulus," in Benjamin D. Paul, ed., *Health, Culture and Community* (New York: Russell Sage Foundation, 1955), 15–42.

41. Joel J. Alpert, John Kosa, and Robert J. Haggerty, "Medical Help and Maternal Nursing Care in the Life of Low-income Families," *Pediatrics,* 39 (May 1967), 749–755; Joel J. Alpert, Melvine D. Levine, and John Kosa, "Public Response to a Poison Management Program," *Journal of Pediatrics,* 71 (December 1967), 890–896.

42. Walter I. Wardwell, "Christian Science Healing," *Journal for the Scientific Study of Religion,* 4 (Spring 1965), 175–181.

43. Eliot Freidson, "Client Control and Medical Practice," *American Journal of Sociology,* 65 (January 1960), 374–382; John D. Stoeckle, Irving K. Zola, and Gerald E. Davidson, "On Going to See the Doctor," *Journal of Chronic Diseases,* 16 (September 1963), 975–989.

44. Sigmund Freud and Joseph Breuer, *Studies in Hysteria* (New York: Nervous and Mental Disorders Publishing Co., 1936).

45. Leon S. Robertson *et al.,* "Family Size and the Use of Medical Resources," in William T. Liu, ed., *Family and Fertility* (Notre Dame, Ind.: University of Notre Dame Press, 1967), pp. 131–144.

46. Kosa, Alpert and Haggerty, "On the Reliability of Family Health Information"; Alpert, Kosa and Haggerty, "A Month of Illness and Health Care."

47. Eliot Freidson, "The Organization of Medical Practice," in Freeman, Levine, and Reeder, *Handbook of Medical Sociology,* pp. 299–320; Irwin M. Rosenstock, "Why People Use Health Services," *Milbank Memorial Fund Quarterly,* 44 (July 1966), 94–124.

48. John Kosa, "Entrepreneurship and Charisma in the Medical Profession," a paper presented at the First International Conference on Social Science and Medicine, 1968.

49. John A. Ryle, *The Natural History of Disease* (London: Cumberlege, 1948).

50. Max B. Clyne, *Night Calls: A Study in General Practice* (London: Tavistock, 1961).

51. Abraham B. Bergman and Robert J. Haggerty, "The Emer-

gency Clinic," *American Journal of Diseases of Children,* 104 (July 1962), 36–44; Joel J. Alpert *et al.,* "A Typology of Users in Hospital Emergency Facilities," a paper presented at the meeting of the American Federation for Clinical Research, 1967.

CHAPTER III—SOCIAL DIFFERENCES IN PHYSICAL HEALTH

1. Daniel F. Sullivan, "Conceptual Problems in Developing an Index of Health," in *Vital and Health Statistics: Data Evaluation and Methods Research,* National Center for Health Statistics, ser. 2, no. 17 (Washington, D.C.: U.S. Government Printing Office, May 1966); Theodore D. Woolsey, *Measurements of the Nation's Health,* address at the meeting of the Washington Chapters of the American Statistical Association and the American Marketing Association, 1967; and Monroe Lerner, discussion of the paper by Theodore D. Woolsey.

2. M. Allen Pond, "Interrelationship of Poverty and Disease," *Public Health Reports,* 76 (November 1961), 967–968.

3. Odin W. Anderson and George Rosen, "An Examination of the Concept of Preventive Medicine," Health Information Foundation, *Research Series,* no. 12 (New York: The Foundation, 1960).

4. Robert M. Woodbury, *Causal Factors in Infant Mortality.* Washington: U.S. Government Printing Office, 1925, p. 148. U.S. Children's Bureau Publication No. 142.

5. Monroe Lerner and Odin W. Anderson, *Health Progress in the United States, 1900–1960* (Chicago: University of Chicago Press, 1963).

6. Various articles by William M. Gafafer cited in Selwyn D. Collins, "Long-Time Trends in Illness and Medical Care," *Public Health Monograph,* no. 48 (Washington, D.C.: U.S. Public Health Service, 1957).

7. Chicago Board of Health, Planning Staff of the Health Planning Project, *A Report on Health and Medical Care in Poverty Areas of Chicago and Proposals for Improvement* (Chicago: Board of Health, 1965); and Mark H. Lepper *et al.,* "Approaches to Meeting Health Needs of Large Poverty Populations," *American Journal of Public Health,* 57 (July 1967), 1153–1157.

8. Evelyn M. Kitagawa and Karl E. Taeuber, eds., *Local Com-*

munity Fact Book, 1960 (Chicago: Community Inventory, University of Chicago, 1963), 324–325.

9. Samuel M. Andelman, "Tuberculosis in Large Urban Centers," address at the meeting of the American Public Health Association, 1965.

10. Lerner and Anderson, *Health Progress in the United States,* pp. 122–130.

11. *Ibid.,* pp. 105–113.

12. Edward G. Stockwell, "Infant Mortality and Socio-Economic Status," *Milbank Memorial Fund Quarterly,* 11 (January 1962), 101–102.

13. Charles V. Willie, "A Research Note on the Changing Association Between Infant Mortality and Socio-Economic Status," *Social Forces,* 37 (March 1959), 225–227.

14. Stockwell, "Infant Mortality and Socio-Economic Status," pp. 110–111.

15. Eleanor P. Hunt and Earl E. Huyck, "Mortality of White and Nonwhite Infants in Major U.S. Cities," *Health, Education, and Welfare Indicators* (January 1966), 1–19.

16. U.S. National Center for Health Statistics, "Disability Days, United States, July 1963–June 1964," *Vital Statistics: Data from the National Health Survey,* ser. 10, no. 24 (Washington, D.C.: U.S. Government Printing Office, November 1965), and "Medical Care, Health Status, and Family Income, United States," *ibid.,* ser. 10, no. 9 (May 1964).

17. U.S. National Center for Health Statistics, "Medical Care, Health Status, and Family Income."

18. Z. M. Stadt *et al.,* "Socio-Economic Status and Dental Caries Experience of 3,911 Five-Year-Old Natives of Contra Costa County, California," *Journal of Public Health Dentistry,* 27 (Winter 1967), 2–6.

19. L. F. Szwejda, "Observed Differences of Total Caries Experience Among White Children of Various Socio-Economic Groups," *Journal of Public Health Dentistry,* 20 (Fall 1960), 59–66.

20. L. F. Szwejda, "Dental Caries Experience by Race and Socio-Economic Level After Eleven Years of Water Fluoridation in Charlotte, North Carolina," *Journal of Public Health Dentistry,* 22 (Summer 1962), 91–98.

21. U.S. National Center for Health Statistics," Medical Care, Health Status, and Family Income."

CHAPTER IV—SOCIAL DIFFERENCES IN MENTAL HEALTH

1. The problem of formulating a useful and highly general definition of mental health for empirical analysis is, of course, no different from the problem of defining physical health, although the use of specific and widely accepted indicators in the field of physical health obscures the underlying normative issue.

2. Erik H. Erikson, "Growth and Crises of the Healthy Personality," *Psychological Issues*, 1 (1959), 50–100; Marie Jahoda, *Current Concepts of Positive Mental Health* (New York: Basic Books, 1958); M. Brewster Smith, "Optima of Mental Health," *Psychiatry*, 13 (1950), 503–510.

3. Michel Foucault, *Madness and Civilization* (New York: Pantheon Books, 1965).

4. Sigmund Freud, *Civilization and Its Discontents* (1930), in *Complete Psychological Works of Sigmund Freud* (standard ed., vol. XXI; London: Hogarth Press, 1961).

5. Ornulv Odegaard, "Current Studies of Incidence and Prevalence of Hospitalized Mental Patients in Scandinavia," in Paul H. Hoch and Joseph Zubin, eds., *Comparative Epidemiology of the Mental Disorders* (New York: Grune and Stratton, 1961), pp. 45–56.

6. Bernard J. Bergen and Claudewell S. Thomas, eds., *Issues and Problems in Social Psychiatry* (Springfield, Ill.: Charles C Thomas, 1966); John Cumming and Elaine Cumming, *Ego and Milieu* (New York: Atherton Press, 1962); Alfred Stanton and Morris Schwartz, *The Mental Hospital* (New York: Basic Books, 1954).

7. Howard E. Freeman and Ozzie G. Simmons, "Feeling of Stigma Among Relatives of Former Mental Patients," *Social Problems*, 8 (1961), 312–321; Freeman and Simmons, "Mental Patients in the Community," *American Sociological Review*, 23 (1958), 147–153; and Simmons and Freeman, "Familial Ex-Patients," *Human Relations*, 12 (1959), 233–242.

8. Emile Durkheim, *Suicide,* trans. John A. Spaulding and George Simpson (Glencoe, Ill.: Free Press, 1951).

9. See Robert E. Clark, "Psychoses, Income and Occupational Prestige," *American Journal of Sociology,* 54 (1949), 433–440; Robert E. Clark, "The Relationship of Schizophrenia to Occupational Income and Occupational Prestige," *American Sociological Review,* 13 (1948), 325–330; John A. Clausen and Melvin L. Kohn, "Relation of Schizophrenia to the Social Structure of a Small City," in Benjamin Pasamanick, ed., *Epidemiology of Mental Disorder* (Washington, D.C.: American Association for Advancement of Science, 1959), pp. 69–95; B. B. Cohen, Ruth Fairbank, and Elizabeth Greene, "Personality Disorder in the Eastern Health District in 1933," *Human Biology,* 11 (February 1939), 112–129; Bruce P. Dohrenwend "Social Status and Psychological Disorder," *American Sociological Review,* 31 (1966), 14–34; J. Warren Dunham, *Community and Schizophrenia* (Detroit: Wayne State University Press, 1965); Robert E. Faris and J. Warren Dunham, *Mental Disorders in Urban Areas* (Chicago: University of Chicago Press, 1939); Robert M. Frumkin, "Occupation and Major Mental Disorders," in Arnold M. Rose, *Mental Health and Mental Disorder* (New York: W. W. Norton, 1955); Robert M. Frumkin, "Occupation and Mental Illness," *Ohio Public Welfare Statistics* (September 1952), 4–13; Edith M. Furbush, "Social Facts Relative to Patients With Mental Disease," *Mental Hygiene,* 6 (1922), 587–611; W. M. Fuson, "Occupation of Functional Psychotics," *American Journal of Sociology,* 48 (1943), 612–613; Donald L. Gerard and Lester G. Houston, "Family Setting and the Social Ecology of Schizophrenia," *Psychiatric Quarterly,* 27 (1953), 19–37; E. M. Goldberg, and S. L. Morrison, "Schizophrenia and Social Class," *British Journal of Psychiatry,* 109 (1963), 785–802; August B. Hollingshead and Frederick C. Redlich, *Social Class and Mental Illness* (New York: John Wiley & Sons, 1958); Robert W. Hyde and Lowell V. Kingsley, "Relation of Mental Disorders to Community Socio-Economic Level," *New England Journal of Medicine,* 231 (October 19, 1944), 543–548; E. Gartly Jaco, *The Social Epidemiology of Mental Disorders* (New York: Russell Sage Foundation, 1960); A. J. Jaffe and E. Shanas, "Economic Differentials in the Probability of Insanity," *American Journal of Sociology,* 44 (1935), 534–539; Eva Johnson, "A Study of Schizophrenia in the Male," *Acta Psychiatrica et Neurologica Scandinavia,* 33 (1958),

Supplement 125; Bert Kaplan, Robert B. Reed, and Wyman Richardson, "A Comparison of the Incidence of Hospitalized and Non-Hospitalized Cases of Psychosis in Two Communities," *American Sociological Review*, 21 (1956), 472–479; Thomas S. Langner, "Environmental Stress and Mental Health," in Paul H. Hoch and Joseph Zubin, eds., *Comparative Epidemiology of Mental Disorders* (New York: Grune and Stratton, 1961), pp. 32–45; R. Lapouse, M. S. Monk, and M. Terris, "The Drift Hypothesis and Socio-Economic Differentials in Schizophrenia," *American Journal of Public Health*, 46 (1956), 978–986; Everett S. Lee, "Socio-Economic and Migration Differentials in Mental Disease," *Milbank Memorial Fund Quarterly*, 41 (1963), 249–268; Dorothea Leighton *et al.*, *The Character of Danger* (New York: Basic Books, 1963); P. Lemkau, C. Tietze and M. Cooper, "Mental Hygiene Problems in an Urban District," *Mental Hygiene*, 26 (1941), 100–119; Ben Z. Locke *et al.*, "Problems in Interpretation of Patterns of First Admissions to Ohio State Public Mental Hospitals for Patients with Schizophrenic Reactions," *Psychiatric Research Reports*, no. 10 (1958); Benjamin Malzberg, *Social and Biological Aspects of Mental Disease* (New York: State Hospitals Press, 1940); Norbert L. Mintz and David T. Schwartz, "Urban Ecology and Psychosis," *International Journal of Social Psychiatry*, 10 (1964), 101–118; W. J. Nolan, "Occupation and Dementia Praecox," *New York State Hospital Quarterly*, 3 (1917), 127–154; Ornulv Odegaard, "Emigration and Insanity," *Acta Psychiatrica et Neurologica* (1932), supplement 4; Benjamin Pasamanick, "A Survey of Mental Disease in an Urban Population, VII," *American Journal of Psychiatry*, 119 (1962), 299–305; Benjamin Pasamanick *et al.*, "A Survey of Mental Disease in an Urban Population, 1," in Benjamin Pasamanick, ed., *Epidemiology of Mental Disorder* (Washington, D.C.: American Association for Advancement of Science, 1959), pp. 183–203; A. J. Rosanoff, "Survey of Mental Disorders in Nassau County, New York," *Psychiatric Bulletin*, 2 (1917), 109–231; Leonard G. Rowntree, Kenneth H. McGill, and Louis P. Hellman, "Mental and Personality Disorders in Selective Service Registrants," *Journal of the American Medical Association*, 128 (Aug. 11, 1945), 1084–1087; C. W. Schroeder, "Mental Disorders in Cities," *American Journal of Sociology*, 48 (1942), 40–47; Ama Sreenivasan and J. Hoenig, "Caste and Mental Hospital Admissions in Mysore State, India," *American Journal of Psychiatry*, 117 (1960), 37–43; Lilli

Stein, "Social Class Gradient in Schizophrenia," *British Journal of Preventive Social Psychiatry,* 11 (1957), 181–195; Dorothy Thomas and Ben A. Locke, "Marital Status, Education and Occupational Differentials in Mental Disease," *Milbank Memorial Fund Quarterly,* 41 (1963), 145–160; Christopher Tietze, Paul Lemkau and Marcia Cooper, "Schizophrenia, Manic-Depressive Psychosis and Social-Economic Status," *American Journal of Sociology,* 47 (1941), 167–175.

10. Rosanoff, "Survey of Mental Disorders"; Nolan, "Occupation and Dementia Praecox."

11. Nolan, "Occupation and Dementia Praecox."

12. Jaco, *The Social Epidemiology;* Locke *et al.,* "Problems in Interpretation of First Admissions."

13. Furbush, "Social Facts Relative to Patients"; Kaplan *et al.,* "A Comparison of the Incidence."

14. Clark, "Psychosis, Income and Occupational Prestige"; Faris and Dunham, *Mental Disorders in Urban Areas;* Frumkin, "Occupation and Mental Illness"; Fuson, "Occupation of Functional Psychotics"; Hollingshead and Redlich, *Social Class and Mental Illness;* Jaco, *The Social Epidemiology;* Odegaard, "Emigration and Insanity"; and Tietze *et al.,* "Schizophrenia, Manic-Depressive Psychosis."

15. Dunham, *Community and Schizophrenia;* Jaco, *Social Epidemiology;* Hollingshead and Redlich, *Social Class and Mental Illness;* Dohrenwend, "Social Status and Psychological Disorder"; Kaplan *et al.,* "A Comparison of Incidence"; Hyde and Kingsley, "Relation of Mental Disorders"; Rowntree *et al.,* "Mental and Personality Disorders."

16. Hollingshead and Redlich, *Social Class and Mental Illness;* O. Eugene Baum, Stanton G. Felzer, and Elaine Shumaker, "Psychotherapy, Dropouts and Lower Socio-Economic Patients," *American Journal of Orthopsychiatry,* 36 (1966), 629–635; Nyla J. Cole, E. H. Hardin Branch, and Roger B. Allison, "Some Relationships Between Social Class and the Practice of Dynamic Psychotherapy," *American Journal of Psychiatry,* 118 (1961), 1004–1012; John A. Clausen, "Ecology of Mental Disorders," in *Symposium on Preventive Social Psychiatry* (Washington, D.C.: Walter Reed Army Institute of Research 1957), 97–109; David Fanshel, "A Study of Caseworkers," *Social Casework,* 39 (1958), 543–551; R. Moore, E. Benedek, and J. Wallace, "Social Class, Schizophrenia and the

Psychiatrist," *American Journal of Psychiatry,* 120 (1963), 149–154; J. Myers, L. Bean and Max P. Pepper, "Social Class and Psychiatric Disorders," *Journal of Health and Human Behavior,* 6 (Summer 1965), 74–79.

17. Dunham, *Community and Schizophrenia;* Dohrenwend, "Social Status and Psychological Disorder"; and Kaplan *et al.,* "A Comparison of Incidence."

18. Durkheim, *Suicide,* p. 243.

19. Louis I. Dublin and Bessie Bunzel, *To Be or Not To Be* (New York: Smith and Haas, 1933).

20. Louis I. Dublin, *Suicide* (New York: Ronald Press, 1963), p. 61.

21. Jack P. Gibbs and Walter Martin, *Status Integration and Suicide* (Eugene: University of Oregon Press, 1964).

22. Peter Sainsbury, *Suicide in London* (London: Chapman and Hall, 1955).

23. Warren Breed, "Occupational Mobility and Suicide Among White Males," *American Sociological Review,* 28 (1963), 179–188; Andrew F. Henry and James F. Short, Jr., *Suicide and Homicide* (New York: Free Press, 1954); Sainsbury, *Suicide in London.*

24. Dublin, *Suicide;* Breed, "Occupational Mobility"; Warren Breed, "Suicide, Migration and Role," *Journal of Social Issues,* 22 (1966), 30–43; Henry and Short, *Suicide and Homicide;* Sainsbury, *Suicide in London;* Elwin H. Powell, "Occupation, Status and Suicide," *American Sociological Review,* 23 (1958), 131–139.

25. Stuart Perry, "The Middle-Class and Mental Retardation in America," *Psychiatry,* 28 (1965), 107–118.

26. J. Wortis, "Prevention of Mental Retardation," *American Journal of Orthopsychiatry,* 35 (1965), 886–895.

27. Hollingshead and Redlich, *Social Class and Mental Illness;* R. Moses and J. Shanan, "Psychiatric Out-patient Clinic," *Archives of General Psychiatry,* 4 (1961), 60–73; Leo Srole *et al., Mental Health in the Metropolis* (New York: McGraw-Hill, 1962); Cohen *et al.,* "Personality Disorder"; Hyde and Kingsley, "Relation of Mental Disorders"; Kaplan *et al.,* "A Comparison of Incidence"; Leighton *et al., The Character of Danger;* Lemkau *et al.,* "Mental Hygiene"; and Rowntree *et al.,* "Mental and Personality Disorders."

28. Cohen *et al.,* "Personality Disorder"; Dohrenwend, "Social Status and Psychological Disorder"; Dunham, *Community and Schizophrenia;* Elmer A. Gardner and Haroutun M. Babigian, "A

Longitudinal Comparison of Psychiatric Services," *American Journal of Orthopsychiatry,* 36 (1966), 818–828; R. W. Hyde and R. M. Chisholm, "The Relation of Mental Disorders to Race and Nationality," *New England Journal of Medicine,* 231 (1944), 612–618; Jaco, *Social Epidemiology of Mental Disorder;* Robert J. Kleiner, Jacob Tuckman and Martha Lavell, "Mental Disorder and Status Based on Race," *Psychiatry,* 23 (1960), 271–274; Judith Lazarus, Ben Z. Locke and Dorothy Thomas, "Migration Differentials in Mental Disease," *Milbank Memorial Fund Quarterly,* 41 (1963), 25–42; Lee, "Socio-Economic and Migration Differentials"; Leighton *et al., The Character of Danger;* Lemkau *et al.,* "Mental Hygiene Problems"; Locke *et al.,* "Problems in Interpretation"; Malzberg, *Social and Biological Aspects;* Pasamanick, "Survey of Mental Disease"; E. S. Pollack *et al.,* "Socio-Economic and Family Characteristics of Patients Admitted to Psychiatric Services," *American Journal of Public Health,* 54 (1964), 506–518; Thomas F. Pugh and Brien MacMahon, *Epidemiologic Findings in United States Mental Hospital Data* (Boston: Little, Brown, 1962); W. F. Roth and F. B. Luton, "The Mental Hygiene Program in Tennessee," *American Journal of Psychiatry,* 99 (1943), 662–675; Rowntree *et al.,* "Mental and Personality Disorders"; Rosanoff, "Survey of Mental Disorders"; Thomas and Locke, "Marital Status, Education"; D. G. Wilson and E. M. Lantz, "The Effect of Culture Change on the Negro Race in Virginia," *American Journal of Psychiatry,* 114 (1957), 25–32.

29. Dohrenwend, "Social Status and Psychological Disorder."

30. Malzberg, *Social and Psychological Aspects;* Pugh and MacMahon, *Epidemiologic Findings.*

31. Malzberg, *Social and Psychological Aspects,* p. 226.

32. Wilson and Lantz, "The Effect of Culture Change."

33. Pollack *et al.,* "Socio-Economic and Family Characteristics."

34. Lee, "Socio-Economic and Migration Differentials"; Lazarus *et al.,* "Migration Differentials"; Thomas and Locke, "Marital Status and Education."

35. Faris and Dunham, *Mental Disorders in Urban Areas;* Donald L. Gerard and Joseph Siegel, "The Family Background of Schizophrenia," *Psychiatric Quarterly,* 24 (1950), 47–73; Gerard and Houston, "Family Setting and Social Ecology"; E. H. Hare, "Family Setting and the Urban Distribution of Schizophrenia," *Journal of Mental Science,* 102 (1956), 753–759; E. H. Hare, "Mental Ill-

ness and Social Conditions in Bristol," *Journal of Mental Science,* 102 (1956), 349–357.

36. Dohrenwend, "Social Status and Psychological Disorder"; Mintz and Schwartz, "Urban Ecology and Psychosis"; Joan L. Burke, Hugh Lafave and Grace Kurtz, "Minority Group Membership as a Factor in Chronicity," *Psychiatry,* 28 (1965), 235–238; Henry Wechsler and Thomas F. Pugh, "Fit of Individual and Community Characteristics and Rates of Psychiatric Hospitalization," *American Journal of Sociology,* 73 (1967), 331–338.

37. Clausen and Kohn, "Relation of Schizophrenia"; Lapouse *et al.,* "The Drift Hypothesis"; Lee, "Socio-Economic and Migration Differentials"; Odegaard, "Emigration and Insanity"; Lazarus *et al.,* "Migration Differentials"; Locke *et al.,* "Immigration and Insanity"; Benjamin Malzberg and Everett Lee, *Migration and Mental Disease* (New York: Social Science Research Council, 1956); F. M. Martin, J. H. F. Brotherston and S. P. W. Chave, "Incidence of Neurosis in a New Housing Estate," *British Journal of Preventive and Social Medicine,* 11 (1957), 196–202; H. B. M. Murphy, "Social Change and Mental Health," in *Causes of Mental Disorders,* (New York: Milbank Memorial Fund, 1961), pp. 280–329; H. B. M. Murphy, "Migration and the Major Mental Disorders," in Mildred Kantor, ed., *Mobility and Mental Health* (Springfield, Ill.: Charles C Thomas, 1965), pp. 5–24; Marc Fried, "Effects of Social Change on Mental Health," *American Journal of Orthopsychiatry,* 34 (1964), 3–28.

38. Jaco, *Social Epidemiology of Mental Disorders.*

39. Lazarus *et al.* "Migration Differentials"; Lee, "Socio-Economic and Migration Differentials"; Thomas and Locke, "Marital Status, Education."

40. Henry S. Shryock, Jr., *Population Mobility Within the United States* (Chicago: Community and Family Study Center, 1964).

41. Basil G. Zimmer, "Participation of Migrants in Urban Structures," *American Sociological Review,* 20 (1955), 218–224.

42. Faris and Dunham, *Mental Disorders.*

43. Gerard and Siegel, "Family Background of Schizophrenia."

44. Mintz and Schwartz, "Urban Ecology and Psychosis."

45. Wechsler and Pugh, "Fit of Individual."

46. Murphy, "Migration and the Major Mental Disorders."

47. Arnold Rose, *Mental Health and Mental Disorder;* Neil A.

Dayton, *New Facts on Mental Disorders* (Springfield, Ill.: Charles C Thomas, 1940); Jaco, *Social Epidemiology;* Locke et al., "Problems in Interpretation"; Malzberg, *Social and Biological Aspects;* Thomas and Locke, "Marital Status, Education."

48. Marc Fried, "Social Problems and Psychopathology," in Leonard J. Duhl, ed., *Urban America and the Planning of Mental Health Services* (New York: Group for the Advancement of Psychiatry, 1964), pp. 403–446.

49. Marc Fried, "Deprivation and Migration: Dilemmas of Causal Interpretation" (to be published).

50. Rowntree et al., "Mental and Personality Disorders."

51. Jaco, *Social Epidemiology.*

52. Dayton, *New Facts on Mental Disorders.*

53. Dublin, *Suicide;* Breed, "Occupational Mobility"; Breed, "Suicide, Migration and Role"; Henry and Short, *Suicide and Homicide;* Sainsbury, *Suicide in London;* and Powell, "Occupation, Status and Suicide."

54. Nyla J. Cole et al., "Socio-Economic Adjustment of a Sample of Schizophrenic Patients," *American Journal of Psychiatry,* 120 (1963), 465–471.

55. *Ibid.*

56. Fried, "Social Problems and Psychopathology."

57. Marc Fried, "The Role of Work in a Mobile Society," in Sam B. Warner, Jr., ed., *Planning for a Nation of Cities* (Cambridge, Mass.: MIT Press, 1966), pp. 81–105; Eugene A. Friedmann et al., *The Meaning of Work and Retirement* (Chicago: University of Chicago Press, 1954); Alex Inkeles, "Industrial Man," *American Journal of Sociology,* 66 (1960), 1–31; Arthur Kornhauser, *Mental Health of the Industrial Worker* (New York: John Wiley & Sons, 1965); Nancy C. Morse and Robert S. Weiss, "The Function and Meaning of Work and the Job," *American Sociological Review,* 20 (1955), 191–198.

58. Kornhauser, *Mental Health of the Industrial Worker.*

59. Faris and Dunham, *Mental Disorders in Urban Areas.*

60. Clausen and Kohn, "Relationship of Schizophrenia"; Dunham, *Community and Schizophrenia;* Gerard and Houston, "Family Background of Schizophrenia"; Goldberg and Morrison, "Schizophrenia and Social Class"; Hare, "Mental Illness and Social Conditions"; Hollingshead and Redlich, *Social Class and Mental Illness;* Jaco, *Social Epidemiology;* Lapouse et al., "The Drift Hypothesis";

Thomas S. Langner and Stanley T. Michael, *Life Stress and Mental Health* (New York: Free Press, 1963); M. H. Lystad, "Social Mobility Among Selected Groups of Schizophrenic Patients," *American Sociological Review*, 22 (1957), 288–292.

61. Clausen and Kohn, "Relationship and Schizophrenia"; Jaco, *Social Epidemiology;* Lapouse *et al.*, "The Drift Hypothesis."

62. Lapouse *et al.*, "The Drift Hypothesis."

63. Gerard and Houston, "Family Setting and Social Ecology."

64. Dunham, *Community and Schizophrenia;* Clausen and Kohn, "Relationship of Schizophrenia."

65. Eli M. Bower, Thomas A. Shellhamer, and John M. Daily, "School Characteristics of Male Adolescents Who Later Became Schizophrenic" *American Journal of Orthopsychiatry*, 30 (1960), 712–729.

66. Goldberg and Morrison, "Schizophrenia and Social Class," p. 786.

67. Dunham, *Community and Schizophrenia.*

68. Cole *et al.*, "Socio-Economic Adjustment."

69. Joseph Kahl and James Davis, "A Comparison of Indexes of Socio-Economic Status," *American Sociological Review*, 20 (1955), 317–325.

70. Warren C. Hagstrom, "The Power of the Poor," in Frank Riessman, Jerome Cohen, and Arthur Pearl, eds., *Mental Health of the Poor* (New York: Free Press of Glencoe, 1964), pp. 205–223.

71. Langner and Michaels, *Life Stress and Mental Health;* Jerome Myers and Bertram Roberts, *Family and Class Dynamics in Mental Illness* (New York: John Wiley & Sons, 1959).

72. Moore *et al.*, "Social Class, Schizophrenia"; Norman Q. Brill and Hugh A. Storrow, "Social Class and Psychiatric Treatment," *Archives of General Psychiatry*, 3 (1960), 340–344; Dewitt L. Crandell and Bruce P. Dohrenwend, "Some Relations Among Psychiatric Symptoms, Organic Illness, and Social Class," *American Journal of Psychiatry*, 123 (1967), 1527–1538.

73. Lloyd H. Rogler and August B. Hollingshead, *Trapped: Families and Schizophrenia* (New York: John Wiley & Sons, 1965).

74. Charles Kadushin, "Social Class and the Experience of Ill Health," in Reinhard Bendix and Seymour M. Lipset, eds., *Class, Status and Power* (New York: Free Press of Glencoe, 1966), pp. 406–412.

75. Howard Freeman and Ozzie G. Simmons, *The Mental Patient*

Comes Home (New York: John Wiley & Sons, 1963); Dunham, *Community and Schizophrenia;* Hollingshead and Redlich, *Social Class and Mental Illness.*

76. William Haase, "The Role of Socio-Economic Class in Examiner Bias," in Riessman, Cohen, Arthur Pearl, eds., *Mental Health of the Poor,* pp. 241–247.

77. Fanshel, "A Study of Caseworkers."

78. Howard T. Blane, Willis F. Overton, and Morris E. Chafetz, "Social Factors in the Diagnosis of Alcoholism," *Quarterly Journal of Studies on Alcoholism,* 24 (1963), 640–663.

79. Hollingshead and Redlich, *Social Class and Mental Illness;* Fanshel, "A Study of Caseworkers"; Moore *et al.,* "Social Class, Schizophrenia"; Brill and Storrow, "Social Class and Psychiatric Treatment."

80. Kadushin, "Social Class."

81. U.S. Department of Health, Education, and Welfare, *Family Income in Relation to Selected Health Characteristics,* National Center for Health Statistics Series 10, no. 2, July 1963; U.S. Department of Health, Education, and Welfare, *Medical Care, Health Status, and Family Income,* National Center for Health Statistics Series 10, no. 9, May 1964; U.S. Department of Health, Education, and Welfare, *Selected Health Characteristics by Occupation,* National Center for Health Statistics Series 10, no. 21, August 1965.

82. Langner and Michaels, *Life Stress and Mental Health.*

83. Dohrenwend, "Social Status and Psychological Disorder"; Edward Zigler and Leslie Phillips, "Psychiatric Diagnosis," *Journal of Abnormal and Social Psychology,* 63 (1961), 607–618.

84. Fried, "Social Problems and Psychopathology."

CHAPTER V—PREVENTION OF ILLNESS AND MAINTENANCE OF HEALTH

1. Stanislav V. Kasl and Sidney Cobb, "Health Behavior, Illness Behavior, and Sick-Role Behavior," *Archives of Environmental Health,* 12 (February 1966), 246–266; and (April 1966), 531–541.

2. Monroe Lerner and Odin W. Anderson, *Health Progress in the United States, 1900–1960: A Report of the Health Information Foundation* (Chicago: University of Chicago Press, 1963); Herman M. Somers and Anne R. Somers, *Doctors, Patients, and Health In-*

surance: The Organization and Financing of Medical Care (Washington, D.C.: Brookings Institution, 1961); U.S. Department of Health, Education, and Welfare, Office of the Secretary, *Health, Education, and Welfare Trends, 1963 Edition* (Washington, D.C.: U.S. Government Printing Office, 1963); U.S. Department of Health, Education, and Welfare, Public Health Service, *Health Statistics From the U.S. National Health Survey: Dental Care, Interval and Frequency of Visits, United States, July 1957–June 1959,* Public Health Service Publication No. 584-B14 (Washington, D.C.: U.S. Government Printing Office, 1960); Stephen S. Kegeles, Stanley Lotzkar, and Lewis W. Andrews, "Predicting the Acceptance of Dental Care by Residents of Nursing Homes," *Journal of Public Health Dentistry,* 26 (Summer 1966), 290–302; U.S. Department of Health, Education, and Welfare, Public Health Service, *Health Statistics From the U.S. National Health Survey: Volume of Physician Visits, United States, July 1957–June 1959,* Public Health Service Publication No. 584-B19 (Washington, D.C.: U.S. Government Printing Office, 1960); U.S. Department of Health, Education, and Welfare, Public Health Service, *Health Statistics From the U.S. National Health Survey, Hospital Discharges and Length of Stay: Short-Stay Hospitals, United States, 1958–1960,* Public Health Service Publication No. 584-B32 (Washington, D.C.: U.S. Government Printing Office, 1962); John D. Stoeckle, Irving K. Zola, and Gerald E. Davidson, "On Going to See the Doctor," *Journal of Chronic Diseases,* 16 (1963), 975–989; Irving K. Zola, "Illness Behavior of the Working Class," in *Blue Collar World,* ed. Arthur B. Shostak and William Gomberg (Englewood Cliffs, N.J.: Prentice-Hall, 1964), pp. 351–361; Eliot Freidson, *Patients' Views of Medical Practice* (New York: Russell Sage Foundation, 1961); Edward A. Suchman, "Social Patterns of Illness and Medical Care," *Journal of Health and Human Behavior,* 6 (Spring 1965), 2–16.

3. Paul N. Borsky and Oswald K. Sagen, "Motivations Toward Health Examinations," *American Journal of Public Health,* 49 (April 1959), 514–527; S. Stephen Kegeles *et al.,* "Survey of Beliefs About Cancer Detection and Taking Papanicolaou Tests," *Public Health Reports,* 80 (September 1965), 815–824; Irwin M. Rosenstock, Mayhew Derryberry, and Barbara K. Carriger, "Why People Fail to Seek Poliomyelitis Vaccination," *Public Health Reports,* 74 (February 1959), 98–103; Godfrey M. Hochbaum, *Public*

Participation in Medical Screening Programs, U.S. Public Health Service Publication No. 572 (Washington, D.C.: U.S. Government Printing Office, 1958); S. Stephen Kegeles, "Some Motives for Seeking Preventive Dental Care," *Journal of the American Dental Association,* 67 (July 1963), 90–98; Fred Heinzelmann, "Determinants of Prophylaxis Behavior with Respect to Rheumatic Fever," *Journal of Health and Human Behavior,* 3 (1962), 73–81; Elizabeth Flack, "Participation in Case Finding Program for Cervical Cancer," administrative report, Cancer Control Program, U.S. Public Health Service (Washington, D.C.: U.S. Government Printing Office, 1960); Howard Leventhal *et al.,* "Epidemic Impact on the General Population in Two Cities," in *The Impact of Asian Influenza on Community Life,* U.S. Public Health Service Publication No. 766 (Washington, D.C.: U.S. Government Printing Office, 1960); S. Stephen Kegeles, "Why People Seek Dental Care," *Journal of Health and Human Behavior,* 4 (Fall 1963), 166–173; Don P. Haefner *et al.,* "Preventive Actions in Dental Disease, Tuberculosis and Cancer," *Public Health Reports,* 82 (May 1967), 451–460; Irwin M. Rosenstock, "Why People Use Health Services," *Milbank Memorial Fund Quarterly,* 44 (July 1966), 94–127.

4. Haefner, "Preventive Actions in Dental Disease, Tuberculosis and Cancer."

5. Charles Kadushin, "Social Class and the Experience of Ill Health," *Sociological Inquiry,* 34 (Winter 1964), 67–80.

6. Kegeles, "Survey of Beliefs about Cancer Detection."

7. *Ibid.*

8. Haefner, "Preventive Actions in Dental Disease, Tuberculosis and Cancer."

9. Kurt Lewin, *A Dynamic Theory of Personality* (New York: McGraw-Hill, 1935).

10. Jerome Bruner and Cecile C. Goodman, "Value and Need as Organizing Factors in Perception," *Journal of Abnormal and Social Psychology,* 42 (1947), 37–39; and Irwin M. Rosenstock and Jean Hendry, "Epidemic Impact on Community Agencies," in *The Impact of Asian Influenza on Community Life,* U.S. Public Health Service Publication No. 766 (Washington, D.C.: U.S. Government Printing Office, 1960).

11. Paul Robbins, "Some Explorations Into the Nature of Anxieties Relating to Illness," *Genetic Psychology Monographs,* No.

66, U.S. Department of Health, Education, and Welfare, Public Health Service, 1962, pp. 91–141.

12. Freidson, *Patients' Views of Medical Practice*, p. 144.

13. Hochbaum, *Public Participation in Medical Screening Programs*.

14. Kegeles, "Some Motives for Seeking Preventive Dental Care."

15. Leon Festinger, *A Theory of Cognitive Dissonance* (Evanston, Ill.: Row Peterson, 1957).

16. Howard Leventhal *et al.*, "Epidemic Impact on the General Population in Two Cities."

17. Kegeles, "Some Motives for Seeking Preventive Dental Care."

18. Irwin M. Rosenstock, "Why People Use Health Services."

19. *Ibid.*

20. Irving K. Zola, "Illness Behavior of the Working Class."

21. Kegeles, "Survey of Beliefs about Cancer Detection."

22. Daniel Rosenblatt and Edward A. Suchman, "Blue-Collar Attitudes and Information Toward Health and Illness," in *Blue-Collar World*, ed. Shostak and Gomberg, pp. 324–333.

23. Irwin M. Rosenstock *et al.*, "Public Knowledge, Opinion and Action Concerning Three Public Health Issues," *Journal of Health and Human Behavior*, 7 (Summer 1966), 91–98.

24. Paul F. Lazarsfeld and Patricia Kendall, "The Communication Behavior of the Average American," in *Mass Communications*, ed., Wilbur L. Schramm (Urbana: University of Illinois Press, 1960), pp. 425–437; Elihu Katz and Paul F. Lazarsfeld, *Personal Influence* (Glencoe, Ill.: Free Press, 1955).

25. Leo Bogart, "The Mass Media and the Blue-Collar Worker," in *Blue-Collar World*, ed. Shostak and Gomberg, pp. 416–428; James W. Swinehart, "Voluntary Exposure to Health Communications," *American Journal of Public Health*, 58 (July 1968), 1265–1275.

26. Earl L. Koos, *The Health of Regionville* (New York: Columbia University Press, 1954).

27. Kadushin, "Social Class and the Experience of Ill Health"; and Gene N. Levine, "Anxiety About Illness: Psychological and Social Bases," *Journal of Health and Human Behavior*, 3 (Spring 1962), 30–34.

28. Ozzie G. Simmons, *Social Status and Public Health*, Social Science Research Council, Pamphlet No. 13 (New York, 1958).

29. U.S. Department of Health, Education, and Welfare, Public Health Service, *Medical Care, Health Status, and Family Income: United States,* Public Health Service Publication No. 1000, series 10, no. 9 (Washington, D.C.: U.S. Government Printing Office, 1965).

30. Elizabeth Herzog, "Some Assumptions About the Poor," *Sociological Service Review,* 37 (December 1963), 389–402; Albert K. Cohen and Harold M. Hodges, Jr., "Characteristics of the Lower-Blue-Collar-Class," *Social Problems,* 10 (Spring 1963), 303–334.

31. Freidson, *Patients' Views of Medical Practice.*

CHAPTER VI—ILLNESS AND CURE

1. David Mechanic, "The Concept of Illness Behavior," *Journal of Chronic Diseases,* 15 (February 1962), 189–194.

2. David Mechanic, "The Sociology of Medicine: Viewpoints and Perspectives," *Journal of Health and Human Behavior,* 7 (Winter 1966), 237–248.

3. David Mechanic, "Some Implications of Illness Behavior for Medical Sampling," *New England Journal of Medicine,* 269 (August 1963), 244–247.

4. Irving Zola, "Problems of Communication, Diagnosis, and Patient Care," *Journal of Medical Education,* 38 (October 1963), 829–838; and "Culture and Symptoms: An Analysis of Patients' Presenting Complaints," *American Sociological Review,* 31 (October 1966), 615–630.

5. David Mechanic, "Response Factors in Illness: The Study of Illness Behavior," *Social Psychiatry,* 1 (August 1966), 11–20.

6. See U.S. National Health Survey, *Medical Care, Health Status, and Family Income,* series 10, no. 9 (Washington, D.C.: U.S. Public Health Service, May 1964).

7. Earl L. Koos, *The Health of Regionville* (New York: Columbia University Press, 1954); Stanley H. King, *Perceptions of Illness and Medical Practice* (New York: Russell Sage Foundation, 1962).

8. Julian Samora *et al.,* "Medical Vocabulary Knowledge Among Hospital Patients," *Journal of Health and Human Behavior,* 2 (Summer 1961), 83–92; Edward Suchman, "Social Patterns of Illness and Medical Care," *Journal of Health and Human Behavior,*

6 (Spring 1965), 2–16; Lois Pratt *et al.*, "Physicians' Views on the Level of Medical Information Among Patients," *American Journal of Public Health*, 47 (October 1957), 1277–1283; Irwin Rosenstock, "Why People Fail to Seek Poliomyelitis Vaccination," *Public Health Reports*, 74 (February 1959), 98–103; Leila Deasy, "Socioeconomic Status and Participation in the Poliomyelitis Vaccine Trial," *American Sociological Review*, 21 (April 1956), 185–191.

9. Koos, *The Health of Regionville.*

10. Irwin Rosenstock, "What Research in Motivation Suggests for Public Health," *American Journal of Public Health*, 50 (March 1960), 295–302.

11. Irving K. Zola, "Illness Behavior of the Working Class," in *Blue-Collar World: Studies of the American Worker*, ed. Arthur Shostak and William Gomberg (Englewood Cliffs, N.J.: Prentice-Hall, 1964).

12. David Mechanic, *Medical Sociology* (New York: Free Press of Glencoe, 1968).

13. Thomas S. Szasz, *The Myth of Mental Illness* (New York: Hoeber-Harper, 1961).

14. See Mechanic, *Medical Sociology.*

15. Eliot Freidson, "Client Control and Medical Practice," *American Journal of Sociology*, 65 (January 1960), 374–382.

16. Edward Suchman, "Stages of Illness and Medical Care," *Journal of Health and Human Behavior*, 6 (Fall 1965), 114–128.

17. *Ibid.*

18. David Mechanic and Edmund Volkart, "Illness Behavior and Medical Diagnoses," *Journal of Health and Human Behavior*, 1 (Summer 1960), 86–94; Howard Freeman and Ozzie Simmons, *The Mental Patient Comes Home* (New York: John Wiley & Sons, 1963); George Brown *et al.*, *Schizophrenia and Social Care* (London: Oxford University Press, 1966); Thomas Scheff, "Users and Non-users of a Student Psychiatric Clinic," *Journal of Health and Human Behavior*, 7 (Summer 1966), 114–121; Mark Lefton *et al.*, "Social Class, Expectations, and Performance of Mental Patients," *American Journal of Sociology*, 68 (July 1962), 79–87; Simon Dinitz *et al.*, "The Posthospital Psychological Functioning of Former Mental Hospital Patients," *Mental Hygiene*, 45 (October 1961), 579–588.

19. Freeman and Simmons, *The Mental Patient Comes Home;* Shirley Angrist *et al.*, "Tolerance of Deviant Behavior, Posthospital

Performance Levels, and Rehospitalization," *Proceedings of the Third World Congress of Psychiatry, 1963,* pp. 237–241.

20. David Mechanic, "Response Factors in Illness."

21. See Pratt *et al.,* "Physicians' Views."

22. Edward Suchman, "Sociomedical Variations Among Ethnic Groups," *American Journal of Sociology,* 70 (November 1964), 319–331; and Suchman, "Social Patterns of Illness and Medical Care."

23. U.S. National Health Survey, *Health Insurance Coverage, July 1962—June 1963,* series 10, No. 11 (August 1964); *Physician Visits,* series 10, No. 19 (June 1965); and *Volume of Dental Visits,* series 10, No. 23 (October 1965) (Washington, D.C.: U.S. Public Health Service).

24. David Mechanic and Edmund Volkart, "Stress, Illness Behavior, and the Sick Role," *American Sociological Review,* 26 (February 1961), 51–58.

25. Michael Balint, *The Doctor, His Patient, and the Illness* (New York: International Universities Press, 1957); Max Clyne, *Night Calls: A Study in General Practice* (London: Tavistock Publications, 1961).

26. August Hollingshead and Frederick C. Redlich, *Social Class and Mental Illness* (New York: John Wiley & Sons, 1958).

27. Suchman, "Stages of Illness and Medical Care."

28. Beatrix Cobb *et al.,* "Patient-Responsible Delay of Treatment in Cancer," *Cancer,* 7 (September 1954), 920–926; Rose Goldsen *et al.,* "Some Factors Related to Patient Delay in Seeking Diagnosis for Cancer Symptoms," *Cancer,* 10 (January–February 1957), 1–7; Barbara Blackwell, "The Literature on Delay in Seeking Medical Care for Chronic Illness," *Health Education Monographs,* 16 (1963); Bernard Kutner and Gerald Gordon, "Seeking Care for Cancer," *Journal of Health and Human Behavior,* 2 (Fall 1961), 171–178; Rose Goldsen, "Patient Delay in Seeking Cancer Diagnosis: Behavioral Aspects," *Journal of Chronic Diseases,* 16 (May 1963), 427–436.

29. Gene Levine, "Anxiety About Illness: Psychological and Social Bases," *Journal of Health and Human Behavior,* 3 (Spring 1962), 30–34.

30. Koos, *The Health of Regionville;* Hollingshead and Redlich, *Social Class and Mental Illness.*

31. Freeman and Simmons, *The Mental Patient Comes Home;*

Lefton *et. al.*, "Social Class, Expectations, and Performance."

32. Frederick Redlich *et. al.*, "Social Class Differences in Attitudes Towards Psychiatry," *American Journal of Orthopsychiatry,* 25 (January 1955), 60–70; Norman Brill and Hugh Storrow, "Social Class and Psychiatric Treatment," *Archives of General Psychiatry,* 3 (October 1960), 340–344.

33. James D. Hardy *et al., Pain Sensations and Reactions* (Baltimore: Williams and Wilkins, 1952); Richard Sternbach and Bernard Tursky, "Ethnic Differences Among Housewives in Psychophysical and Skin Potential Responses to Electric Shock," *Psychophysiology,* 1 (January 1965), 241–246.

34. John Clausen and Marian Yarrow, eds., "The Impact of Mental Illness on the Family," *Journal of Social Issues,* 11 (1955), entire issue.

35. Marian Yarrow *et al.*, "The Psychological Meaning of Mental Illness in the Family," *Journal of Social Issues,* 11 (1955), 25–32.

36. Lionel Lewis and Joseph Lopreato, "Arationality, Ignorance, and Perceived Danger in Medical Practices," *American Sociological Review,* 27 (August 1962), 508–514; Paul B. Cornely and Stanley K. Bigman, "Acquaintance with Municipal Government Health Services in a Low-Income Urban Population," *American Journal of Public Health,* 52 (November 1962), 1877–1886.

37. Redlich *et al.*, "Social Class Differences"; Brill and Storrow, "Social Class and Psychiatric Treatment."

38. Rosenstock, "What Research in Motivation Suggests for Public Health."

39. Koos, *The Health of Regionville,* p. 37.

40. Ann Cartwright, *Patients and Their Doctors: A Study of General Practice* (New York: Atherton Press, 1967).

41. National Center for Health Statistics, *Cycle 1 of the Health Examination Survey: Sample and Response,* series 11, no. 1 (April 1964) (Washington, D.C.: U.S. Public Health Service); and Commission on Chronic Illness, *Chronic Illness in a Large City* Cambridge, Mass.: Harvard University Press, 1957).

42. Frank Riessman *et al.*, eds., *Mental Health of the Poor* (New York: Free Press of Glencoe, 1964).

43. Hollingshead and Redlich, *Social Class and Mental Illness;* Jerome Myers and Leslie Schaffer, "Social Stratification and Psychiatric Practice: A Study of an Outpatient Clinic," *American*

Sociological Review, 19 (June 1954), 307–310; Brill and Storrow, "Social Class and Psychiatric Treatment."

44. Mark Zborowski, "Cultural Components in Responses to Pain," *Journal of Social Issues,* 8, no. 4 (1952), 16–30.

45. *Ibid.,* pp. 27–28.

46. Sternbach and Tursky, "Ethnic Differences Among Housewives."

47. Sidney Croog, "Ethnic Origins, Educational Level, and Responses to a Health Questionnaire," *Human Organization,* 20 (Summer 1961), 65–69.

48. David Mechanic, "Religion, Religiosity, and Illness Behavior," *Human Organization,* 22 (Fall 1963), 202–208.

49. Charles Kadushin, "The Friends and Supporters of Psychotherapy," *American Sociological Review,* 31 (December 1966), 786–802; Scheff, "Users and Non-users"; Charles Kadushin, "Social Distance Between Client and Professional," *American Journal of Sociology,* 67 (March 1962), 517–531.

50. Odin Anderson, "Infant Mortality and Social and Cultural Factors," in *Patients, Physicians and Illness,* ed. E. G. Jaco (Glencoe, Ill.: Free Press, 1958).

51. Suchman, "Sociomedical Variations Among Ethnic Groups."

CHAPTER VII—THE TREATMENT OF THE SICK

1. Henry F. Howe, ed. *The Physician's Career* (Chicago: American Medical Association, 1967), pp. 26, 48.

2. Robert E. Coker, Jr., John Kosa, and Bernard G. Greenberg, "Medical Careers in Public Health," *Milbank Memorial Fund Quarterly,* 44 (April 1966), Part I, 147–258; Frances S. McConnell, John Kosa, and Robert E. Coker, Jr., "The Selection of the Field of Public Health," *American Journal of Public Health,* 56 (May 1966), 764–775; John D. Stoeckle and Irving K. Zola, "After Everyone Can Pay for Medical Care," *Medical Care,* 2 (January 1964), 36–41.

3. John Kosa, "Entrepreneurship and Charisma in the Medical Profession," paper presented at the International Conference on Social Science and Medicine, 1968.

4. Leon S. Robertson *et al.,* "Race, Status, and Medical Care," *Phylon,* 28 (Winter 1967), 353–360.

5. Richard I. Feinbloom *et al.*, "The Physician's Knowledge of Low-income Families," Paper presented at the meeting of the American Public Health Association, 1967.

6. Leon S. Robertson, "On the Intraurban Ecology of Primary Care Physicians" (mimeographed, 1968).

7. Health Manpower Study Commission, *Health Manpower for the Upper Midwest* (Saint Paul, Minn., June, 1966); John Kosa, "The Foreign-trained Physician in the United States," *Journal of Medical Education*, 44 (January 1969), 46–51.

8. Robert R. Cadmus and John H. Ketner, *Organizing Ambulance Services in the Public Interest* (Chapel Hill, N.C., January 1965).

9. Sheldon Lowry and Donald G. Hay, *Acceptance of Voluntary Health Insurance in Sampson County, North Carolina* (North Carolina Agricultural Experiment Station, 1955).

10. Bert Ellenbogen, Charles E. Ramsey, and Robert A. Danley, "Health Need, Status, and Subscription to Health Insurance," *Journal of Health and Human Behavior*, 7 (Spring 1966), 63.

11. Jerry Solon, "Patterns of Medical Care," *American Journal of Public Health*, 50 (December 1960), 1905–1913.

12. Joel J. Alpert *et al.*, "Types of Families Using an Emergency Clinic"; Joel J. Alpert, John Kosa, and Robert J. Haggerty, "A Month of Illness and Health Care Among Low-income Families," *Public Health Reports*, 82 (August 1967), 705–713.

13. See E. R. Weinerman *et al.*, "Yale Studies in Ambulatory Medical Care," *American Journal of Public Health*, 56 (July 1966), 1036–1056; Abraham B. Bergman and Robert J. Haggerty, "The Emergency Clinic," *American Journal of Diseases of Children*, 104 (1962), 36–44; Jerry Solon, "Sociocultural Variations Among a Hospital's Outpatients," *American Journal of Public Health*, 56 (June 1966), 884–895; Leon S. Robertson *et al.*, "Anticipated Acceptance of Neighborhood Health Clinics by the Urban Poor," *Journal of the American Medical Association*, 205 (September 16, 1968), 815–818.

14. Robert J. Haggerty, "Family Medicine," *Journal of Medical Education*, 37 (June 1962), 531–580; Robert R. Huntley, "Epidemiology of Family Practice," *Journal of the American Medical Association*, 185 (July 20, 1963), 175–178; Lynn P. Carmichael, "A Program of Instruction in Family Medicine," *Journal of Medical Education*, 40 (April 1965), 370–375; George A. Silver, *Family*

Medical Care (Cambridge, Mass.: Harvard University Press, 1963).

15. Kosa, "Entrepreneurship and Charisma in the Medical Profession."

16. John Kosa et al., "Crisis and Stress in Family Life," *Wisconsin Sociologist*, 4 (Summer 1965), 11–19.

17. Martin K. White, Joel J. Alpert and John Kosa, "Hard-to-reach Families in a Comprehensive Care Program," *Journal of the American Medical Association*, 201 (September 11, 1967), 801–806.

18. Margaret C. Heagarty, "The Use of the Telephone in Pediatric Practice," in Robert J. Haggerty and Morris Green, eds., *Ambulatory Pediatrics* (Philadelphia: W. B. Saunders Company, 1968), pp. 136–138.

19. Margaret C. Heagarty *et al.*, "Use of the Telephone by Low-income Families," *Journal of Pediatrics*, 73 (November 1968), 740–744.

20. "Comprehensive Health Planning," a symposium of articles in the *American Journal of Public Health*, 58 (June 1968), 1015–1089.

21. Joel J. Alpert *et al.*, "Effective Use of Comprehensive Pediatric Care," *American Journal of Diseases of Children*, 116 (November 1968), 529–533.

22. J. Whitney Brown, "The Content of General Practice," unpublished manuscript.

23. Marcel A. Fredericks, John Kosa, and Leon S. Robertson, "The Doctor and the Poor," paper presented at the meeting of the Eastern Sociological Society, 1969.

24. Julius A. Roth *et al.*, "Who will Treat the Poor?" paper presented at the meeting of the American Sociological Association, 1967.

25. Earl L. Koos, *The Health of Regionville* (New York: Columbia University Press, 1954), pp. 88–94; Lyle Saunders, *Cultural Difference and Medical Care* (New York: Russell Sage Foundation, 1954), pp. 79–87; Harold D. McDowell, "Osteopathy: A Study of a Semi-Orthodox Healing Agency and the Recruitment of its Clientele," unpub. Master's thesis, University of Chicago, 1950.

26. See Marvin B. Sussman *et al.*, *The Walking Patient* (Cleveland: Western Reserve University Press, 1967); Malcolm W. Klein

et al., "Problems of Measuring Patient Care in the Out-Patient Department," *Journal of Health and Human Behavior,* 2 (Summer 1961), 138–144; Norman H. Berkowitz, Mary F. Malone, and Malcolm W. Klein, "Patient Care as a Criterion Problem," *Journal of Health and Human Behavior,* 3 (Fall 1962), 171–176; Joel J. Alpert, John Kosa, and Leon Robertson, "A Typology of Users of Hospital Emergency Facilities," *Clinical Research,* 15 (April 1967), 341.

27. Howard S. Becker *et al., Boys in White* (Chicago: University of Chicago Press, 1961), especially chap. 16.

28. Statements on emergency wards are taken from an unpublished study by Julius A. Roth and Dorothy J. Douglas.

29. Herbert E. Klarman, "Characteristics of Patients in Short-Term Hospitals in New York City," *Journal of Health and Human Behavior,* 3 (Spring, 1962), 46–52.

30. Anthony M. Lowell, *Socio-Economic Conditions and Tuberculosis Prevalence: New York City* (New York: Tuberculosis and Health Association, 1956); Leonard J. Duhl and Margaret Schubert, "Research Report on Mass X-ray Survey" (Contra Costa County, Calif., X-ray Survey Corporation, 1952).

31. Personal communication from Walter Klink.

32. *The TB Clinic Attitudes, Management, and Standards* (New York: National Tuberculosis Association, 1967), p. 10.

33. The information is taken from the author's studies of tuberculosis hospitals. See his "Behavior Control in Tuberculosis," *T: International Union Against Tuberculosis* (July 1963), 17–23.

34. Dorothy Miller and Michael Schwartz, "County Lunacy Commission Hearings," *Social Problems,* 14 (Summer 1966), 26–35; Thomas J. Scheff, "The Societal Reaction to Deviance," *Social Problems,* 11 (Spring 1964), 401–413.

35. August B. Hollingshead and Frederick G. Redlich, *Social Class and Mental Illness* (New York: John Wiley & Sons, 1958); Jerome K. Myers, Lee L. Bean, and Max P. Pepper, "Social Class and Psychiatric Disorders," *Journal of Health and Human Behavior,* 6 (Summer 1965), 74–79; Raymond G. Hunt, Orville Gurrslin, and Jack L. Roach, "Social Status and Psychiatric Service in a Child Guidance Clinic," *American Sociological Review,* 23 (February 1958), 81–83; Georges Sabagh *et al.,* "Social Class and Ethnic Status of Patients Admitted to a State Hospital for the Retarded," *Pacific Sociological Review,* 2 (Fall 1959), 76–80.

36. Hollingshead and Redlich, *Social Class and Mental Illness,* p. 295; Sabagh *et al.,* "Social Class and Ethnic Status"; Robert Hardt and Sherwin Feinhandler, "Social Class in Mental Hospitalization Prognosis," *American Sociological Review,* 24 (December 1959), 815–821.

37. Julius A. Roth and Elizabeth M. Eddy, *Rehabilitation for the Unwanted* (New York: Atherton Press, 1967).

38. *Ibid.*

CHAPTER VIII—READJUSTMENT AND REHABILITATION OF PATIENTS

1. Marvin B. Sussman, "Use of the Longitudinal Design in Studies of Long-Term Illness: Some Advantages and Limitations," *Gerontologist,* 2, Part II (June 1964), 25–29.

2. Robert A. Scott, *The Itinerant Client* (forthcoming); Thomas J. Scheff, "Typification in the Diagnostic Practices of Rehabilitation Agencies," Robert A. Scott, "Comments About Interpersonal Processes of Rehabilitation," and Albert F. Wessen, "The Rehabilitation Apparatus and Organization Theory," in Marvin B. Sussman, ed., *Sociology and Rehabilitation* (Washington D,.C.: American Sociological Association, 1966), pp. 132–178; Elliott A. Krause, "After the Rehabilitation Center," *Social Problems,* 14 (Fall 1966), 197–206; Gideon Sjoberg *et al., The Bureaucracy Problem* (New York: McGraw-Hill Book Company), forthcoming.

3. Robert A. Scott, "The Selection of Clients by Social Welfare Agencies: The Case of the Blind," *Social Problems,* 14 (Winter 1967), 248–257; Peter H. Rossi, "Boobytraps and Pitfalls in the Evaluation of Social Action Programs," paper presented at the meeting of the American Statistical Association, 1967.

4. Charles Kadushin, "Social Class and the Experience of Ill Health," *Sociological Inquiry,* 34 (Winter 1964), 67–80; and Aaron Antonovsky, "Social Class and Illness: A Reconsideration," *Sociological Inquiry,* 37 (Spring 1967), 311–322. See further Charles Kadushin, "Social Class and Ill Health: The Need for Further Research. A Reply to Antonovsky," *Sociological Inquiry,* 37 (Spring 1967), 323–332.

5. Zahava D. Blum, personal communication.

6. Marie R. Haug and Marvin B. Sussman, "Social Class Measurement: Some Problems and Proposals" (unpublished).

7. Martin Dishart, *The Incidence of Disability in Maryland* (College Park, Md.: Bureau of Educational Research and Field Services, University of Maryland, 1967).

8. Frank Reissman and Sylvia Scribner, "The Under-Utilization of Mental Health Services by Workers and Low Income Groups," *American Journal of Psychiatry,* 121 (February 1965), 798–801.

9. *Ibid.*

10. Elliott A. Krause, *Factors Related to Length of Mental Hospital Stay* (Boston: Massachusetts Department of Mental Health, 1967).

11. *Ibid.*

12. Benjamin Pasamanick, Frank R. Scarpitti, and Simon Dinitz, *Schizophrenics in the Community* (New York: Appleton-Century-Crofts, 1967).

13. Simon Dinitz, Mark Lefton, Shirley Angrist, and Benjamin Pasamanick, "Psychiatric and Social Attributes as Predictors of Case Outcome in Mental Hospitalization," *Social Problems,* 8 (Spring 1961), 322–328.

14. F. T. Kolouch, "Computer Shows How Patient Stays Vary," *Modern Hospital,* 105 (November 1965), 130–134.

15. Morris W. Stroud, III, *et al.,* "Rehabilitation Patients' Needs: A Five-Year Follow-Up Study" (in process).

16. Marvin B. Sussman *et al., Rehabilitation and Tuberculosis: Predicting the Vocational and Economic Status of Tuberculosis Patients* (Cleveland: Western Reserve University, 1964).

17. D. M. Kissen, "Relapse in Pulmonary Tuberculosis Due to Special Psychological Causes," *Health Bulletin* (Department of Health for Scotland) 15, no. 1 (1957); and D. M. Kissen, "Some Psychological Aspects of Pulmonary Tuberculosis," *International Journal of Social Psychiatry,* 3, no. 4 (1958).

18. Charles M. Wylie, "Delay in Seeking Rehabilitation After Cerebrovascular Accidents," *Journal of Chronic Disease,* 14 (October 1961), 442–451.

19. Stroud *et al.,* "Rehabilitation Patients' Needs."

20. C. W. Tempel *et al.,* "An Analysis of Hospital Records of Patients Discharged from a Large Tuberculosis Service," *U.S. Armed Forces Medical Journal,* 4 (December 1953), 1719–1733;

W. B. Tollen, "Irregular Discharge: The Problem of Hospitalization of the Tuberculous," *Public Health Reports,* 63 (November 1948), 1441–1473.

21. Louis J. Moran *et al.,* "The Use of Demographic Characteristics in Predicting Response to Hospitalization for Tuberculosis," *Journal of Counseling Psychology,* 19, 1 (1955), 65–70.

22. Sussman *et al., Rehabilitation and Tuberculosis.*

23. Sidney Katz and Austin Chinn, "Multidisciplinary Studies of Illness in Aged Persons," *Journal of Chronic Disease,* 13 (1961), 453–464.

24. Daniel Rosenblatt and Edward A. Suchman, "The Underutilization of Medical-Care Services by Blue-Collarites," and "Blue-Collar Attitudes and Information Toward Health and Illness," in Arthur B. Shostak and William Gomberg, eds., *Blue-Collar World: Studies of the American Worker* (Englewood Cliffs, N.J.: Prentice-Hall, 1964), pp. 324–349.

25. L. Schneiderman, "Social Class, Diagnosis, and Treatment," *American Journal of Orthopsychiatry,* 35 (January 1965), 99–105.

26. Sussman, *Sociology and Rehabilitation,* pp. 179–222.

27. Marvin B. Sussman *et al., The Walking Patient: A Study in Outpatient Care* (Cleveland: Western Reserve University Press, 1967).

28. See Eliot Freidson, "Disability as Social Deviance," in Sussman, *Sociology and Rehabilitation,* pp. 71–99; and A. S. Yerby, "The Disadvantaged and Health Care," *American Journal of Public Health,* 56 (January 1966), 5–9.

29. George James, "Poverty as an Obstacle to Health Progress in Our Cities," *American Journal of Public Health,* 55 (November 1965), 1757–1771.

30. Jack T. Conway, "The Beneficiary, The Consumer," *American Journal of Public Health,* 55 (November 1965), 1784.

31. Erving Goffman, *Stigma* (Englewood Cliffs, N.J.: Prentice-Hall, 1963).

32. George A. Streeter, "Phantasies of Tuberculosis Patients," *Psychosomatic Medicine,* 19 (July–August 1957), 287–292.

33. Scheff, "Typification in the Diagnostic Practices," p. 141.

34. Michael Balint, *The Doctor, His Patient, and the Illness* (New York: International Universities Press, 1957), p. 216.

35. Stroud *et al.,* "Rehabilitation Patients' Needs."

36. Howard E. Freeman and Ozzie G. Simmons, "Social Class

and Posthospital Performance Levels," *American Sociological Review*, 24 (June 1959), 345–351.

37. Marvin B. Sussman, William B. Weil, and Alan J. Crain, "Family Interaction, Diabetes, and Sibling Relationships," *International Journal of Social Psychiatry*, 12 (Winter 1966), 35–43; and "Effects of a Diabetic Child on Marital Integration and Related Measures of Family Functioning," *Journal of Health and Human Behavior*, 7 (Summer 1966), 122–127; Morris W. Stroud *et al.*, "Rehabilitation Patients' Needs"; Reuben Hill, "Social Stresses on the Family," *Social Casework*, 39 (1958), 139–150.

38. Robert Maisel, "The Ex-Mental Patient and Rehospitalization," *Social Problems*, 15 (Summer 1967), 18–24.

39. Edward A. Suchman, "Medical 'Deprivation,'" *American Journal of Orthopsychiatry*, 36 (July 1966), 665–672; and "Social Patterns of Illness and Medical Care," *Journal of Health and Human Behavior*, 6 (1965), 2–16; Rodney M. Coe and Albert F. Wessen, "Social-Psychological Factors Influencing the Use of Community Health Resources," *American Journal of Public Health*, 55 (July 1965), 1024–1031.

CHAPTER IX—THE FUTURE OF POVERTY

1. Michael Harrington, *Poverty, Family Planning, and the Great Society* (New York: Planned Parenthood Federation, 1966), p. 5; Arthur Shostak and William Gomberg, eds., *New Perspective on Poverty* (Englewood Cliffs, N.J.: Prentice-Hall, 1965), pp. 50–57; Mary F. Waldrop and Richard Q. Bell, "Effects of Family Size and Density on Newborn Characteristics," *American Journal of Orthopsychiatry*, 36 (April, 1966), 544–550; Mary F. Waldrop and Richard Q. Bell, "Relation of Preschool Dependency Behavior to Family Size and Density," *Child Development*, 35 (December 1964), 1187–1195.

2. Mollie Orshansky, as reported in *Planned Parenthood News*, June 1966, p. 3. See also President's National Advisory Commission on Rural Poverty, *The People Left Behind* (Washington, D.C.: Government Printing Office, 1967), pp. 75–84.

3. *Planned Parenthood News*, March 1967, p. 1.

4. *Evening Bulletin* (Philadelphia), January 15, 1967, p. 7.

5. *News*, Spring 1967, Association for Voluntary Sterilization, New York.

6. Robert Coles, "Abortion and the Laws of the States," *New Republic*, June 10, 1967, p. 11; "The Indignity of Abortion," *Village Voice*, July 13, 1967, pp. 5, 29; David T. Smith, ed., *Abortion and the Law* (Cleveland: Case Western Reserve University Press, 1968).

7. Alice S. Rossi, "Abortion Laws and Their Victims," *Trans-Action* (September–October 1966), 8.

8. Paul H. Gebhard *et al.*, *Pregnancy, Birth, and Abortion* (New York: Harper & Bros., 1958).

9. Phil Kerby, "Abortion Laws and Attitudes," *The Nation*, June 12, 1967, p. 754; Herman Schwartz, "A Survey of Abortion Law Reform," *Humanist*, 27 (July–August 1967), 123–126; Harold M. Schmeck, Jr., "Doctors Critical of Abortion Laws," *New York Times*, April 29, 1967, p. 27.

10. George Varky, *Profile of U.S. Women in the Reproductive Ages Needing Family Planning Assistance* (New York: Planned Parenthood—World Population, 1966); Harry C. Bredemeier, "The Lower-Class Family of Procreation," in Bernard Goldstein, ed., *Low Income Youth in Urban Areas* (New York: Holt, Rinehart and Winston, 1967).

11. Frederick S. Jaffe, "Family Planning and Public Policy," paper presented at the meeting of the American Sociological Association, 1967; Herbert Gans, "Poverty and Culture: Some Basic Questions about Methods of Studying Life-Styles of the Poor," (unpublished).

12. Mark R. Arnold, "U.S. Expands its Birth-Control Services to the Poor," *National Observer*, November 21, 1966, pp. 1, 16; George N. Lindsay, *Closing the Gap* (New York: Planned Parenthood Federation, 1966); *The People Wheel* (New York: Planned Parenthood Federation, 1966).

13. Frederick S. Jaffe, "A Strategy for Implementing Family Planning Services," *Studies in Family Planning*, no. 17, February 1967; Harold L. Sheppard, *The Effects of Family Planning on Poverty in the U.S.* (Washington, D.C.: Senate Sub-Committee on Employment, Manpower, and Poverty, 1967); Community Action Program, *Community Action for Health: Family Planning* (Washington, D.C.: Office of Economic Opportunity, 1967); Edwin M.

Schur, ed., *The Family and the Sexual Revolution* (Bloomington: Indiana University Press, 1964).

14. Sanford Kravitz, "Community Action Programs," *American Child,* 46 (November 1965), 1–6; Sargent Shriver, "New Weapons in Fighting Poverty," *Public Welfare,* 24 (January 1966), 9–14; Frank Riessman and Martin Rein, "The Third Force Ideology: An Anti-Poverty Ideology," *American Child* (November 1965), 10–14; Harry Caudill, "Reflections on Poverty in America," in Shostak and Gomberg, eds., *New Perspectives on Poverty,* pp. 3–8.

15. Office of Economic Opportunity, *Community Action Workbook* (Washington, D.C.: OEO, 1965), Part III, A-7.

16. See "Participation of the Poor," *Yale Law Journal,* 74 (no. 4, 1966), 598–629; Elinor Graham, "Poverty and the Legislative Process," in Ben B. Seligman, ed., *Poverty as a Public Issue* (New York: Free Press of Glencoe, 1966), pp. 251–271; Peter Morris and Martin Rein, *Dilemmas of Social Reform* (New York: Atherton Press, 1967); George A. Brager and Francis P. Purcell, *Community Action Against Poverty* (New Haven: College and University Press, 1967); Allan R. Talbot, *The Mayor's Game* (New York: Harper & Row, 1967).

17. Mark R. Arnold, "Revolt of Spokesmen for the Poor," *National Observer,* May 9, 1966, p. 6; Erwin Knoll and Jules Witcover, "Fighting Poverty and City Hall," *Reporter,* June 3, 1965, pp. 19–22; Herbert Krosney, *Beyond Welfare: Poverty in the Supercity* (New York: Holt, Rinehart & Winston, 1966).

18. Arthur B. Shostak, "Containment, Co-optation or Co-determination," *American Child,* 46 (November 1965), 15–19; and Shostak, "Urban Politics and Poverty," paper presented at the meeting of the American Sociological Association, 1966.

19. David B. Truman, *The Governmental Process* (New York: Alfred A. Knopf, 1951; Nelson W. Polsby, *Community Power and Political Theory* (New Haven: Yale University Press, 1963).

20. Kenneth B. Clark, "A Relevant War Against Poverty: Some Problems of Community Action Programs" (statement read before the Clark Subcommittee, March 18, 1967); Earl Raab, "What War and Which Poverty," *The Public Interest* (Spring 1966), 45–56.

21. Richard A. Cloward and Richard M. Elman, "Poverty, Injustice and the Welfare State," *The Nation,* March 7, 1966, pp. 264–268; Robert Morris and Robert H. Binstock, *Feasible Planning*

for Social Change (New York: Columbia University Press, 1966); Peter Kong-Ming New and J. Thomas May, "Alienation and Communication Among Urban Renovators," *Human Organization,* 25 (Winter 1966), 352–358.

22. Arthur B. Shostak and C. P. Wolf, "New Roles and Old Realities: Spokesmen for the Poor," paper presented at the meeting of the Eastern Sociological Society, 1968; R. M. Kramer and C. Denton, "Organization of a Community Action Program," *Social Work,* 15 (October 1967), 69–80.

23. Daniel P. Moynihan, "The Professionalization of Reform," *The Public Interest* (Fall 1965), 13; Richard Cloward and Richard Elman, "Advocacy in the Ghetto," *Trans-Action* (December 1966), 21–27; Richard Flacks, "On the Uses of Participatory Democracy," *Dissent,* 16 (November–December 1966), 701–708.

24. Paul Bullock, "Morality and Tactics in Community Organizing," in Jeremy Larner and Irving Howe, eds., *Poverty: Views from the Left* (New York: William Morrow, 1968), pp. 137–148.

25. Nan Robertson, "Should the Poor Lead the Poor?" *New York Times,* March 21, 1967, p. 16; Melvin Seeman, "Antidote to Alienation," *Trans-Action* (May–June 1966), 35–39.

26. Harry C. Bredemeier, "The Politics of the Poverty Cold War," *Urban Affairs Quarterly,* 2 (June 1968), 34.

27. See James Tobin, "Conquering Poverty in the U.S. by 1977," *New Republic,* June 3, 1967, pp. 14–18.

28. Reece McGee, "Welfare in Affluence," *The Nation,* February 14, 1966, pp. 174–180; Eleanor P. Wolf and Charles N. Lebeaux, "Class and Race in the Changing City," in Leo F. Schnore and Henry Fogin, eds., *Urban Research and Policy Planning* (Beverly Hills, Calif.: Sage Publications, 1967), pp. 99–130.

CHAPTER X—THE FUTURE OF HEALTH CARE

1. Michael M. Davis, Jr., *Clinics, Hospitals, and Health Centers* (New York: Harper & Bros., 1927); Irwin M. Rosenstock, "Why People Use Health Services," *Milbank Memorial Fund Quarterly,* 44 (July 1966), 94–127; Rene Sand, *The Advance to Social Medicine* (London: Staples, 1952); George A. Rosen, *A History of Public Health* (New York: MD Publications, 1958).

2. Anselm L. Strauss, "Medical Ghettos," *Trans-Action,* 4 (May

1967), 7–16; John D. Stoeckle, "The O.P.D. as Ambulatory Care at the Hospital," in A. Lillienfeld and A. Gifford, eds., *Chronic Diseases and Public Health* (Baltimore: Johns Hopkins Press, 1966), pp. 221–228; Gordon Marmerstedt and Alice L. Spillane, "Family Doctor or School Physician: A Study of Who Does Physical Examinations," *Journal of School Health*, 32 (June 1962), 215–221.

3. See the "Chadwick Clinics," in Massachusetts carrying out case-finding surveys for tuberculosis in the schools in the 1920's. *A Century of Tuberculosis Control in Massachusetts, 1850–1950* (Boston: Massachusetts Tuberculosis and Health League, 1951); Howard Freeman, "Social Change and the Organization of Mental Health Care," *American Journal Orthopsychiatry*, 35 (July 1965), 717–722.

4. George James, "Poverty and Public Health," *American Journal of Public Health*, 55 (November 1965), 1757–1771; William H. Stewart, "New Dimensions of Public Health," *American Journal of Public Health*, 57 (April 1967), 584–588.

5. Talcott Parsons, "Definition of Health and Illness in the Light of American Values and Social Structure," in E. G. Jaco, ed., *Patients, Physicians, and Illness* (Glencoe, Ill.: Free Press, 1958), pp. 165–187.

6. Margaret Olendzki, Charles H. Goodrich, and George G. Reader, "The Significance of Welfare Status in the Case of Indigent Patients," *American Journal of Public Health*, 53 (October 1963), 1676–1684; Charles H. Goodrich, Margaret Olendzki, and George G. Reader, "A Progress Report on an Experiment in Welfare Medical Care," *American Journal of Public Health*, 55 (January 1965), 88–93.

7. "Private Health Insurance—Self Appraisal," Health Insurance Council, *Health Insurance Viewpoints*, 7, no. 1 (February 1967).

8. I. S. Falk, "Medical Care and Social Policy," *American Journal of Public Health*, 55 (April 1965), 522–528.

9. "Volume of Physician Visits, July, 1957–June, 1959," *Health Statistics*, U.S. National Health Survey, series B, no. 19 (Washington, D.C.: U.S. Department of Health, Education and Welfare, 1960); U.S. National Center for Health Statistics, *Current Estimates from Health Interview Survey*, July, 1963–June, 1964, series 10, no. 13 (Washington, D.C.: Government Printing Office, 1964); Maurice E. Odoroff and Leslie Morgan Abbee, "Use of General

Hospitals: Factors in Outpatient Visits," *Public Health Reports*, 72 (June 1957), 478–483.

10. *Preliminary Report on Patterns of Medical and Health Care in Poverty Areas in Chicago* (Chicago: Chicago Board of Health Medical Care Report, 1966).

11. Karl Singer, *Charlestown and the Health of the People*, unpublished manuscript.

12. Jerry A. Solon, Cecil G. Sheps, and Sidney S. Lee, "Patterns of Medical Care: A Hospital's Outpatients," *American Journal of Public Health*, 50 (December 1960), 1905–1913.

13. Raymond C. Lerner and Corinne Kirchner, *Municipal General Hospital Outpatient Population Study in New York City Outpatient Departments, VII Utilization of Clinics and Other Sources of Medical Care* (New York: School of Public Health and Administrative Medicine, Columbia University, 1967).

14. Series 10, no. 18, National Center for Health Statistics, 1964.

15. Massachusetts Department of Public Welfare, Bureau of Research and Statistics, *Report on Vendor Payments for Medical Care Classified by Vendor* (Boston: Department of Public Welfare, 1966).

16. Barbara Blackwell, "The Literature on Delay in Seeking Medical Care for Chronic Illness," *Health Education Monographs*, no. 16 (1963), 3–32.

17. *Preliminary Report on Patterns of Medical and Health Care in Poverty Areas in Chicago* (Chicago: Chicago Board of Health Medical Care Report, 1966).

18. Leon Robertson, John Kosa, Joel J. Alpert, "Race, Status and Medical Care," paper at the Society for the Study of Social Problems, 1967; Joseph Dorsey, personal communication; Membership, Massachusetts Medical Society, Local Directories Massachusetts Medical Society, 1925, 1930, 1940, 1950, 1965.

19. C. E. Phillibert, personal communication.

20. H. Jack Geiger, "The Neighborhood Health Center," *Archives of Environmental Health*, 14 (June 1967), 912–916; Count D. Gibson, "The Columbia Point Health Center and Health Association," paper presented at the American Public Health Association, 1966; Luther J. Carter, "Rural Health," *Science*, 156 (June 16, 1967), 1466–1468; Ralph Memlo, "Family Doctor to a Community," *Boston* (March 1967), 53–57; Elinor Langer, "Medicine for the Poor: A New Deal in Denver," *Science*, 153 (July 29, 1966),

508–512; "OEO's Neighborhood Health Center: Social Intervention in the Alliance of Poverty and Disease," *Labor Rehabilitation Report,* 5 (May 1967), 14–15.

21. Consultative Council on Medical and Allied Services, *Interim Report on the Future Provision of Medical and Allied Services* (London: His Majesty's Stationery Office, 1920).

22. Medical Planning Commission, "Draft Interim Report," *British Medical Journal,* 1 (June 1942), 749–750; *Health Centres Report* (London: Medical Practitioner's Union, October, 1960).

23. C. Taylor *et al.,* "Health Centres of Harlow," *Lancet,* 269 (October 1955), 863–870; "Health Centres of Tomorrow," *Lancet,* 252 (January 1947), 32–33, 78–79, 114–116, 154–156, 189–190, 228–230; A. B. Stewart *et al.,* "Health Centres of Today," *Lancet,* 250 (March, April, May 1946), 392–395, 471–473, 515–516, 550–551, 586–587, 665–667; Stephen Taylor, "Haygarth House, Harlow, Building a Health Centre," *Lancet,* 262 (February 1952), 253–257; R. C. Wolfinden and R. H. Perry, "Bristol's New Health Centre," *Lancet,* 262 (June 1952), 1297–1300; "Health Centres or Medical Centres," editorial, *Lancet* (January 21, 1961), 149–150; "Annotations," *Lancet* (May 21, 1960), 1120; Lord Taylor and S. Chave, *Mental Health and Environment* (London: Longmans, 1964); "Report on Health Centres," *British Medical Journal,* 2 (August 1956), 89–91 (supplement); "Survey of Health Centres," *British Medical Journal,* 2 (October 1960), 175–177; *Health and Welfare, The Development of Community Care, Revision to 1973–74 Plans for the Health and Welfare Services of Local Authorities in England and Wales* (London: Her Majesty's Stationery Office, 1964).

24. Henry E. Sigerist, *Socialized Medicine in the Soviet Union* (New York: W. W. Norton, 1937); M. Cristina Vera and Alfred Yankauer, "National Health Service of Chile," *Physician's Forum* (June 1967).

25. Ira V. Hiscock, "Development of Neighborhood Health Services," *Milbank Memorial Fund Quarterly,* 13 (January 1935), 30–52; Alfred Yankauer, "An Historical Analysis of Programs for the Reduction of Early Childhood Mortality in Latin America," *Journal of Tropical Pediatrics,* 12 (September 1966), 26–31; S. W. Wynne, "Neighborhood Health Center Development in the City of New York," *Milbank Memorial Fund Quarterly,* 9 (April 1931), 37–45; Michael M. Davis, "Health Center Idea," *Public Health Nurse* (January 1916).

26. Charles F. Wilinsky, "The Blossom Street Health Unit," *Nation's Health*, 6 (June 1924), 397–398; Charles F. Wilinsky, "The Health Center," *American Journal of Public Health*, 17 (July 1927), 677–682; Charles F. Wilinsky, "Dovetailing Health Work," *Modern Hospital*, 47 (September 1936), 1–3.

27. Charles F. Wilinsky, personal communication.

28. *The Health Units of Boston*, 1924–1933 and 1924–1944 (Boston: City of Boston Printing Department, 1933, 1945).

29. William Foley, personal communication; *Annual Reports*, Boston City Health Department.

30. Norman R. Ingraham, "Planning for Healthful Communities: The Neighborhood Health Center," *American Journal of Public Health*, 56 (December 1966), 1987–1989; C. E. A. Winslow and S. Zimand, *Health Under the El* (New York: Harper & Bros., 1937); "Bellevue-Yorkville Health Building Dedicated in New York City," *Milbank Memorial Fund Quarterly*, 5, no. 1 (1927), 13–15; Michael M. Davis, Jr., "Public Health Work, Health Center in Cleveland," in *Immigrant Health and the Community* (New York: Harper & Bros., 1921), pp. 376–390; James A. Tobey, "Health Center Movement in United States," *Modern Hospital*, 19 (March 1920), 212–214; "Symposium on the Health Centers," *American Journal of Public Health*, 11 (March 1921), 212–233.

31. Child Health Centers, *A Survey Committee on Medical Care for Children*, White House Conference on Child Health and Protection, Medical Service I (New York: Century, 1932).

32. J. L. Pomeroy, "Health Center Development in Los Angeles County," *Journal of the American Medical Association*, 93 (1929), 1546–1550; J. L. Pomeroy, "County Health Administration in Los Angeles County," *American Journal of Public Health*, 11 (September 1921), 796–800.

33. Rosen, *A History of Public Health*.

34. Sand, *The Advance to Social Medicine*.

35. Howard Brown and Raymond S. Alexander, "The Gouverneur Ambulatory Care Unit: A New Approach to Ambulatory Care," *American Journal of Public Health*, 54 (October 1964), 1661–1665.

36. Davis, *Clinics, Hospitals and Health Centers*.

37. Herbert Gans, *The Urban Villagers* (New York: Free Press of Glencoe, 1962).

38. V. M. Hoge, "Health Centers in the United States," *Lancet*,

246 (January 1944), 131–132; Otis L. Anderson, "Health Centers," *Military Medicine* 123 (August 1958), 103–107.

39. Frederick D. Mott and Milton I. Roemer, *Rural Health and Medical Care* (New York: McGraw-Hill, 1948); John B. Grant, "Health Centers and Regionalization," *American Journal of Public Health*, 43 (January 1953), 9–13; C. E. A. Winslow, *Health on the Farm and in the Village* (New York: Macmillan Company, 1931); C. E. A. Winslow, *A City Set On A Hill* (New York: Doubleday, 1934); "New York Health Demonstrations," *Milbank Memorial Fund Quarterly Bulletin*, 2, nos. 1, 2, 3 (April, July, October, 1924), 1–22; Milton Terris, "Herman Biggs' Contribution to the Modern Concept of Health Centres," *Bulletin History of Medicine*, 20 (October 1946), 387–412; Caldwell B. Esselstyn, "Group Practice with Branch Centers in a Rural County," *New England Journal of Medicine*, 248 (March 1953), 488–493.

40. "Health Service Areas: Requirements for General Hospitals and Health Centers," *Public Health Bulletin*, no. 292 (1945), in *Selected Papers of Joseph W. Mountin* (Washington, D.C.: Joseph W. Mountin Memorial Committee, 1956), pp. 181–183; Joseph W. Mountin and August Hoenack, "The Health Center," *Public Health Reports*, 61 (September 1946), 1369–1379; *The Nation's Health Facilities: Ten Years of Hill-Burton Hospital and Medical Facilities Program, 1946–1956*, Public Health Service Publication No. 616, (1955).

41. Alan A. Taeloar and Don Chill, *Patient Care Facilities: Construction Needs and Hill-Burton Accomplishments*. Chicago: American Hospital Association, 1961.

42. *European Conference on Rural Hygiene, Minutes*, vol. II (Geneva: League of Nations Health Organization, 1931); Sidney Kark and John Cassel, "The Phoela Health Centre," *South African Medical Journal*, 26 (February 1952), 101–104; Conrad Seipp, personal communication; Conrad Seipp, ed., *Selected Papers of John B. Grant*, chap. 3 (Baltimore: Johns Hopkins University Press, 1963), pp. 21–24.

43. Harbans S. Takulia *et al.*, *The Health Center Doctor in India* (Baltimore: Johns Hopkins University Press, 1967).

44. Kark and Cassel, "The Phoela Health Centre"; Sidney L. Kark and G. W. Stewart, eds., *A Practice of Social Medicine: A South African Team's Experiences in Different African Communities* (Edinburgh: Livingstone, 1962).

45. G. W. Gale, "Government Health Centres in the Union of South Africa," *South African Medical Journal*, 23 (July 1943), 630–636; H. Sutherland Gear, "South African Native Health and Medical Service," *ibid.*, 17 (June 1943), 167–172; G. W. Gale, "Native Medical Ideas and Practices in Relation to Native Medical Services," *ibid.*, 8 (October 1934), 748–753; G. W. Gale, "Health Centre Practice, Promotive Health Services and the Development of the Health Centres Scheme," *ibid.*, 20 (June 1946), 326–330.

46. Innes H. Pearse and Lucy H. Crocker, *The Peckham Experiment* (London: Allen and Unwin, 1943).

47. George A. Silver, *Family Medical Care* (Cambridge, Mass.: Harvard University Press, 1963); George A. Silver, "Beyond General Practice: The Health Team," *Yale Journal of Biology and Medicine*, 31 (September 1958), 29–39.

48. Parnie S. Snoke and E. Richard Weinerman, "Comprehensive Programs in University Medical Centers," *Journal of Medical Education*, 40 (July 1965), 625–657; Joel J. Alpert, John Kosa, Robert J. Haggerty, "A Study of Health Care of Low Income Families," paper, Massachusetts Public Health Association, 1965.

49. William A. MacColl, *Group Practice and Prepayment of Medical Care* (Washington, D.C.: Public Affairs Press, 1966).

50. Ray H. Elling, "The Design and Evaluation of Planned Change in Health Organizations," in A. Shostak, ed., *Sociology in Action* (Homewood, Ill.: Dorsey Press, 1966), pp. 292–302; Earl Siegel, "Migrant Families: Health Problems of Children," *Clinical Pediatrics*, 5 (October 1966), 635–640; Robert Coles, "The Lives of Migrant Farm Workers," *American Journal of Psychiatry*, 122 (September 1965), 271–285.

51. George Baehr, "The Hospital as the Center of Community Care," *American Journal of Public Health*, 54 (October 1964), 1653–1660.

52. A. H. Anderson, "Space as a Social Cost," *Journal of Farm Economics*, 32 (August 1950), 411–450.

53. Lisbeth Bamberger, "Health Care and Poverty," *Bulletin of the New York Academy of Medicine*, 42 (December 1966), 1140–1149; Martin K. White, Joel J. Alpert, John Kosa, "Hard-to-Reach Families in a Comprehensive Care Program," *Journal of the American Medical Association*, 201 (September 11, 1967), 123–128.

54. John D. Stoeckle and Irving K. Zola, "Views, Problems and Potentialities of the Clinic," *Medicine*, 43 (May 1964), 413–422;

John P. Connelly, John B. Stoeckle, and Edna S. Lepper, "The Physician and Nurse: Their Interprofessional Work in Office and Hospital Ambulatory Settings," *New England Journal of Medicine,* 275 (October 1966), 765–769.

55. Caldwell B. Esselstyn, "The Outlook for Group Practice," paper at Michigan State Medical Society, 1966.

56. Ward Darley and Anne R. Sommers, "Medicine, Money and Manpower," *New England Journal of Medicine,* 276 (June 1967), 1234–1238.

57. Sir Geoffrey Vickers, "Community Medicine," *Lancet,* (April 29, 1967), 944–947.

58. Osler L. Peterson *et al.,* "What is Value for Money in Medical Care?" *Lancet* (April 8, 1967), 771–776.

59. Stephen S. Kegeles, "Why People Seek Dental Care: A Test of Conceptual Formulation," *Journal of Health and Human Behavior,* 4 (Fall 1965), 141–147; Howard E. Freeman and Camille Lambert, Jr., "Preventive Dental Behavior of Urban Mothers," *Journal of Health and Human Behavior,* 6 (Fall 1965), 166–173; Camille Lambert, Jr., *et al.,* "Public Clinic Care and Eligibility," *American Journal of Public Health,* 53 (August 1963), 1196–1204.

60. Jules V. Coleman and Paul Errara, "The General Hospital Emergency Room and Its Psychiatric Problems," *American Journal of Public Health,* 53 (August 1963), 1294–1301; Maurice E. Chafetz, Howard T. Blane and James J. Muller, "Acute Psychiatric Services in the General Hospitals," *American Journal of Psychiatry,* 123 (December 1966), 664–669.

61. Alfred Yankauer and Ruth A. Lawrence, "A Study of Periodic School Medical Examinations," *American Journal of Public Health,* 45 (January 1955), 71–78; D. B. Nyswander, *Solving School Health Problems: The Astoria Demonstration Study,* conducted by the Health Department and Board of Education of New York City (New York: Commonwealth Fund, 1942).

62. I. M. Moriyama, "Present Status of Infant Mortality Problems in the United States," *American Journal of Public Health,* 56 (April 1966), 623–626.

63. D. Baird, "The Epidemiology of Prematurity," *Journal of Pediatrics,* 65 (December 1964), 909–924.

64. Conrad Seipp, ed., *Selected Papers of John B. Grant* (Baltimore: Johns Hopkins University Press, 1963).

CHAPTER XI—HEALTH AND POVERTY
RECONSIDERED

1. See the articles by Aaron Antonovsky, "Social Class and Illness," *Sociological Inquiry*, 37 (Spring 1967), 311–322; "Social Class, Life Expectancy and Overall Mortality," *Milbank Memorial Fund Quarterly*, 45 (April 1967), 67–75; and "Social Class and the Major Cardiovascular Diseases," *Journal of Chronic Diseases*, 21 (May 1968), 65–106. For the opposing view see Charles Kadushin, "Social Class and the Experience of Ill Health," *Sociological Inquiry*, 34 (Winter 1964), 67–80; and John A. Ross, "Social Class and Medical Care," *Journal of Health and Human Behavior*, 3 (Spring 1962), 35–41.

2. Suchman, however, found that both high and low socio-economic groups show the same amount of concern about their illnesses. Edward Suchman, "Stages of Illness and Medical Care," *Journal of Health and Human Behavior*, 6 (Fall 1965), 114–128.

3. Irving K. Zola, "Illness Behavior of the Working Class," in Arthur Shostak and William Gomberg, eds., *Blue-Collar World* (Englewood Cliffs, N.J.: Prentice-Hall, 1964).

4. See, for example, Vaun A. Newill, "Distribution of Cancer Mortality Among Ethnic Subgroups of the White Population of New York City," *Journal of the National Cancer Institute*, 26 (February 1961), 405–417; Haitung King *et al.*, "Cancer Mortality and Religious Preference," *Milbank Memorial Fund Quarterly*, 43 (July 1965), 349–358; Ann Hallman Pettigrew and Thomas F. Pettigrew, "Race, Disease and Desegregation," *Phylon*, 24 (Winter 1963), 315–333; "Centennial Conference on the Health Status of the Negro," College of Medicine, Howard University, Washington, D.C., March 1967 (mimeographed).

5. Mark Zborowski, "Cultural Components in Responses to Pain," *Journal of Social Issues*, 8 (1952), 16–30; Clyde Z. Nunn, John Kosa and Joel J. Alpert, "Causal Locus of Illness and Adaptation to Family Disruptions," *Journal for the Scientific Study of Religion*, 7 (Fall 1968), 210–218.

6. See Edward Suchman, "Sociomedical Variations Among Ethnic Groups," *American Journal of Sociology*, 70 (November 1964), 319–331.

7. Odin W. Anderson, "Infant Mortality and Social and Cultural

Factors," in E. Gartly Jaco, ed., *Patients, Physicians, and Illness* (Glencoe, Ill.: Free Press, 1958), pp. 10–24.

8. Joel J. Alpert *et al.*, "Types of Families Using an Emergency Clinic," *Medical Care*, 7 (Jan.–Feb. 1969), 55–61.

9. Bernard G. Greenberg and H. Bradley Wells, "Linear Discriminant Analysis in Perinatal Mortality," *American Journal of Public Health*, 53 (April 1963), 594–602.

10. Edward S. Rogers, "Public Health Asks of Sociology," *Science*, 159 (February 2, 1968), 506–508. See the rejoinder by Leon S. Robertson, "Sociology Stretches Its Goals," *Science*, 160 (April 26, 1968), 375–376.

11. Helen C. Chase, "Perinatal and Infant Mortality in the United States and Six West European Countries," *American Journal of Public Health*, 57 (October 1967), 1735–1748.

12. John Kosa, "Entrepreneurship and Charisma in the Medical Profession," paper presented at the International Conference on Social Science and Medicine, 1968.

13. American Public Health Association, Medical Care Section Newsletter, no. 60, April 1968, p. 5.

14. Richard D. Lyons, "Foreign Physicians, Many Unqualified, Fill Vacuum in U.S.," *New York Times*, September 29, 1967; John Kosa, "The Foreign-trained Physician in the United States," *Journal of Medical Education*, 44 (January 1969), 46–51.

APPENDIX

1. Adopted from a comparable section in Mortimer Spiegelman, *Significant Mortality and Morbidity Trends in the United States since 1900*, rev. ed. (Bryn Mawr, Pa.: American College of Life Underwriters, 1966).

2. *International Conference for the Sixth Revision of the International Lists of Diseases and Causes of Death* (Paris: April 1948).

3. Monroe Sirken, James W. Pifer, and Mortimer L. Brown, *Design of Surveys Linked to Death Records* (Washington, D.C.: U.S. Public Health Service, National Vital Statistics Division, September 1962).

4. Harold F. Dorn and Iwao M. Moriyama, "Uses and Significance of Multiple Cause Tabulations for Mortality Statistics," *American Journal of Public Health*, 54 (March 1964), 400–406.

5. U.S. National Center for Health Statistics, *Selected Family Characteristics and Health Measures Reported in the Health Interview Survey*, U.S. Public Health Service Publication No. 1000, series 3, no. 7 (January 1967).

6. Claire Selltiz *et al.*, *Research Methods in Social Relations* (New York: Holt, Rinehart and Winston, 1964).

7. Jack Elinson, "Methods of Sociomedical Research," in Howard E. Freeman, Sol Levine and Leo G. Reeder, eds., *Handbook of Medical Sociology* (Englewood Cliffs, N.J.: Prentice-Hall, 1963), pp. 449–472.

8. Joseph Zubin, "Classification of the Behavior Disorders," *Annual Review of Psychology*, 18 (1967), 373–406.

9. John J. Weber, Jack Elinson and Leonard M. Moss, "The Application of Ego Strength Scales to Psychoanalytic Clinic Records," *Proceedings of the 20th Anniversary Conference of the Columbia Psychoanalytic Clinic for Training and Research*, October 1965, pp. 215–273.

10. Lee J. Cronbach and Paul E. Meehl, "Construct Validity in Psychological Tests," *Psychological Bulletin*, 52 (July 1955), 281–302. See also *Standards for Educational and Psychological Tests and Manuals* (Washington, D.C.: American Psychological Association, 1966).

11. Selltiz *et al.*, *Research Methods in Social Relations*.

12. Elinson, "Methods of Sociomedical Research."

13. *Ibid.*; and Jacob J. Feldman, "The Household Interview Survey as a Technique for the Collection of Morbidity Data," *Journal of Chronic Diseases*, 11 (May 1960), 535–557.

14. Iwao M. Moriyama *et al.*, "Inquiry into Diagnostic Evidence Supporting Medical Certifications of Death," *American Journal of Public Health*, 48 (October 1958), 1376–1387.

15. *Ibid.*

16. Iwao M. Moriyama, "Factors in Diagnosis and Classification of Deaths from CVR Diseases," *Public Health Reports*, 75 (March 1960), 189–195.

17. Kurt Pohlen and Haven Emerson, "Errors in Clinical Statements of Causes of Death," *American Journal of Public Health*, 33 (May 1943), 505–516; and Robert H. Gruver and Edward D. Fries, "A Study of Diagnostic Errors," *Annals of Internal Medicine*, 47 (July 1957), 108–120.

18. George James, Robert E. Patton, and A. Sandra Heslin, "Ac-

curacy of Cause-of-Death Statements of Death Certificates," *Public Health Reports,* 70 (January 1955), 39–51.

19. H. William Mooney, *Methodology in Two California Health Surveys,* Public Health Monograph No. 70, Public Health Publication No. 942, 1962.

20. Arthur Pearl, Robert Buechley, and Wendell R. Lipscomb, "Cirrhosis Mortality in Three Large Cities," in David J. Pittman and Charles R. Snyder, eds., *Society, Culture and Drinking Patterns* (New York: John Wiley & Sons, 1962), pp. 345–352; and Wendell R. Lipscomb and Elaine Sulka, "Some Factors Affecting the Geographic Comparisons of Alcoholism Prevalence Rates," *Quarterly Journal of Studies on Alcohol,* 22 (December 1961), 588–596.

21. Metropolitan Life Insurance Company, "Alcoholism: A Growing Medical-Social Problem," *Statistical Bulletin,* 48 (April 1967), 7–10.

22. Lipscomb and Sulka, "Some Factors Affecting the Geographic Comparisons of Alcoholism Prevalence Rates."

23. Dorn and Moriyama, "Uses and Significance of Multiple Cause Tabulations."

24. Robert S. Myers, "The Audit Makes 'Evaluation' Meaningful," *Modern Hospital,* 87 (July 1956), 96–108.

25. U.S. National Center for Health Statistics, *Comparison of Hospitalization Reporting in Three Survey Procedures,* Public Health Service Publication No. 1000, series 2, no. 8 (July 1965).

26. Norman Kreitman, "The Reliability of Psychiatric Diagnosis," *Journal of Mental Science,* 107 (September 1961), 876–886.

27. Lester Breslow, "Uses and Limitations of the California Health Survey Studying the Epidemiology of Chronic Disease," *American Journal of Public Health,* 47 (February 1957), 168–172.

28. Harold F. Dorn, "Methods of Measuring Incidence and Prevalence of Disease," *American Journal of Public Health,* 41 (March 1951), 271–278.

29. Ray E. Trussell and Jack Elinson, *Chronic Illness in a Rural Area* (Cambridge, Mass.: Harvard University Press, 1959); and Commission on Chronic Illness, *Chronic Illness in a Large City* (Cambridge, Mass.: Harvard University Press, 1959).

30. Trussell and Elinson, *Chronic Illness in a Rural Area.*

31. Commission on Chronic Illness, *Chronic Illness in a Large City.*

32. *Ibid.*, p. 326.

33. Jack Elinson and Ray E. Trussell, "Some Factors Relating to Degree of Correspondence for Diagnostic Information Obtained by Household Interviews and Clinical Examinations," *American Journal of Public Health*, 47 (March 1957), 311–321. See also Sidney Cobb *et al.*, "On the Measurement of Prevalence of Arthritis and Rheumatism from Interview Data," *Journal of Chronic Diseases*, 3 (February 1956), 134–139; Dean E. Krueger, "Measurement of Prevalence of Chronic Disease by Household Interviews and Clinical Evaluations," *American Journal of Public Health*, 47 (August 1957), 953–960; and Donovan J. Thompson and Joseph Tauber, "Household Survey, Individual Interview, and Clinical Examination to Determine the Prevalence of Heart Disease," *American Journal of Public Health*, 47 (September 1957), 1311–1340.

34. Cobb *et al.*, "On the Measurement of Prevalence," p. 139.

35. U.S. National Center for Health Statistics, *Three Views of Hypertension and Heart Disease*, Public Health Service Publication No. 1000, series 2, no. 22 (March 1967).

36. American Medical Association, Council on Medical Service, *A Study of Multiple Screening*, rev. ed. (Chicago, 1955); Gordon S. Siegel, *Periodic Health Examination*, Public Health Service Publication No. 1010 (1963); Barkev S. Sanders, "Completeness and Reliability of Diagnoses in Therapeutic Practice," *Journal of Health and Human Behavior*, 5 (Summer 1964), 84–94.

37. Kendall A. Elsom *et al.*, "Nature and Distribution of Newly Discovered Disease in Executives," *Journal of the American Medical Association*, 172 (January 1956), 5–10.

38. Bernard Kutner, Henry B. Makover and Abraham Oppenheim, "Delay in the Diagnosis and Treatment of Cancer," *Journal of Chronic Diseases*, 7 (February 1958), 95–120.

39. U.S. National Health Survey, *Cooperation in Health Examination Surveys*, Health Statistics, Series D-2, Public Health Service Publication No. 584-D2 (June 1960); and U.S. National Health Survey, *Attitudes toward Cooperation in a Health Examination Survey*, Health Statistics, Series D-6, Public Health Service Publication No. 584-D6 (July 1961).

40. Sidney Cobb, Stanley King, and Edith Chen, "Differences between Respondents and Nonrespondents in a Morbidity Survey Involving Clinical Examination," *Journal of Chronic Diseases*, 6 (August 1957), 95–108.

41. Joel J. Alpert *et al.,* "Acceptance and Rejection of a Comprehensive Pediatric Care Program by Low-Income Families," paper presented at the meeting of the American Public Health Association, 1965.

42. U.S. National Center for Health Statistics, *Health Interview Responses Compared with Medical Records,* Public Health Service Publication No. 1000, series 2, no. 7 (July 1965).

43. Mooney, *Methodology in Two California Health Surveys.*

44. Nedra B. Belloc, "Validation of Morbidity Survey Data by Comparison with Hospital Records," *Journal of the American Statistical Association,* 49 (December 1954), 832–846.

45. Mooney, *Methodology in Two California Health Surveys.*

46. Trussell and Elinson, *Chronic Illness in a Rural Area.*

47. U.S. National Center for Health Statistics, *Comparison of Hospitalization Reporting.*

48. U.S. National Center for Health Statistics, *Reporting on Hospitalization in the Health Interview Survey,* Public Health Service Publication No. 1000, series 2, no. 6 (July 1965).

49. Barkev S. Sanders, "How Good are Hospital Data from a Household Survey?" *American Journal of Public Health,* 49 (December 1959), 1596–1606.

50. Jerry Alan Solon *et al.,* "Patterns of Medical Care: Validity of Interview Information on Use of Hospital Clinics," *Journal of Health and Human Behavior,* 3 (Spring 1962), 21–29.

51. John Kosa, Joel J. Alpert, and Robert J. Haggerty, "On the Reliability of Family Health Information," *Social Science and Medicine,* 1 (July 1967), 165–181.

52. Belloc, "Validation of Morbidity Survey Data."

53. U.S. National Center for Health Statistics, *Health Interview Responses.*

54. U.S. National Health Survey, *A Study of Special Purpose Medical-History Techniques,* Health Statistics, Series D-1, Public Health Service Publication No. 584-D1 (January 1960).

55. Kosa, Alpert, and Haggerty, "On the Reliability of Family Health Information."

56. Feldman, "The Household Interview Survey."

57. Mooney, *Methodology in Two California Health Surveys.*

58. Geoffrey Beall and Sidney Cobb, "The Frequency Distribution of Episodes of Rheumatoid Arthritis as Shown by Periodic

Examination," *Journal of Chronic Diseases,* 14 (September 1961), 291–310.

59. Lester Breslow, Editorial, *Journal of Chronic Diseases,* 14 (September 1961), 289–290.

60. Margaret B. Bailey, Paul W. Haberman, and Jill Sheinberg, "Identifying Alcoholics in Population Surveys," *Quarterly Journal of Studies on Alcohol,* 27 (June 1966), 300–315.

61. Paul W. Haberman, "Differences between Families Admitting and Denying an Existing Drinking Problem," *Journal of Health and Human Behavior,* 4 (Summer 1963), 141–145.

62. Bruce P. Dohrenwend and Barbara S. Dohrenwend, "The Problem of Validity in Field Studies of Psychological Disorder," *Journal of Abnormal Psychology,* 70 (February 1965), 52–69.

63. Leo Srole *et al., Mental Health in the Metropolis: The Midtown Study,* vol. 1 (New York: McGraw-Hill Book Company, 1962). See also Thomas S. Langner, "A Twenty-Two Item Screening Score of Psychiatric Symptoms Indicating Impairment," *Journal of Health and Human Behavior,* 3 (Winter 1962), 269–276.

64. Paul W. Haberman, "An Analysis of Retest Scores for an Index of Psycho-Physiological Disturbance," *Journal of Health and Human Behavior,* 6 (Winter 1965), 257–260.

65. Bruce P. Dohrenwend, "Social Status and Psychological Disorder," *American Sociological Review,* 31 (February 1966), 14–34.

66. Dohrenwend and Dohrenwend, "The Problem of Validity in Field Studies."

67. Sidney Cobb and Joseph Rosenbaum, "A Comparison of Specific Symptom Data Obtained by Nonmedical Interviewers and by Physicians," *Journal of Chronic Diseases,* 4 (September 1956), 245–252.

68. U.S. National Health Survey, *A Study of Special Purpose Medical-History Techniques.*

69. Daniel G. Horvitz, "Sampling and Field Procedures of the Pittsburgh Morbidity Survey," *Public Health Reports,* 67 (October 1952), 1003–1012.

70. U.S. Public Health Service, *A Health Study in Kit Carson County, Colorado,* Public Health Service Publication No. 844 (1962).

71. Trussell and Elinson, *Chronic Illness in a Rural Area.*

72. U.S. National Health Survey, *A Study of Special Purpose Medical-History Techniques.*

73. Mooney, *Methodology in Two California Health Surveys,* p. 48.

74. Kosa, Alpert, and Haggerty, "On the Reliability of Family Health Information."

75. U.S. National Health Survey, *Evaluation of a Single-Visit Cardiovascular Examination,* Health Statistics, Series D-7, Public Health Service Publication No. 584-D7 (December 1961).

76. Charles Y. Glock *et al.,* "Variability of Daily Blood Pressure Measurements in the Same Individuals Over a Three-Week Period," *Journal of Chronic Diseases,* 4 (November 1956), 469–476.

77. Bernard Schlesinger, "Errors of Diagnosis in Pediatrics," *British Medical Journal,* no. 4910 (February 12, 1955), 369–371.

78. J. Frederick Sparling, "Measuring Medical Care Quality," *Hospitals,* 36 (March 16, 1962), 62–68.

79. L. Henry Garland, "Studies on the Accuracy of Diagnostic Procedures," *American Journal of Roentgenology,* 82 (July 1959), 25–38.

80. Jacob Yerushalmy *et al.,* "An Evaluation of the Role of Serial Chest Roentgenograms in Estimating the Progress of Disease in Patients with Pulmonary Tuberculosis," *American Review of Tuberculosis,* 64 (September 1951), 225–248.

81. Garland, "Studies on the Accuracy of Diagnostic Procedures," p. 37.

82. Jacob Yerushalmy *et al.,* "The Role of Dual Reading in Mass Radiogram," *American Review of Tuberculosis,* 61 (April 1950), 443–464.

83. Kreitman, "The Reliability of Psychiatric Diagnosis."

84. Norman Kreitman *et al.,* "The Reliability of Psychiatric Assessment," *Journal of Mental Science,* 107 (September 1961), 887–908.

85. F. William Sunderman and Frederick Boerner, *Normal Values in Clinical Medicine* (Philadelphia: W. B. Saunders, 1949).

86. Regina Loewenstein, John Colombotos, and Jack Elinson, "Interviews Hardest-to-Obtain in an Urban Health Survey," *Proceedings of the Social Statistics Section of the American Statistical Association* (1962), 160–166.

87. Ann Cartwright, "The Families and Individuals Who Did Not Cooperate in a Sample Survey," *Milbank Memorial Fund Quarterly,* 37 (October 1959), 347–368.

88. Jacob J. Feldman, "Barriers to the Use of Health Survey Data

in Democratic Analysis," *Milbank Memorial Fund Quarterly,* 36 (July 1958), 203–221.

89. See Spiegelman, *Significant Mortality and Morbidity Trends.*

90. Herbert Goldhamer and Andrew Marshall, *Psychosis and Civilization* (Glencoe, Ill.: Free Press, 1949).

91. Richard J. Plunkett and John E. Gordon, *Epidemiology and Mental Illness* (New York: Basic Books, 1960).

92. Ernest M. Gruenberg and David S. Sanders, "Mental Health," in Hugh R. Leavell and F. Gurney Clark, eds., *Preventive Medicine for the Doctor in his Community* (New York: McGraw-Hill Book Company, 1965), 394–423.

93. M. N. Pai, "Some Mistaken Diagnoses," *Practitioner,* 172 (June 1954), 673–681.

94. Benjamin Pasamanick, ed., *Epidemiology of Mental Disorder* (Washington, D.C.: American Association for the Advancement of Science, 1959), pp. 183–201.

95. August B. Hollingshead and Frederick C. Redlich, *Social Class and Mental Illness* (New York: John Wiley & Sons, 1958).

96. David Mechanic and Margaret Newton, "Some Problems in the Analysis of Morbidity Data," *Journal of Chronic Diseases,* 18 (June 1965), 569–580.

Index

Contributors

Aaron Antonovsky is Senior Research Associate, Israel Institute of Applied Social Research, and Teaching Associate, Department of Social Medicine, Hebrew University-Hadassah Medical School, Jerusalem, Israel.

Marc Fried is Research Professor at the Institute of Human Sciences, Boston College, Chestnut Hill, Massachusetts.

Paul W. Haberman is Research Associate, Division of Sociomedical Sciences, Columbia University School of Public Health and Administrative Medicine, New York, New York.

John Kosa is Director, Medical Care Research Unit, and Lecturer in Sociology at Harvard Medical School, Boston, Massachusetts.

Monroe Lerner is Associate Professor, Department of Medical Care and Hospitals, School of Hygiene and Public Health, Johns Hopkins University, Baltimore, Maryland.

David Mechanic is Professor and Chairman, Department of Sociology, University of Wisconsin, Madison, Wisconsin.

Leon S. Robertson is Research Associate, Harvard Medical School and Children's Hospital Medical Center, Boston, Massachusetts.

Irwin M. Rosenstock is Professor of Public Health Administration, School of Public Health, University of Michigan, Ann Arbor, Michigan.

Julius A. Roth is Professor, Department of Sociology, University of California, Davis, California.

Arthur Shostak is Associate Professor, Department of Social Sciences, Drexel Institute of Technology, Philadelphia, Pennsylvania.

John Stoeckle, M.D., is Assistant Professor of Medicine, Harvard Medical School and Massachusetts General Hospital, Boston, Massachusetts.

Marvin B. Sussman is Professor and Chairman, Department of Sociology, Case Western Reserve University, Cleveland, Ohio.

Irving Kenneth Zola is Associate Professor, Department of Sociology, Brandeis University, Waltham, Massachusetts.